1.26.88

Cardiopulmonary Bypass

Principles and Management

Cardiopulmonary Bypass

Principles and Management

Edited by

KENNETH M. TAYLOR
MD, FRCS, FRCSE, FSA

Professor of Cardiac Surgery
Royal Postgraduate Medical School
Hammersmith Hospital, London

Baltimore
WILLIAMS & WILKINS

First published in 1986 by
Chapman and Hall Ltd

Distributed in the U.S., its dependencies the
Philippine Islands and Canada by
Williams and Wilkins
428 East Preston Street, Baltimore, MD 21202

ISBN 0–683–08105–5

Printed and bound in Great Britain
at the University Press, Cambridge

Accurate indications, adverse reactions, and dosage schedules for drugs are provided in this book, but it is possible that they may change. The reader is urged to review the package information data of the manufacturers of the medications mentioned.

Library of Congress Cataloging in Publication Data

Cardiopulmonary bypass
Includes bibliographies and index
1. Cardiopulmonary bypass methods
I. Taylor, K.M.
WG168 C266
RD598C354 1986 617'.412 86-9265

ISBN 0-683-08105-5

Contents

Contributors

W. H. Bain MD FRCS, Professor of Cardiac Surgery, Western Infirmary, Glasgow, G11 6NT, UK

L. S. Berman, Senior Scientist, Pall Biomedical Corporation, 30, Sea Cliff Avenue, Glen Cove, NY 11542, USA

D. W. Bethune, Consultant Anaesthetist, Thoracic Surgical Unit, Papworth Hospital, Papworth Everard, Cambridge, UK

M. V. Braimbridge, Consultant Cardiothoracic Surgeon, St Thomas's Hospital, London, UK

D. Bregman MD, Professor and Chairman, Dept. of Surgery, St Joseph's Hospital and Medical Center, Paterson, NJ, USA

K. G. Davidson, Consultant Cardiothoracic Surgeon, Royal Infirmary, Glasgow, G4 0SF, UK

M. de Leval, Consultant Cardiac Surgeon, Hospital for Sick Children, Great Ormond Street, London, UK

J. Donald Hill MD, Professor and Chairman, Dept. of Cardiovascular Surgery, Pacific Medical Center, San Francisco, CA, USA

E. Iatridis MS, Perfusion Specialties, Presbyterian Hospital, Pacific Medical Center, San Francisco, CA, USA

P. Kaskel BA, Dept. of Surgery, Columbia Presbyterian Medical Center, New York, USA

F. Marin, Pall Biomedical Corporation, 30, Sea Cliff Avenue, Glen Cove, NY, 11542, USA

A. D. McLaren MB ChB DObst RCOG FFARCS, Consultant Anaesthetist, Western Infirmary, Glasgow, G11 6NT, UK

D. G. Melrose MA BM BCh MRCP FRCS, Emeritus Professor of Surgical Science, Royal Postgraduate Medical School, Hammersmith Hospital, London, UK

D. C. Miller FFARCS, Consultant Anaesthetist, Royal Hospital for Sick Children, Glasgow, G3 8SJ, UK

D. T. Pearson MB FRCP FFARCS, Consultant Cardiothoracic Anaesthetist, Regional Cardiothoracic Centre, Freeman Hospital, High Heaton, Newcastle-upon-Tyne, NE7 7DN, UK

E. C. Peirce 2nd, Henry Kaufmann Professor of Hyperbaric Surgery, Mount Sinai School of Medicine, New York, USA

B. Sethia BSc FRCS, Senior Registrar, Dept. of Cardiac Surgery, Royal Infirmary, Glasgow, UK

J. C. Simpson, Consultant Anaesthetist, National Heart Hospital, Westmoreland Street, London, UK

K. M. Taylor, Dept. of Cardiac Surgery, Postgraduate Medical School, Hammersmith Hospital, London, UK

M. A. Tobias, Consultant Anaesthetist, Wythenshawe Hospital, Manchester, M23 9LT, UK

D. J. Wheatley MD ChM FRCS, British Heart Foundation Professor of Cardiac Surgery, Dept. of Cardiac Surgery, Royal Infirmary, Glasgow, UK

D. R. Wheeldon HNC MIBiol., Research Assistant, Papworth Hospital, Cambridge, UK

G. Wright BA MSc PhD RMN, W. E. Dunn Unit of Cardiology, University of Keele and North Staffordshire Hospital Centre, UK

Foreword

It is a great pleasure to introduce this new volume on cardiopulmonary bypass skilfully edited by Professor Kenneth Taylor. Little more than 30 years have passed since Gibbon's report of the first successful cardiac repair with cardiopulmonary bypass. This accomplishment transformed cardiac surgery and facilitated practical application of advances in surgical technique, physiology, myocardial protection, and immunology. Since this seminal achievement, dramatic progress has been made, with ever-increasing emphasis on minimizing physiologic derangement associated with bypass of the heart and lungs. In modern cardiac surgery, thorough and current understanding of the mechanical, physiological, and pathophysiological aspects of cardiopulmonary bypass is essential, and this excellent work will serve as a background and reference resource for the surgeon or anaesthesiologist in training and for the established practitioner.

Norman E. Shumway, MD
John C. Baldwin, MD

Preface

It is surely a sign of progress when attention in cardiac surgical practice turns from mortality to morbidity. The development of acceptably safe and reliable techniques for cardiopulmonary bypass have in past years allowed the very considerable development and refinement in surgical techniques for congenital, valvular and ischaemic heart disease. Open heart surgery is now undertaken with the expectation of excellent patient survival and improvement in the quality of life postoperatively. There is however an undeniable morbidity associated with conventional open-heart surgical techniques. It is generally true that the more sensitive and persistent the search, the higher the yield in terms of demonstrable morbidity. There is clearly a necessary balance to be achieved between turning the blind eye like Nelson at Trafalgar, and on the other hand scrutinizing every aspect of clinical practice, as if with an electron microscope.

There is no doubt that the current phase in cardiac surgical development is one in which refinement and improvement in cardiopulmonary bypass techniques feature to a large extent. Much work has been done in the past few years in order to determine the physiology and pathophysiology of conventional techniques of perfusion and oxygenation, and also to examine the effects of exposing blood to the artificial materials of the extracorporeal circuit. This scientific endeavour and various aspects of improvement in clinical perfusion practice set the scene for this textbook. There is a strong emphasis on physiology and pathophysiology, and this is right. An appreciation of these underlying mechanisms will undoubtedly lead to improvement in patient management.

Cardiopulmonary bypass is a multidisciplinary area. It involves surgeons, physicians, anaesthetists, biochemists, perfusionists, physiologists and many more. The authors have been selected for their broad appreciation of the subjects under discussion. The chapters review current thinking, the spectrum of present clinical practice, and the likely future developments in each area of interest. It is to be hoped that this textbook will both educate and stimulate all who are involved in this fascinating area of medicine.

K.M.T.

1
A history of cardiopulmonary bypass

D. G. MELROSE

It is, perhaps, invidious to select from the many who recognized in the 1930s that perfusion techniques used by physiologists to study organ function might be adapted to gain access to the interior of the human heart, but one who put it succinctly was O'Shaughnessy writing in the *Lancet* of 1939. Tragically he was to be killed a year later at the beginning of World War II. In his paper on the 'Future of Cardiac Surgery' he quotes Levine (1937) and writes,

> 'the real key to further advance in the surgical treatment of established cardiac defects will only be provided by the provision of some simple and efficient method of maintaining cerebral circulation while the heart is temporarily out of commission. Naturally there are many other problems of a local nature for solution . . . but so long as the surgeon is faced with the certainty of irreparable cerebral damage if he interrupts the circulation for any appreciable period he has little incentive to devise operative procedures that he cannot carry out'.

As if in answer to this plea Gibbon (1937) had published an account of the first elective cardiopulmonary bypass carried out in the cat. He was able to occlude the pulmonary artery for 25 minutes while shunting the cardiac output through an assembly of pumps and an oxygenator, his aim being to make pulmonary embolectomy possible. It is fitting therefore that Gibbon (1954) was also to report the first successful complete bypass of the heart and lungs in a human, though we must wait until 1953 for that. World War II intervened and though it delayed progress at the time it also acted as a powerful stimulus when it had ended. Many surgeons had successfully dealt with intrathoracic wounds, including those of the heart itself, and the pressure to treat surgically cardiac abnormalities became a real force, stimulating research in several countries. Crafoord and Andersen in Sweden produced the rotating disc oxygenator which Bjork (1948) described in his thesis. Jongbloed (1949) in Holland, Thomas and Beaudouin (1951) in France and Melrose (1953) in England, joined several American colleagues, Dennis *et al.* (1951), Dodrill *et al.* (1953), Helmsworth *et al.* (1953), Kantrowitz and Kantrowitz (1950), Mustard *et al.* (1954), Clowes (1951) and Miller, Gibbon and Gibbon (1951) in describing equipment used successfully in the experimental laboratory. But whilst the first tentative steps were being taken to apply these machines clinically, Lillehei and Varco (1955) at the University of Minnesota began using cardiopulmonary bypass in infants and young children with a simple pump and a donor adult as an oxygenator. They were able to use their cross circulation technique because they circulated only between 10% and 25% of the normal cardiac output of the patient, accepting the evidence of Andreasen and Watson (1952) that a dog would survive a period of 30 minutes of occlusion of the superior and inferior vena cava provided the azygos vein was patent, thus providing about 10% of the normal venous inflow to the heart. Ethical and other difficulties eventually persuaded them to abandon the use of donors but not before they had carried out elective cardiac surgery for several congenital anomalies. When Kirklin *et al.* (1955) at the Mayo Clinic confirmed their results, using a modified version of Gibbon's machine and a flow rate which was close to the normal cardiac output, modern cardiac surgery really began.

1.1 EQUIPMENT

1.1.1 Pumps

Inevitably, when equipment was scaled up to allow the whole circulation to be carried rather than small proportions of it, it evolved by simple development of the tools of physiology. Virtually all organ perfusion systems included a pump capable of a variable pulsatile output imitating the natural pulse contour. The best known was that of Dale and Schuster (1928). Modifications of this pump or of the principle behind it initiated virtually all of the early whole body perfusion experiments, including those of Gibbon and some of the first human perfusions were carried out with it. Such pulsatile pumps would have continued to dominate the field for pulsatile flow is normal and we must assume that the body is adapted to such a flow. Indeed sophisticated examples of such pumps continued to be used successfully for several years (Melrose, 1955). But, practical as well as theoretical considerations came to govern choice in the absence of any really conclusive evidence of the role of the pulse in the circulation. A very attractive alternative was available in the form of the occlusive roller pump. Henry and Jouvelet (1934) in France and De Bakey (1934) in the USA had given their names to two examples of this type in the same year and both had devised these pumps to facilitate direct blood transfusion. Enlarged to allow flows in excess of 5 litres a minute they had many advantages at the time. Mention must also be made of the Sigmamotor pump (DeWall, 1956) which substituted compressing fingers for rollers to occlude progressively the tube within it and, though it did not survive as flowrates increased it has an important historical place.

Each of the two basic types had merits and demerits. Both shared the useful attribute of allowing the inexpensive disposal of all material with which blood had come in contact and both had eliminated the interference to flow of internal valves. But the roller pump was, undoubtedly, much simpler to set up and use, was easy to drive by hand in the event of power failure, and the low amplitude pulse produced was much more manageable through the relatively small bore peripheral cannulae used at that time. It deservedly won the day.

It is interesting to note that the controversy between continuous and pulsatile flow pumps continues to this day (Taylor, 1984). Much new evidence has, of course, sharpened the debate since Wesolowski (1953) and Melrose (1958) discussed the problem in the 1950s and today there is a considerable and rapidly growing literature on the subject. Two recent reviews indicate that the matter is by no means settled yet (Edmunds, 1982; Philbin *et al.*, 1982).

1.1.2 Oxygenators

When we turn to imitation of the function of the lungs, scaling up primitive oxygenators proved more complex than pumps. Four solutions were initially available and two of these have survived to this day.

Mention has already been made of cross-circulation from a living donor, a technique quickly abandoned, but for many years a variety of homologous or heterologous natural lungs were incorporated into bypass systems and some were even used clinically. Never very successful, the complexity of preparation and unpredictability of performance mitigated against biological oxygenators and in spite of theoretical advantages they are most unlikely ever to be considered again.

The second line of development which is no longer used involved the exposure of blood directly to gas while spread over an arrangement of surfaces. Many and various were the mechanical solutions chosen, the principle involved having a long history from its introduction by von Frey and Gruber in 1885. Two references are useful in following the progress of this line of development: the monograph of Galleti and Brecher (1962) and a review by Hewitt and Creech (1966). Though superseded, the screen and disc oxygenators can rightfully claim pride of place in the 'popularization' of cardiopulmonary bypass. When Dennis *et al.* (1951) performed the first total bypass in man they used rotating screens, and when Gibbon (1954) performed the first successful total bypass in man he used vertical stationary screens. Developments of the rotating disc oxygenator by Melrose (1953) and by Cross *et al.* (1956) dominated the 1960s as cardiac surgery spread widely around the world.

The problems of the time were best handled by reusable filming oxygenators, complex and difficult to clean though they were, but already the inexorable advance of simple disposable equipment was making itself felt. Most of the tubing was already being discarded after a single use and one by one each durable component was challenged by a disposable alternative. A rather petulant comment at the time reads 'Not only must the actual efficiencies and effectiveness of each of these methods be taken into account, but a study of their practicality will often reject an excellent solution on grounds of complexity, expense, difficulty in maintenance or cleaning. While fully disposable systems have the most appeal they may be prohibitively expensive. It is sometimes better to clean thoroughly a well made item than to risk possible defects in manufacture in a replacable one.' Another comment on this subject was made by Osborn (1958) 'I think disposability is important. When you can get something clean and sterile ready to use and then throw it away afterwards that is important. You have to make a lot of compromises if you want disposability.'

Just as the simple roller pump came to exclude the more elaborate early pulsatile pumps so the third of the alternatives, the disposable bubble oxygenator replaced the filming devices.

The principle of oxygenating blood by the direct injection of gas into its substance in the form of bubbles has, if anything, the longest history of all. Von Schroder is credited with the introduction of the method in 1882 and in several laboratories it became the standard method for organ perfusion. The modern form is derived from the work of Clark *et al.* (1950). They advocated dispersion of oxygen through a sintered-glass filter directly into venous blood and they also introduced the concept of reducing the surface tension of blood after oxygenation by bringing it into contact with siloxane antifoaming agents thus enabling the foam to be more easily debubbled. However it was the disposable helical reservoir bubble oxygenator, originated and described in 1956 by De Wall *et al.* which pointed the way to the future. It was deceptively simple, and though an immediate success in many centres, it proved disappointingly difficult to use in others. New designs followed rapidly, the most widely distributed being that of Rygg and Kyvsgaard (1958), introduced in Denmark and a similar type by Hyman (1956) in the USA. There is no doubt that such devices work much more efficiently on low viscosity blood since it is much easier to defoam, and the ability to select a sterile pack, assemble the machine, and use it without donor blood even in an emergency had obvious merit. But the belief that fresh blood, taken into heparin, was necessary to prevent disastrous bleeding problems waned slowly and it was not until a more general acceptance of the safety of haemodilution that the bubble oxygenator came into its own. It is perhaps an interesting historical detail that the first completely successful animal perfusions carried out by Melrose *et al.* (1953) were done with a priming solution of 6% dextram saline, rather than with blood which had caused persistent hypotension during the initial experiments. Regrettably when the first patients were operated on clinicians ignored this demonstrably safer technique and, reverting to normal clinical practice, used fresh blood with its attendant difficulties. Now that mass production of efficient and reliable bubble oxygenators is the norm it is proper to pay tribute to the pioneering engineers who brought them to the present state of excellence.

Notwithstanding the present world-wide dominance of bubble oxygenators there remains a persistent suspicion that direct exposure of blood to gas is damaging to blood and that it is better to avoid the additional danger of gas embolism by not creating bubbles in the first place. In the 1950s this suspicion was a great deal stronger and led to the development of membrane oxygenators whereby a semipermeable membrane was interposed between blood and gas. The pioneers in this area were Kolff and Clowes. In 1944, Kolff and Berk had observed arterialization of blood as it passed through the cellophane chambers of the artificial kidney and later Kolff and Balzer (1955) used a coil dialyser as an oxygenator in successful animal experiments. Clowes *et al.* (1956) were most persistent in overcoming the very considerable technical problems of the time and by 1958 were able to report clinical use in adults though the oxygenator required over 25 m^2 of membrane area to support the necessary gas exchange.

Subsequent progress was frustratingly slow. The two fundamental aspects of design: suitable membranes on the one hand, and a suitable structure to support them on the other have both proved to be inherently very complex problems. Nature's ability to grow structures of great complexity and to supply blood to them by the branching of tubes of decreasing size is not capable of imitation. The smallest artificial capillaries we have been able to manufacture of synthetic material are of the order of 20–50 times the diameter of natural ones and as the time needed to oxygenate a film of blood varies as the square of its thickness these relatively large passages are extremely inefficient as diffusion sites. Difficulties attend the even delivery of blood to an array of such tubes, assembled as they must be into manifolds or header chambers. The same strictures apply to designs of sandwich type in which closely opposed pairs of membrane sheets conduct blood between alternating oxygen spaces. Such devices necessarily incorporate some method of establishing a uniform planar flow between the flat membranes and these usually take the form of spaces with grooves of similar surface irregularities designed to encourage even spreading and some mixing on the surface of the membranes. For even were the membrane to impose a truly negligible resistance to gas diffusion there exists adjacent to the surface a slowly moving boundary layer which impedes convection of the blood to the exchange surface and greatly limits gas transfer. In natural capillaries this boundary layer diffusion resistance is small because their size is small. Blocked by our inability to achieve these dimensions the only solution remains to promote vigorous lateral mixing within the blood passages in artificial membrane lungs and thus to promote increased convection which facilitates diffusion.

Suitable membranes now exist which have excellent gas diffusion properties. The discovery by Kammermeyer (1957) that silicone elastomers could be made with exceptionally high permeability both to oxygen and carbon dioxide whilst being biologically inert provided the impetus to Bramson *et al.* (1965), Kolobow and Bowman (1963), Landé *et al.* (1969) and others to design devices suitable for routine clinical use and commercial production. Improved membranes and better blood distribution reduced the necessary area tenfold from the 25 m^2 of Clowes to 2.5 m^2. Now even this bench mark of efficiency has been exceeded by the substitution of micro-porous teflon or polypropylene membranes for silicone and by active mixing techniques which allow complete adult gas exchange to be achieved in a device whose surface area is only 0.8 m^2 (Melrose and Fleming, 1980).

Essentially the exacting criteria required of an ideal artificial lung can now be met. The membranes available and the configuration in which they are used can be made to produce a closed-circuit device of remarkable efficiency, without sacrifice of safety or simplicity in use, of atraumatic performance over long periods, and of acceptable cost.

Further, the pioneering fluid dynamic analyses of Weissman and Mockros (1968) and of Drinker (1972) and Drinker *et al.* (1969) which led to these increases in efficiency indicate that we are not yet at the end of this development.

1.1.3 Intracardiac suction

Little need be said about other items of equipment used in cardiopulmonary bypass. Gradual improvement in the quality and design of cannulae, tubing and reservoirs has inevitably accompanied the expansion in demand for these products and inevitably they are disposable. But one issue which still causes concern is the handling of blood seeping into the open heart or spilling into the pericardial cavity itself, for there is little doubt that a most destructive element in the extracorporeal circuit is the recovery of this blood.

Too little attention has been paid to this aspect. Osborn *et el.* (1962) pointed out the contribution that careful design of the actual sucker tip can make and Benzing *et al.* (1966) indicated that meticulous control of suction pressure gradient and rate of withdrawal can ensure much gentler handling. But most are content to use a system of roller pumps under relatively crude control. Recently, an interesting paper by de Jong *et al.* (1980) emphasized that there is little relevance in using a membrane oxygenator instead of the haematologically more destructive bubble oxygenator when all the benefits so gained are counteracted by uncontrolled suction. They further point out that such control can be achieved and a significant improvement in haemostasis gained. Perhaps at last with modern electronics a method simple and reliable enough for everyday use will eliminate the clumsy and traumatic methods which have changed little during the last quarter century.

1.2 HYPOTHERMIA AND MYOCARDIAL PRESERVATION

No history of the development of bypass techniques can be complete without considering the place of hypothermia and of elective cardiac arrest. From the outset there were those who believed that manipulation of the body temperature might of itself be sufficient to provide the necessary operating time. Certainly the hibernating animal has always excited great interest and when Bigelow *et al.* (1949) proved that the period during which an animal would withstand circulatory arrest could be greatly prolonged by reducing the body temperature he reawakened biological interest leading to clinical application. McQuiston (1949) noted the protective effect of mild hypothermia in the operative management of cyanotic heart disease; Lewis and Taufic (1953) and Swan and Zeavin (1954) reported various successful intracardiac operations using direct vision under hypothermia even before Gibbon's important first case. When Andjus and Smith (1955) demonstrated that it was possible to maintain the non-hibernating rat without respiration or heart-beat for more than an hour at a core temperature close to 0°C it seemed that the future was assured.

But it was not to be. Man is not a hibernator and cannot maintain energy-exchange processes during the long periods required to bring about cooling to and rewarming from low temperatures. The nearest we have come to it has been the technique of Drew (1959) who used extracorporeal pumps to maintain the circulation through these periods to provide complete circulatory arrest for an hour at temperatures below 10°C. The technique helped provide evidence of safe time limits but proved too complex to replace conventional bypass procedures and like so many hopeful alternatives it has been abandoned.

However, hypothermia remains inextricably linked with bypass technique. The ability to control tissue temperature and thus influence its metabolism by controlling the temperature of the circulating blood is a fundamental component of all present day cardiac surgery. Fashions change and the ideal body temperature for cardiac surgery has fluctuated to and fro from the normal 37°C down to as low as 20°C. Most are content with modest alterations which are easy to control and which provide well-understood advantages.

The heart itself is a special case. Since it became evident that even a satisfactory perfusion of the whole body did not necessarily provide good surgical access to the heart unceasing attention has been directed to this problem. The goal is a flaccid heart from which all blood flow is excluded and whose metabolism is so reduced that no irreversible damage occurs during surgery. The first attempts to achieve this were proposed in 1955.

Melrose *et al.* (1955) suggested that deliberate manipulation of the ionic environment of the myocardium might provide the answer. Using potassium citrate to exaggerate the effect described by Ringer in 1883, where potassium inhibited and calcium stimulated the heart, they were able to demonstrate in several animal species a reliable method of stopping and starting the heart. Lam *et al.* (1955) described the use of acetylcholine injected into the root of the aorta to achieve a similar but less-dramatic effect. In both techniques simply flushing out the coronary system with blood from the heart–lung machine restored normal function.

The potassium citrate method was widely accepted and by 1957 was in general use. Acetylcholine did not find favour to the same extent and faded from the scene. Sadly, however, the obvious combination of potassium citrate elective arrest and myocardial hypothermia was not exploited at the time though experimental evidence was available to suggest the advantages of this (Baker *et al.*, 1957). Had it been so history would have been different, for potassium arrest at normal temperature only extended the safe period of ischaemia for a relatively short period and as surgical problems increased in complexity and acquired disease brought problems of myocardial inadequacy the technique was found wanting.

Cross (1957) showed that a very cold heart withstood ischaemia much better than a warm one and then showed that initial arrest with potassium citrate followed by washout with oxygenated blood at close to 0°C further reduced oxygen consumption. But this and several other promising lines of research were cut off as elective arrest was abandoned in favour of a variety of alternatives. Several schools emerged; simple anoxia, individual coronary perfusion at normal temperature or at varying degrees of hypothermia, surface cooling of the heart without perfusion and of course combinations of these. None was so obviously successful as to displace the others and history was to confirm the initial idea, elective cardiac arrest now called cardioplegia returning to complete the full circle in a generation.

It returned because it had been kept alive in Germany. Holscher (1967) had continued to study induced arrest throughout the 1960s but it was the work of Bretschneider (1964) which ushered in the new wave of cold cardioplegia. They substituted sodium-poor, calcium-free, procaine-containing solutions for those previously used. Sondergaard and Senn (1967) took these up clinically in Aarhus with excellent experimental results. Kirsch *et al.* (1972) in Hamburg and Hearse *et al.* (1976) in London devised original solutions after painstaking analysis of the effect of individual components in the light of much greater knowledge of the metabolism of the heart. They also produced excellent clinical results. Roe *et al.* (1977), Tyers *et al.* (1974) and Buckberg (1979) in the United States all made powerful contributions and today it is unusual for cardiac surgery to proceed without cardioplegia. However, only time will tell whether this time the biochemists, physiologists and surgeons have got it right.

The history of the safe entry into the cavities of the living human heart to allow surgical repair is a short one but one full of fascination. For it spans also the entry into medicine of the enormous power of technology. My own experience in this field commenced when the only aids to clinical acumen were the X-ray machine, the microscope, the test-tube, the electrocardiogram and the cardiac catheter. The art of medicine was not yet accompanied by the science of medicine. Perhaps the present is best exemplified by the many national and international societies of artificial organs. These associations have brought together experts from all the appropriate disciplines.

Countless people live without natural kidneys, a man has lived without a natural heart for several months, every organ is under scrutiny for replacement. While advance in cardiopulmonary bypass will be less spectacular than in the heady 1960s it will be relentless and based more securely on a wealth of confirmed fact. The prospect is wonderful.

REFERENCES

Andjus, R. K. and Smith, A. N. (1955) Reanimation of adult rats from body temperatures between 0 and +2°C. *J. Physiol.*, **128**, 446.

Andreasen, A. T. and Watson, F. (1952) Experimental cardiovascular surgery. *Br. J. Surg.*, **39**, 548–51.

Baker, J. B. E. *et al.* (1957) Arrest of isolated heart with potassium citrate. *Lancet*, **ii**, 555–9.

Benzing, G. 3rd, De Forest, D. and Kaplan, S. (1966) Multiple line single-reservoir automatic cardiotomy return system. *J. Thorac. Cardiovasc. Surg.*, **51**, 238.

Bigelow, W. B. *et al.* (1949) Hypothermia; its possible role in cardiac surgery investigation of factors governing survival in dogs at low body temperatures. *Anaesthesiology*, **10**, 590.

Bjork, V. O. (1948) Brain perfusions in dogs with artificially oxygenated blood. *Acta Chir. Scand.*, **96** (Suppl. 137), 1–122.

Bramson, M. L., Osborn, J. J., Main, F. B. *et al.* (1965) A new disposable membrane oxygenator with integral heat exchanger. *J. Thorac. Cardiovasc. Surg.*, **50**, 391.

Bretschneider, H. J. (1964) Uberlebanzeit under Wiederbelebungszeit des Herzen bei Normo- und Hypothermia. *Verh. Dtsch. Ges. Kreislanfforsch*, 30, 11.

Buckberg, G. D. (1979) A proposed 'solution' to the cardioplegia controversy. *J. Thorac. Cardiovasc. Surg.*, 77, 803.

Clark, L. C. *et al.* (1950) The oxygenation of blood by gas dispersion. *Science*, **III**, 85.

Clowes, J. H. A. Jr (1951) Experimental procedures for entry into the left heart to expose mitral valve. *Ann. Surg.*, **134**, 957–68.

Clowes, G. H. A. Jr *et al.* (1956) An artificial lung dependent upon diffusion of oxygen and carbon dioxide through plastic membranes. *J. Thorac. Surg.* **32**, 630.

Cross, F. S. (1958) Discussion on cardiac arrest in *Extracorporeal Circulation* (ed. J. G. Allen), Charles C. Thomas, Springfield Ill., p. 491.

Cross, F. S. *et al.* (1956) Evaluation of a rotating disc type reservoir oxygenator. *Proc. Soc. Exp. Biol. Med.*, **93**, 210–14.

Dale, H. H. and Schuster, E. H. J. (1928) A double perfusion pump. *J. Physiol.*, **64**, 356–64.

De Bakey, M. E. (1934) Simple continuous-flow blood transfusion instrument. *New Orleans Med. S. J.*, **87**, 386–9.

de Jong, J. C. F. *et al.* (1980) Hematologic aspects of cardiotomy suction in cardiac operations. *J. Thorac. Cardiovasc. Surg.*, **79**, 227.

Dennis, C. *et al.* (1951) Development of a pump-oxygenator to replace the heart and lungs: an apparatus applicable to human patients and application in one case. *Ann. Surg.*, **134**, 709–21.

DeWall, R. A. *et al.* (1956) A simple, expendable artificial oxygenator for open heart surgery. *Surg. Clin. N. Am.*, **36**, 1025–34.

Dodrill, F. D. *et al.* (1953) Pulmonary valvuloplasty under direct vision using the mechanical heart for a complete bypass of the right heart in a patient with congenital pulmonary stenosis. *J. Thorac. Surg.*, **26**, 584–97.

Drew, C. E. (1959) Profound hypothermia. *Lancet*, **i**, 745.

Drinker, P. A. (1972) Progress in membrane oxygenator design. *Anaesthesiology*, **37**, 242.

Drinker, P. A., Bartlett R. H., Bialer R. M. *et al.* (1969) Augmentation of membrane gas transfer by induced secondary flows. *Surgery*, **66**, 775.

Edmunds, L. H. Jr (1982) Pulseless cardio-pulmonary bypass. *J. Thorac. Cardiovasc. Surg.*, **84**, 800–4.

Galetti, P. M. and Brecher, G. A. (1962) *Heart–Lung Bypass*, Grune and Stratton, New York.

Gibbon, J. H. Jr (1937) Artificial maintenance of circulation during experimental occlusion of pulmonary artery. *Arch. Surg.*, **34**, 1105–31.

Gibbon, J. H. Jr (1954) Application of a mechanical heart and lung apparatus to cardiac surgery. *Minnesota Med.*, **37**, 171–85.

Hearse, D. J., Stewart, D. A., Braimbridge, M. V. *et al.* (1976) Cellular protection during myocardial ischaemia: The development and characterization of a procedure for the induction of reversible ischaemic arrest. *Circulation*, **54**, 193.

Helmsworth, J. A. *et al.* (1953) An oxygenator-pump for use in total bypass of heart and lungs. *J. Thorac. Surg.*, **26**, 617.

Henry, H. and Jouvelet, P. (1934) Appareil à transfusion du sang. *Bull. Acad. de Med. Paris*, **111**, 312–19.

Hewitt, R. L. and Creech, O. Jr (1966) History of the pump oxygenator. *Arch. Surg.*, **93**, 680–96.

Holscher, B. (1967) Studies by electron microscopy on the effects of magnesium chloride–procainamide or potassium citrate on the myocardium in induced cardiac arrest. *J. Cardiovasc. Surg.* (*Torino*), **8**, 136.

Hyman, E. S. (1956) Simple, disposable, autoclavable plastic unit to substitute for heart and lungs. *Trans. Am. Soc. Art. Int. Organs*, **2**, 1.

Jongbloed, J. (1949) The mechanical heart lung system. *Surg. Gynec. Obstet.*, **89**, 684–91.

Kammermeyer, K. (1957) Silicone rubber as a selective barrier. *Ind. Eng. Chem.*, **49**, 1685.

Kantrowitz, A. and Kantrowitz, A. (1950) Experimental left heart to permit surgical exposure of the mitral valve in cats. *Proc. Soc. Exp. Biol.*, **74**, 193.

Kirklin, J. W. *et al.* (1955) Intracardiac surgery with aid of mechanical pump-oxygenator system (Gibbon type) report of 8 cases. *Proc. Staff Meeting Mayo Clinic*, **30**, 201.

Kirsch, U., Rodewald, G. and Kalmúr, P. (1972) Induced ischaemic arrest. Clinical experience with cardioplegia in open-heart surgery. *J. Thorac. Cardiovasc. Surg.*, **63**, 121.

Kolff, W. J. and Balzer, R. R. (1955) Artificial coil lung. *Trans. Am. Soc. Artif. Int. Organs*, **1**, 39.

Kolff, W. J. and Berk, H. T. Jr (1944) Artificial kidney: a dialyser with a great area. *Acta Med. Scand.*, **117**, 121.

Kolobow, T. and Bowman, R. L. (1963) Construction and evaluation of an alveolar membrane artificial heart lung. *Trans. Am. Soc. Artif. Int. Organs.*, **9**, 238.

Lam, C. R. *et al.* (1955) Induced cardiac arrest for intracardiac surgical procedures. *Ann. Surg.*, **146**, 439.

Landé, A. J., Fillmore, S. J., Subramanian *et al.* (1969) 24 hour veno-arterial perfusions of awake dogs with a simple membrane oxygenator. *Trans. Am. Soc. Artif. Int. Organs.*, **15**, 181.

Lewis, F. J. and Taufic, M. (1953) Closure of atrial septal defects with the aid of hypothermia. Experimental accomplishments and the report of one successful case. *Surgery*, **33**, 52.

Lillehei, C. W. and Varco (1955) The results of direct vision closure of ventricular septal defects in eight patients by means of controlled cross circulation. *Surg. Gynae. Obstet.*, 447–66.

McQuiston, W. O. (1949) Anaesthetic problems in cardiac surgery in children.

Melrose, D. G. (1953) A mechanical heart–lung machine for use in man. *Br. Med. J.*, **2**, 57.

Melrose, D. G. (1955) A heart–lung machine for use in man. *J. Physiol.*, **127**, 51–3.

Melrose, D. G. (1958) Continuous and pulsatile flow pumps in *Extracorporeal Circulation* (ed.) J. G. Allen, Charles C. Thomas, Springfield, Ill., pp. 14–19.

Melrose, D. G. and Fleming, J. (1980) The extracorporeal 'Interpulse' Tm membrane oxygenator. *Proc. Eur. Soc. Art. Organs*, **VII**, 245.

Melrose, D. G. *et al.* (1953) Experimental physiology of a heart–lung machine in parallel with normal circulation. *Br. Med. J.* **2**, 62.

Melrose, D. G. *et al.* (1955) Elective cardiac arrest. *Lancet*, **ii**, 21.

Miller, B. J., Gibbon, J. H. Jr and Gibbon, M. H. (1951) Recent advances in the development of a mechanical heart and lung apparatus. *Ann. Surg.*, **134**, 694.

Mustard, W. T. *et al.* (1954) A surgical approach to transposition of the great vessels with extracorporeal circuit. *Surgery*, **36**, 39–51.

Osborn, John J. (1958) Discussion on oxygenators in *Extracorporeal Circulation* (ed. J. G. Allen), Charles C. Thomas, Springfield, Ill., pp. 105–6.

Osborn, J. J. *et al.* (1962) Haemolysis during perfusion. Sources, means of reduction. *J. Thorac. Cardiovasc. Surg.*, **43**, 459.

O'Shaughnessy, L. (1939) Future of cardiac surgery. *Lancet*, **2**, 969–71.

Philbin, D. M. *et al.* (1982) Should we pulse? *J. Thorac. Cardiovasc. Surg.*, **84**, 805–6.

Ringer, S. (1883) *J. Physiol.*, **4**, 29.

Roe, B. B., Hutchinson, J. C., Fishman, N. H. *et al.* (1977) Myocardial protection with cold, ischaemic, potassium-induced cardioplegia. *J. Thorac. Cardiovasc. Surg.* **73**, 366–74.

Rygg, I. H. (1958) Discussion of oxygenators, in *Extracorporeal Circulation* (ed. J. G. Allen), Charles C. Thomas, Springfield, Ill., p. 108.

Sondergaard, T. and Senn, A. (1967) Klinische Erfahrungen mit der Kardioplegie nach Bretschneider. *Laugenbecks. Arch. Chir.*, **319**, 661.

Swan, H. and Zeavin (1954) Cessation of circulation in general hypothermia: Technics of intracardiac surgery under direct vision. *Ann. Surg.*, **139**, 385.

Taylor, K. M. (1984) The statuo of pulsatile pefusion. *Current Med. Lit.*, **3**, 66–9.

Thomas, J. A. and Beaudouin, P. (1951) Characteristiques physiologiques du coeur–poumon artificial pour la perfusion au sang du corps humain. *J. Physiol., Paris*, **43**, 311.

Tyers, G. F., Hughes, H. C. Jr, Todd, G. J. *et al.* (1974) Protection from ischaemic cardiac arrest by coronary perfusion with cold Ringer's lactate solution. *J. Thorac. Cardiovasc. Surg.*, **67**, 411.

Von Frey, M. and Gruber, M. (1885) Ein Respirations-apparat fur Isolirte Organe. *Arch. Physiol.*, **9**, 519–32.

Von Schroder, W. (1882) Uber die Bildungsstatte des Harnstoffs. *Arch. Path. Pharm.*, **15**, 364–402.

Weissman, M. H. and Mockros, L. F. (1968) Gas transfer to blood flowing in coiled circular tubes. *J. Eng. Mech. Div., ASCE* **93** No Em6, Proc. paper 6007, p. 857, June.

Wesolowski, S. A. *et al.* (1953) Perfusion of the pulmonary circulation by non-pulsatile flow. *Surgery* **33**, 370–5.

2

Measurement and monitoring for cardiopulmonary bypass

W. H. BAIN

Intelligent management of cardiopulmonary bypass and the subsequent smooth take-over of the circulation by the heart, requires the measurement, display and informed response to certain indices of cardiovascular function and to biochemical changes. Monitoring commences in the anaesthetic room, with acquisition and display of the ECG and arterial blood pressure (using a non-invasive technique prior to the induction of anaesthesia). After the patient is anaesthetized, the necessary vascular cannulations and intubations are done, to permit further measurements, blood sampling etc.

The factors usually monitored include:

ECG and heart rate Arterial blood pressure Central venous pressure Arterial pump flow rate Suction pump flow rate Core temperature Peripheral temperature Blood temperature (in arterial line) Coolant temperature (in heat exchanger) Modified ECG	continuously
Arterial blood gases (PO_2, PCO_2) pH, base deficit Haematocrit Plasma potassium concentration Urine flow Myocardial temperature Left atrial pressure	intermittently

2.1 ELECTROCARDIOGRAM (ECG)

The ECG display will indicate the presence of heart rhythm changes and also of myocardial ischaemia. This latter function is especially valuable in patients with coronary artery disease during the induction of anaesthesia and preparation for bypass. A read-out of heart rate is normally available continuously. A print of the pre-bypass ECG pattern should be retained for comparison with the early post-bypass trace. When cardiopulmonary bypass has been established, the ECG serves as an indicator of adequate coronary perfusion. When elective cardioplegia is induced, the ECG should rapidly become isoelectric. The reappearance of any electrical activity while the aorta remains cross-clamped indicates the need for more cardioplegic solution and/or myocardial cooling. When heart action has been restored and a pulsatile pump is being used in the counterpulsation mode, a 'clean' ECG signal is required to trigger the pump.

2.2 ARTERIAL BLOOD PRESSURE

In patients with precarious ventricular function, non-invasive blood pressure monitoring (e.g. an automated sphygmomanometer) should be commenced before the patient is anaesthetized. Subsequently a cannula (18 or 20 gauge) will be introduced into a radial artery and connected to a pressure transducer.

Patency of the cannula is maintained by heparinized saline (1000 units heparin per 500 ml normal saline) from a pressurized reservoir, connected to the cannula through a slow-drip regulator (Intra-flo). The cannula and the saline-filled line which connects it to the transducer must be of semi-rigid materials which will not distort the blood pressure wave form.

The system is calibrated as follows:

The line to the arterial cannula is occluded temporarily, the transducer is opened to atmospheric pressure, and 'zero' is set on the display. A saline-filled column 136 cm in height is then connected to the transducer, and the amplifier again adjusted until the display registers 100mm Hg (13.3 kPa). The calibration and zeroing taps on the transducer are closed and the arterial line re-opened. The display should now read the arterial pressure. An approximate check on the accuracy of an intra-arterial blood pressure display can be made using a conventional mercury or anaeroid sphygmomanometer, with its pneumatic cuff applied to the arm in which the radial cannula is inserted. The cuff is inflated to a pressure which just occludes the brachial artery; this is the point where the pulsatile character of the BP display is abolished. The sphygmomanometer cuff pressure at this point registers the systolic BP.

When cardiopulmonary bypass is instituted, the arterial BP falls and then slowly rises to normal or above-normal levels during the period of bypass. The 'ideal' arterial pressure during bypass has not been defined, and probably should vary from patient to patient according to the state of their peripheral and cerebral vasculature. Controversy exists as to when intervention to raise or lower the arterial pressure is necessary. A mean pressure of less than 30 mmHg (4 kPa) is below the critical closing pressure of some vascular beds, and significant underperfusion of these areas may result. A supra-normal mean pressure implies an elevated total systemic resistance with the probability of underperfusion of some vascular beds.

The systemic BP should be interpreted with two physiological facts in mind:

(1) The arterial blood pressure represents the product of cardiac output (or pump output) and peripheral vascular resistance,
(2) Left ventricular oxygen consumption is directly related to the systolic blood pressure.

Thus a systolic blood pressure which is above the normal range is probably a consequence of an increased peripheral vascular resistance, and will require an increased O_2 supply to the left ventricle. In the immediate post-bypass period, when the myocardium is recovering from cardioplegia, the ventricular myocardium will recover more quickly if its work is minimized while O_2 supply, i.e. coronary flow, is maximized. This can be achieved by reducing the systolic blood pressure and left atrial pressure while maintaining diastolic blood pressure, by the selective use of peripheral vasodilator agents.

Informed interpretation of the systemic blood pressure is of crucial importance at the time of weaning from cardiopulmonary bypass, and during the first few hours thereafter. It is during this period that manipulation of the systemic vascular resistance and capacitance by vasodilator drugs can be most useful. The objective is to optimize the oxygen supply/demand ratio for the left ventricle (Fig. 2.1). The work demand of the left ventricle can be equated with the area under the aortic pressure pulse during systole, measurable as the systolic pressure-time index (SPI), or as tension-time index (TTI) (Sarnoff *et al.*, 1958). Oxygen supply in the myocardium (i.e. coronary flow) can be related to area under the diastolic portion of the aortic pressure pulse minus the left ventricular diastolic pressure, measurable as the diastolic pressure index (DPI).

The therapeutic objective is to minimize the energy demand whilst ensuring a maximum energy supply, and at the same time ensuring an adequate cardiac output. Sarnoff's work in 1958 showed that the increased left ventricular work associated with increasing cardiac output demanded relatively little increase in energy (oxygen) supply, provided the increase in output was not accompanied by a rise in systemic pressure (Fig. 2.2).

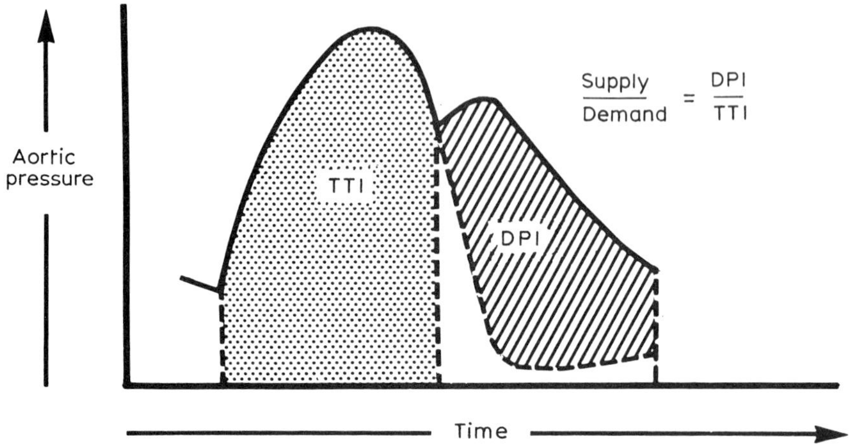

Fig. 2.1 A diagram relating the myocardial supply/demand ratio to the areas under the systolic and diastolic portions of the aortic pressure wave form. Coronary flow (Supply) occurs mainly in diastole. Ventricular work (Demand) occurs mainly in systole. TTI = Tension-time index; DPI = diastolic pressure index (i.e. area under aortic diastolic pressure minus left ventricular diastolic pressure).

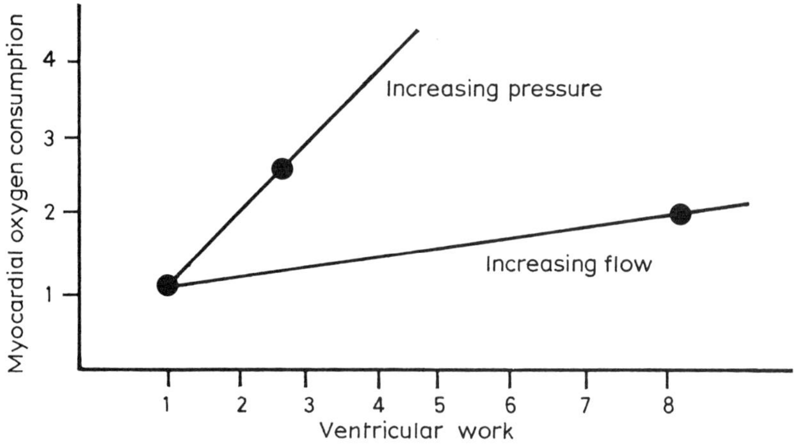

Fig. 2.2 The relationship between ventricular work and myocardial oxygen consumption: (i) where the workload is associated predominantly with increased blood pressure; (ii) where work is associated with increased blood flow (or cardiac output). (Sarnoff *et al.* 1958).

2.3 CENTRAL VENOUS PRESSURE

Central venous pressure (CVP) is monitored through a long cannula introduced into an internal jugular or subclavian vein, with its tip in the superior vena cava (Fig. 2.3). The use of a percutaneous catheter introducing set (e.g.

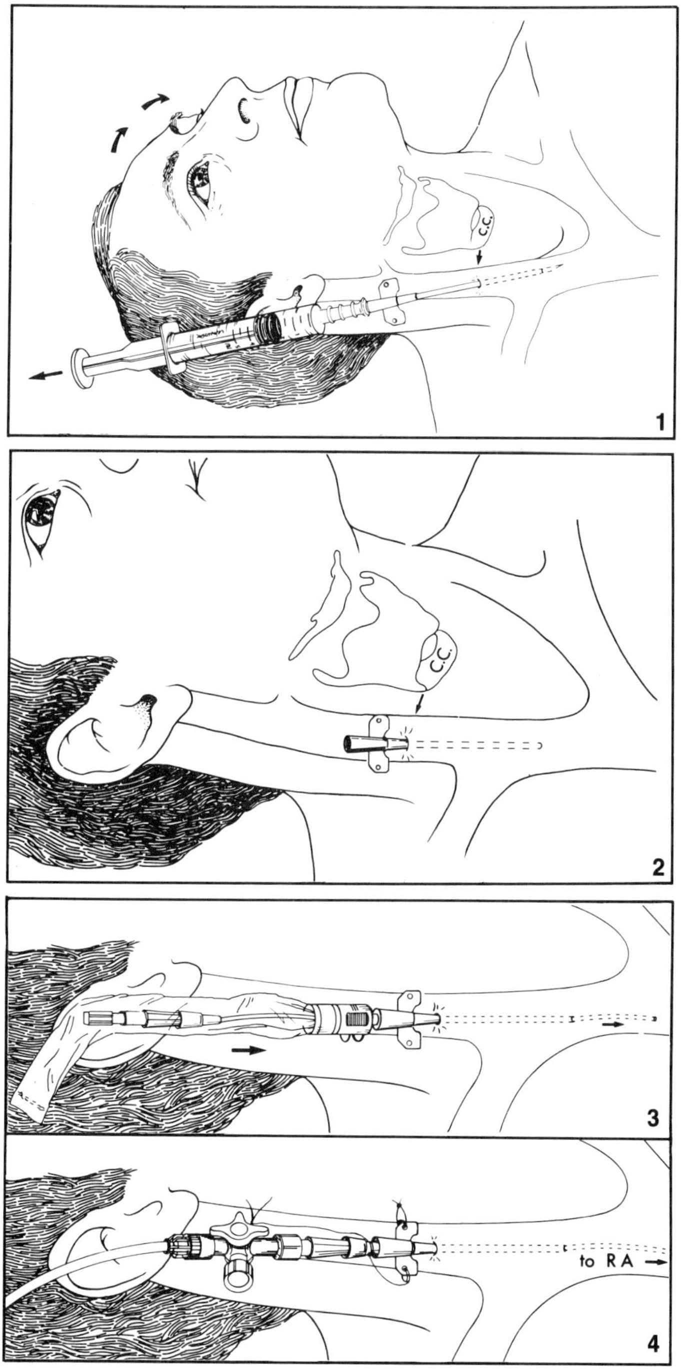

Fig. 2.3 (1, 2, 3 and 4) Steps in the insertion of a long cannula into the superior vena cava, via the right internal jugular vein.

USCI Hemaquet) allows the introduction of a 'sleeve' into a central vein which can serve the dual purpose of central pressure monitoring and as a route for the rapid introduction of a Swan–Ganz catheter in the postoperative period. Central venous cannulae are used as a route for intravenous fluid and electrolyte infusion, but the cannula used for pressure monitoring should not be used to administer powerful vasoactive drugs. Flushing such a multiple-use cannula could inadvertently administer a bolus of a vasoactive drug with dangerous results. The zero reference point for the central venous pressure is the right atrium, and care should be taken to ensure that the venous pressure transducer is located at this level at all times. If the transducer is just 6 inches above mid-thorax, the apparent central venous pressure will be 11.4 mmHg (1.52 kPa) lower than the actual central venous pressure. The normal central venous pressure in an anaesthetized patient on intermittent positive pressure ventilation is around 5–10 mmHg (0.67–1.3 kPa); but pressures ranging up to and beyond 20–25 mmHg (2.6–3.3 kPa) will be found in patients with cardiac failure associated with reduced right ventricular compliance or tricuspid valve malfunction.

During cardiopulmonary bypass the venous pressure falls to zero unless there is some obstruction to venous outflow. A rapid rise in central venous pressure accompanied by a fall in extracorporeal volume signals an obstructed venous outflow line. A sustained elevation of pressure in the superior vena cava (SVC) can cause cerebral oedema, and monitoring of SVC pressure is particularly valuable when the SVC has been taped around a small venous cannula to gain access to a sinus venosus defect or an anomalous right upper pulmonary vein.

At the end of bypass, with normal circulation restored, the response of the central venous pressure to increments of blood volume is a guide to the adequacy of volume replacement. In most circumstances however, the use of the left atrial pressure for this purpose is more appropriate, and this is easily achieved by needle puncture while the heart is exposed in theatre. The right and left atrial pressure will usually rise in parallel in response to an increase in blood volume, as long as they remain within the normal range. Dysfunction of either ventricle will distort this relationship however, and the use of the central venous pressure to infer left atrial pressure is unreliable and not advised.

Central venous pressure monitoring is normally continued through the early postoperative period, and the rate of change of the central venous pressure during transfusion is a useful guide to blood volume restitution. A progressive sustained rise in central venous pressure in this period, in the absence of colloid infusion, is due to cardiac failure, peripheral vasoconstriction, or pericardial tamponade. A fixed rise will accompany atrial arrhythmias associated with loss of normal atrial contraction.

The base-line central venous pressure in a well-sedated patient on intermittent positive pressure ventilation during the first few hours postoperatively, is usually 4–5 mmHg (0.5–0.67 kPa) higher than that noted peri-operatively in theatre. This difference in central venous pressure is most marked in patients who show marked peripheral vasoconstriction in the early post-operative period. Abrupt transient rises in central venous pressure are most likely to be due to restlessness or breath-holding in a ventilated patient.

2.4 LEFT ATRIAL PRESSURE AND PULMONARY WEDGE PRESSURE MEASUREMENT

A knowledge of the left atrial pressure in conjunction with the systemic arterial pressure, yields the most valuable information about the functional status of the left ventricle.

While the heart is exposed at operation, the left atrial pressure can be measured directly by needle puncture. In patients whose left ventricular function is suspect and in whom manipulation of pre-load, after-load and myocardial contractility will be required postoperatively, the left atrial pressure can be monitored for several days through a cannula introduced into the left atrium as shown in Fig. 2.4.

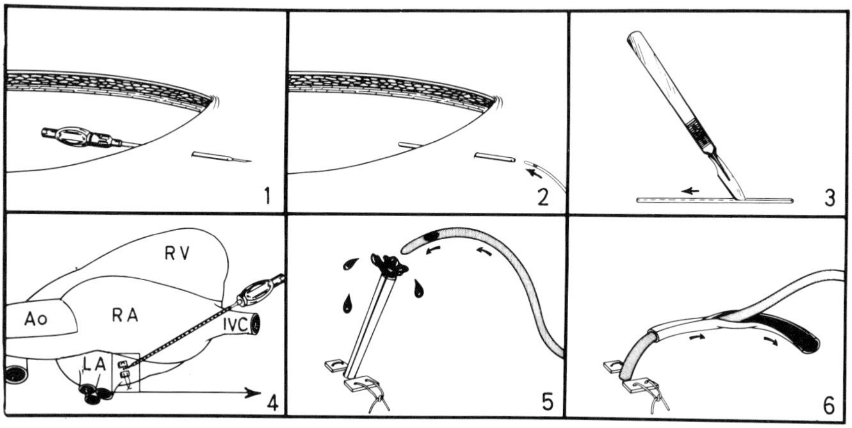

Fig. 2.4 A method of introducing a left atrial cannula during exposure of the heart (see text for details).

A purse-string stitch incorporating two teflon felt pledgets is placed in the left atrial wall close to the junction of the right superior pulmonary veins. A Wallace catheter (size 16 g) is passed through the skin and rectus muscle at the lower end of the sternotomy wound, by piercing these structures with a Medicut cannula from within out, then passing the Wallace catheter through it. The Medicut cannula is then removed, and cut length-wise with a scalpel. This modified cannula and its needle are then used to enter the left atrium through the purse-string stitch; the needle is removed; the Wallace catheter is introduced through the Medicut into the left atrial cavity; the Medicut sleeve is withdrawn and peeled off the Wallace catheter; finally the purse-string is tightened and tied.

Where measurement of left atrial pressure is desirable pre-operatively as well as during and after surgery, a Swan–Ganz balloon-tipped catheter (Fig. 2.5) can be introduced prior to surgery into the pulmonary artery to measure pulmonary artery pressure, and in the wedged position, the pulmonary capillary wedge pressure (PWP) as an index of left atrial pressure. Suitable pulmonary artery catheters will also allow thermodilution measurements of cardiac output.

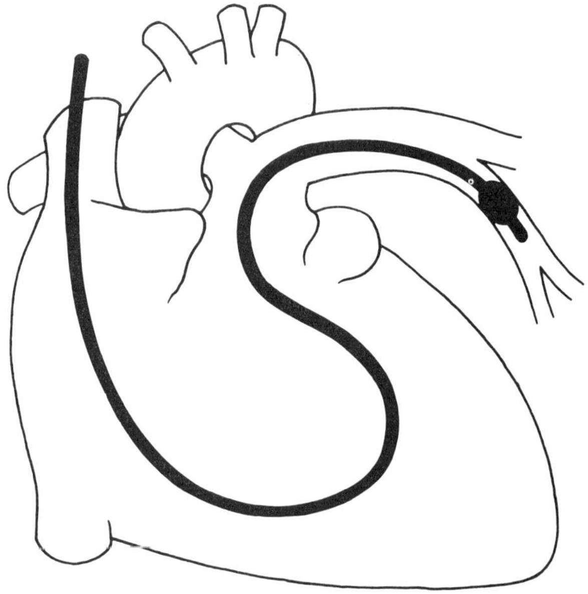

Fig. 2.5 Principles of the flow directed Swan-Ganz pulmonary artery balloon catheter. Balloon deflated – pulmonary arterial pressure. Balloon inflated – left atrial pressure.

Assuming competence and normal function of the mitral valve, the mean left atrial pressure reflects the left ventricular diastolic pressure, and is a readily available marker of left ventricular function. A mean left atrial pressure in the range 5–15 mmHg (0.67–2 kPa), in the presence of an adequate cardiac output and systemic blood pressure, denotes acceptable left ventricular function. The left atrial pressure in an individual patient, after open-heart surgery will be determined by the volume of blood presenting to the left ventricle, and the ability of the ventricle to forward it to the systemic circulation. Thus the principal determinants of left atrial pressure are circulating blood volume, left ventricle compliance and contractility, and systemic arteriolar resistance. Systemic venomotor tone will affect left atrial pressure through its capacitance function, by affecting circulating blood volume.

The left atrial pressure is a particularly useful index of myocardial function during the period when the patient is being weaned off heart–lung bypass. It is common practice to restore the circulating volume by adding increments of 100–200 ml of blood whilst observing the consequent rise in left atrial pressure, and systemic blood pressure. One is, in effect, seeking the optimum point on the Frank–Starling curve (Fig. 2.6) for that individual, at that time (Braunwald *et al.*, 1967).

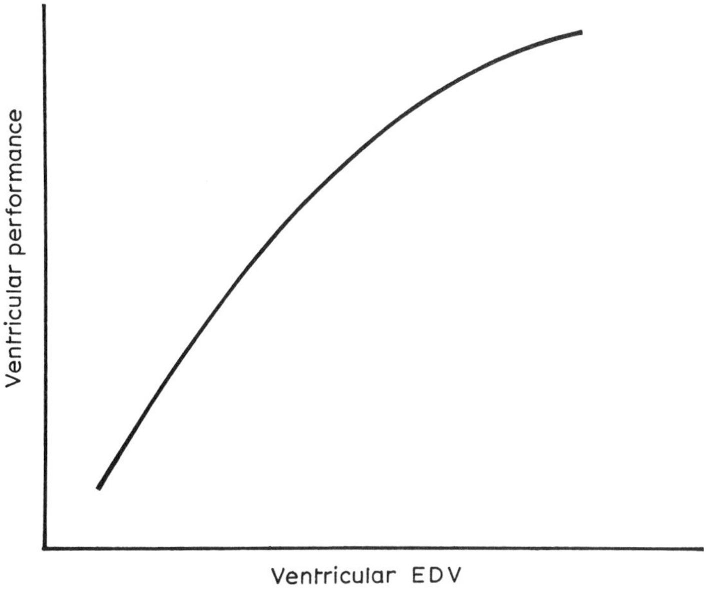

Fig. 2.6 The simplified relationship between indices of ventricular filling (end-diastolic volume, end-diastolic pressure, or left atrial pressure) and ventricular performance. (The Frank–Starling curve.) EDV = End diastolic volume.

2.5 ARTERIAL PUMP FLOW RATE

The arterial input from the pump is normally monitored continuously, and most teams pre-select a flow rate of $2.4\,l\,m^{-2}$ BSA min^{-1} (Moffitt *et al.*, 1962). There is good evidence that higher flows do not improve tissue perfusion, while on the other hand they are associated with more mechanical blood damage and a greater risk of embolism with microbubbles. The almost universal use of moderate hypothermia allows the safe use of lower pump flow rates. Reduction of the core (naso-pharyngeal) temperature to 28°C is associated with a 50% reduction in oxygen requirements, and a flow rate of $1.8\,l\,m^{-2}\,min^{-1}$ will meet perfusion demands at this temperature (see Chapter 6).

During the past five years, evidence has accumulated to show that most organs and the micro-vasculature prefer a pulsatile form of blood flow (Taylor *et al.*, 1982). This is best achieved by using a modified pump system which imparts a truly pulsatile flow and pressure quality to arterial perfusion. A pulse pressure of at least 25 mmHg (3.3 kPa) should consistently be achieved at normal flow rates. This type of arterial pump has the added advantage of offering a counterpulsation facility for use when weaning off bypass, to reduce ventricular work while improving coronary blood flow (Powell *et al.*, 1970).

2.6 SUCTION PUMP FLOW

The flow rate through cardiotomy suction pumps and those attached to intracardiac vents, should be no more than is necessary to provide a clear operative field, or to decompress the heart and pulmonary circuit. The pumping of a blood/air mixture is the principal source of haemolysis and protein denaturation during cardiopulmonary bypass (Pruit *et al.*, 1971).

2.7 TEMPERATURE

The central and peripheral body temperatures are monitored during, and for some hours after cardiopulmonary bypass. In addition the monitoring of blood temperature downstream from the heat exchanger, and of water temperature in the heat-exchanger is necessary.

The central or core temperature is usually measured with a nasopharyngeal probe, since this relatively accurately reflects this temperature.

Peripheral temperature is measured from the skin of a toe or finger exposed to the room air. The gap between the central and peripheral temperatures offers useful information about tissue perfusion. A progressively widening gap usually signifies increasing peripheral vasoconstriction.

Myocardial temperature may be measured with a needle-probe in the interventricular septum as a guide to the adequacy of selective myocardial cooling techniques. A myocardial temperature of 15°C or less should be achieved during cold cardioplegia. It must be appreciated, however, that uneven cooling may occur where coronary artery disease affects regional myocardial perfusion. The reduction of body (core) temperature to 28°C or below, has become a routine adjunct to cardiopulmonary bypass in most centres. The advantages are:

(1) A smaller gradient between the selectively cooled heart (where cold cardioplegia has been used) and its surroundings.
(2) Pump flow rate can be reduced, reducing collateral return to the heart, while maintaining adequate metabolic supply to vital organs.
(3) Safe circulatory arrest time can be extended to 10–12 minutes in the event of heart–lung machine breakdown.

It should be noted however, that it may take up to 35 minutes for conventional cardiopulmonary bypass circuits to reduce the nasopharyngeal temperature to 28°C (Fig. 2.7).

2.8 BIOCHEMISTRY

The blood gas tensions, pH, and plasma potassium levels should be monitored during cardiopulmonary bypass. Though in-line sensors for PO_2, oxygen saturation, PCO_2 and pH are in limited use and the focus of much development, intermittent blood sampling remains the standard technique at least for the present. Modern oxygenators have been refined to the point where they can be relied upon to maintain the arterial PO_2 and PCO_2 at safe levels, provided the blood/gas flow ratios are appropriate. Periodic measurement is prudent however, and a PaO_2 between 100 and 200 mmHg (13.3 and 26.6 kPa) is the aim. Higher PaO_2 levels are unnecesary and may cause small vessel constriction and a risk of micro bubble formation.

An arterial PCO_2 of around 40 mmHg (5.3 kPa) should be maintained during normothermic cardiopulmonary bypass. At the beginning of bypass the gas-flow required to achieve this may produce excessively high levels of PO_2, where the oxygenator is ventilated with 100% oxygen. A better method is to employ two sources of gas for the oxygenator; one comprising 100% oxygen, and the other a mixture of 95% oxygen and 5% carbon dioxide. By varying the proportions of these gases flowing through the oxygenator, a more appropriate arterial PCO_2 can be maintained. CO_2 build-up may occur in the rewarming phase, particularly when high-efficiency bubble oxygenators are used (see Chapter 15).

Blood pH tends to fall slightly during bypass, due to an increased production of lactic acid. The inclusion of 50 mmols sodium bicarbonate in the prime usually suffices to correct this, but measurement of pH half-hourly throughout bypass may call for additional bicarbonate. The appropriate pH for various degrees of hypothermia has been controversial for 20 years. The consensus at present suggests that a mild alkalosis achieved by a reduction of PCO_2 to between 30 and 35 mmHg (4–4.7 kPa) is correct (Rahn *et al.*, 1975).

Plasma potassium levels should be measured during and after cardiopulmonary bypass, and kept within the range of 4.5–5.5 mmol l^{-1}. Defibrillation is more difficult and ventricular arrhythmias are more frequent, if the

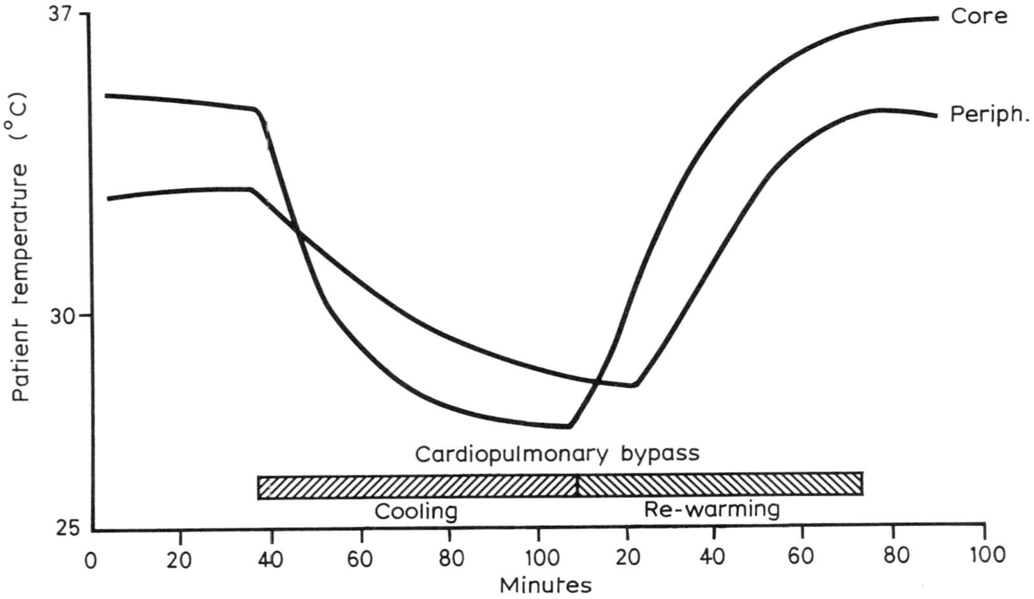

Fig. 2.7 The core (nasopharyngeal) and peripheral temperature during cardiopulmonary bypass with cooling to 28°C. The curves represent the mean temperatures from 20 consecutive patients, using the Cobe Optiflo II integral heat-exchanger with coolant temperature at 27°C during cooling and 38–40°C during rewarming.

plasma potassium level is allowed to fall below 4.5 mmol l^{-1}. Excessive elevations in the plasma potassium levels after cardiopulmonary bypass rarely reflect a true total body hyperkalaemia, but more often reflect a sodium–potassium redistribution, with massive movement of intracellular potassium into the extacellular fluid.

2.9 CEREBRAL FUNCTION

Modified electroencephalography is being used to monitor the amplitude and frequency of electrical activity in the brain during bypass, as an early warning of cerebral underperfusion. Our own experience confirms previous work in observing a flattening of brain waves when the arterial pressure on bypass falls to low levels (<35 mmHg (4.7 kPa)). We have not, however, been able to correlate changes in the intra-operative record of a cerebral function monitor with subsequent clinical evidence of neurological damage. The perfusion pressure at which flattening of the trace occurs varies from patient to patient, and it seems likely that calibre and vaso-activity of the cerebral vessels are important determinants of cerebral perfusion during bypass in older patients.

The reduction of body temperature to 25–28°C also modifies the electroencephalogram, and lessens the value of a cerebral function monitor during elective total-body cooling. Nevertheless, cerebral dysfunction of varying degrees remains a principal cause of morbidity after cardiopulmonary bypass, and any device which may reduce the incidence of this problem should be carefully evaluated. Recent studies with evoked potential responses, and with biochemical markers of brain injury may prove more sensitive.

2.10 COMPUTER-LINKED MONITORING

The capacity of a computer or microprocessor to handle vast quantities of data with great rapidity makes it a useful adjunct to a monitoring network. Thus a computer linked on-line to the various monitors used in the theatre and intensive care area, can sample all the measurements at very frequent intervals, and generate accurate and detailed information about the patient's course. Suitably programmed, the output of such a computer can take the form of trend graphs, cumulative blood and fluid balances, lists of laboratory reports, and a chronological listing of surgical and nursing interventions. This output can be displayed on command for individual patients, or can be plotted/printed at regular intervals as a shift-report for the records (Fig. 2.8). The storage capacity of the computer can be used to collate the trends in certain measurements from many patients to yield a valuable teaching aid.

The computer can also be programmed to aid decision-making, and even to implement therapy. Such 'closed-loop' systems have been used in a few

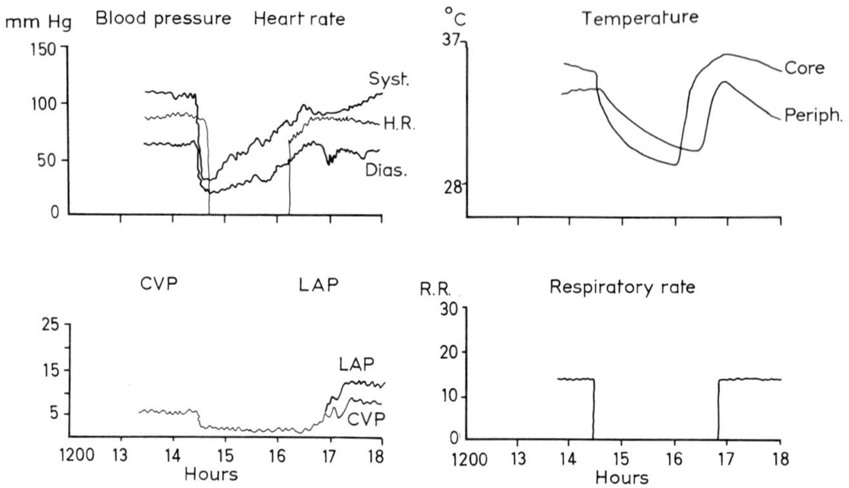

Fig. 2.8 Re-drawn from a computer print-out of the intra-operative course of a patient undergoing cardiopulmonary bypass with hypothermia and cardioplegia. The monitors were connected to the patient in theatre between 1320 hours and 1330, and the patient transferred to ITU at 1800 hours. (DEC 11/23 computer; S & W monitors; sampling rate – every 60 seconds; Calcomp flat-bed plotter.)

centres for several years (Robicsek *et al.*, 1977, Sheppard and Kouchoukos, 1977).

The recent rapid developments in microprocessor technology are now offering a tool to solve the problems described by Lewis in 1967. 'For monitoring, the surgeon needs a perceptive and sensitive assistant capable of performing repetitive and monotonous observations without exhaustion or error, and capable of carrying out useful and logically consistent analysis of these observations' (Lewis, 1967).

REFERENCES

Braunwald, E., Ross, J. and Sonnenblick, E. H. (1967) Mechanisms of contraction of the normal and failing heart. *N. Engl. J. Med.*, **277**, 794.

Lewis, F. J. (1967) Computer techniques in the care of surgical patients. *Surgery*, **62**, 630.

Moffit, E. A., Kirklin, J. W. and Theye, R. A. (1962) Physiologic studies during whole body perfusion in Tetralogy of Fallot. *J. Thorac. Cardiovasc. Surg.*, **44**, 180.

Powell, W. J. Jr, Daggett, W. M., Magro, A. E., Bianco, J. A., Buckley, M. J., Sanders, C. A., Kantrowitz, A. R. and Austen, W. G. (1970) Effects of intra-aortic balloon counterpulsation on cardiac performance, oxygen consumption, and coronary blood flow in dogs. *Circ. Res.*, **26**, 753.

Pruit, K. M., Stroud, R. M. and Scott, J. W. (1971) Blood damage in the heart–lung machine. *Proc. Soc. Exp. Biol. Med.*, **137**, 714.

Rahn, H., Reeves, R. B. and Howell, B. J. (1975) Hydrogen ion regulation, temperature, and evolution. *Am. Rev. Resp. Dis.*, **112**, 165.

Robicsek, F., Masters, T. N., Reichert, P. L., Daugherty, H. K. and Cook, J. W. (1977) Three years experience of computer-based Intensive Care of patients. *Col. Works Cardiopulm. Dis.*, **21**, 48.

Sarnoff, S. J., Braunwald, E., Welch, G. H. Jr *et al.* (1958) Haemodynamic determinants of oxygen consumption of the heart with special reference to the tension-time index. *Am. J. Physiol.*, **192**, 48.

Sheppard, L. C. and Kouchoukos, N. T. (1977) Automation of measurements and interventions in the systematic care of post-operative cardiac surgical patients. *Med. Instrument.*, **11**, 296.

Taylor, K. M., Bain, W. H., Davidson, K. G. and Turner, M. A. (1982) Comparative clinical study of pulsatile and non-pulsatile perfusion in 350 consecutive patients. *Thorax*, **37**, 324.

3

Anaesthesia for cardiopulmonary bypass in adults

ALEXANDER D. McLAREN

Anaesthesia for the cardiac surgical patient presents an interesting challenge to the anaesthetist. Drugs used to produce sleep, analgesia, and muscle relaxation (the classical triad of anaesthesia) often have a detrimental effect on the cardiovascular system. Patients with a damaged myocardium as a result of ischaemic heart disease or altered haemodynamics due to valvular disease are in a particularly hazardous situation. An awareness of the potential problems, and their remedies, a knowledge of the physiology, pathology and pharmacology of the cardiovascular system, expertise in the handling of the special equipment involved in cardiopulmonary bypass, and an ability to tolerate the caprices of cardiac surgeons are prerequisites for the anaesthetist providing a cardiac surgical service.

The responsibilities of the cardiac surgical anaesthetist do not differ from those associated with other forms of anaesthesia and can be divided into five main sections:

(1) Pre-operative assessment
(2) Premedication
(3) Monitoring
(4) Anaesthesia and the maintenance of cardiovascular stability for cardiopulmonary bypass
(5) Postoperative care
  (a) Analgesia
  (b) Airway management

3.1 PRE-OPERATIVE ASSESSMENT

All patients scheduled for elective cardiac surgery have been subjected to an exhaustive medical and biochemical work-up. Factors which may adversely affect the outcome of surgery, e.g. body weight, smoking, hypertension, diabetes, will have been identified and advice given or therapy instituted to ensure that the patient presents for surgery in the optimum possible condition.

A pre-operative visit is vital in order that the anaesthetist may establish rapport with the patient and familiarize himself with the clinical situation. A detailed medical history, clinical evaluation, examination of electrocardiogram and chest X-ray, and scrutiny of the results of laboratory tests (haematology, biochemistry, respiratory function tests) form the basis of the anaesthetic assessment. The results of cardiac catheterization, angiograms, and echocardiography are usually available and yield invaluable information to forewarn of patients who may present particular problems to the anaesthetist.

Pre-operative drug therapy in the cardiac patient should be closely examined. Any history of allergies or adverse reactions to anaesthetic agents must be noted. Patients presenting for coronary artery surgery are almost invariably on β-adrenergic blocking drugs. The inadvisability of discontinuing such therapy prior to surgery is well established due to the high incidence of rebound hypertension and angina (Harrison and Alderman, 1976). The effects of such drugs may indeed be beneficial in the intra-operative period where prevention of tachycardia and hypertension is all important in preventing an increased myocardial oxygen demand. Other antihypertensive drugs, e.g. methyldopa, nifedipine, should also be continued until the day of surgery as they may contribute to a reduced incidence of pre- or intra-operative hypertension.

Digoxin is normally discontinued 48 h prior to surgery. Though this may help to reduce digoxin-induced arrhythmias it may also result in a more rapid ventricular response to atrial fibrillation and it may be necessary to administer digoxin or a β-adrenergic blocker intra-operatively. Depletion of total body potassium is common in patients who have been on prolonged diuretic therapy. Hypokalaemia must be corrected pre-operatively as a deficiency of this ion may result in arrhythmias at the induction of anaesthesia.

3.2 PREMEDICATION

Cardiac surgery represents a major traumatic experience in a patient's life. Patients with ischaemic heart disease are susceptible to anginal attacks brought on by the tachycardia and hypertension associated with emotion. Such attacks may increase in frequency following admission to hospital for surgery. The aim of premedication should be to reduce the patients' anxiety and reduce the effect of potentially stressful stimuli, e.g. the visits of the surgeon, anaesthetist, physiotherapist, and close relatives, to a minimum.

The idea that anxiety starts one to two hours prior to surgery is obviously fallacious.

The author's practice is to use heavy oral sedation in patients about to undergo surgery for ischaemic heart disease. This entails seeing the patients two to three days prior to surgery in order to prescribe routine day and night sedation. Despite the recent introduction of newer benzodiazepine drugs, e.g. lorazepam, temazepam, the standard drug remains diazepam. A dose of 2–5 mg thrice daily will produce a tranquil, co-operative patient unaffected by the often worrying stimuli experienced in the days prior to surgery. Night sedation is routinely prescribed in order that patients are guaranteed sleep in their unaccustomed environment.

Oral benzodiazepines are our standard premedicant drugs. Diazepam (10–30 mg) or nitrazepam (5–20 mg) are given orally two hours prior to surgery, usually with a cup of tea. The avoidance of narcotic drugs as premedicants ensures that such premedication, including the tea, will have left the stomach by the time of induction (Todd and Nimmo, 1983).

Anticholinergic drugs, e.g. atropine or hyoscine, are not required in the premedication of cardiac surgery patients. Bronchial secretions are not a problem and the patient is saved the unpleasant experience of a dry mouth and the potentially undesirable effect of tachycardia. If vagolytic therapy should be required during operation small incremental doses of atropine can be given to achieve the desired effect.

Topical nitroglycerin is a useful adjunct to sedation in patients with unstable or nocturnal angina. Application at the time of premedication may help to prevent anginal attacks during the pre-operative and induction periods (Miner and Conti, 1978).

Heavy pre-operative sedation may be hazardous to patients with valvular heart disease. The risk of emotionally induced imbalance between myocardial oxygen supply and demand is less significant. A suitable dose of benzodiazepine, e.g. diazepam 5–15 mg given two hours pre-operatively, provides a sedated patient, amnesic for the period leading up to induction of anaesthesia. In poor risk cases it is a wise safeguard to give oxygen from the time of premedication in order that arterial hypoxaemia be avoided.

3.3 MONITORING (see Chapter 2)

It is our routine practice to monitor:

(1) Electrocardiogram
(2) Arterial blood pressure
(3) Central venous pressure
(4) Urine output
(5) Nasopharyngeal (core) and peripheral temperature

(6) Blood gas analysis and acid–base status
(7) Serum potassium
(8) Haematocrit
(9) Activated clotting time to determine both the adequacy of heparinization and its reversal by protamine
(10) Cerebral function monitor

We are not convinced, except in patients who are extremely ill, of any advantage in inserting our intravascular monitoring cannulae prior to induction of anaesthesia.

Pulmonary artery flotation cannulae, which allow measurement of pulmonary capillary wedge pressure, central venous pressure, and cardiac output, are not inserted routinely as the vast majority of cases can be managed perfectly well without introducing this expensive, invasive, and potentially hazardous monitor into routine practice. They do, however, provide extremely useful information in patients who:

(1) Are known to have poor left ventricular function (left ventricular end diastolic pressure $\geq$14 mmHg (1.9 kPa) or ejection fraction $\leq$40%).
(2) Are demonstrated to have abnormal ventricular wall motion at angiography.
(3) Have had a recent myocardial infarction or episode of congestive cardiac failure.
(4) Have severe pulmonary hypertension.

A recent innovation is the percutaneous pulmonary artery catheter introducer sheath with haemostasis valve. This can be used as a means of fluid administration during operation and if an indication arises a pulmonary artery catheter can be readily inserted.

3.4 ANAESTHESIA AND MAINTENANCE OF CARDIOVASCULAR STABILITY

The multiplicity of induction techniques recommended by cardiac surgical centres without demonstrable difference in intra- or postoperative morbidity or mortality leads one to suspect that the expertise of the individual anaesthetists involved is a more important factor in anaesthetic safety than the cocktails used.

Certain considerations must be borne in mind. All important is the maintenance of myocardial oxygen balance, i.e. at all times myocardial oxygen supply must be greater than myocardial oxygen demand. Factors which influence the myocardial oxygen balance are indicated in Table 3.1. Any increase in heart rate or blood pressure (or both) will result in an increased myocardial oxygen demand and if this demand cannot be met, e.g.

Table 3.1 Factors affecting myocardial oxygen balance

Oxygen supply	*Oxygen demand*
1 Coronary blood flow	1 Heart rate (rhythm)
2 Oxygen delivery	2 Preload
a O_2 saturation	3 Afterload
b Haematocrit	4 Contractility

in a heart with an obstructed coronary circulation, then myocardial hypoxia is the inevitable result.

A useful concept attempting to relate myocardial oxygen supply and demand is that suggested by Hoffman and Buckberg (1975). The area under the left ventricular systolic ejection curve, which represents the integrated left ventricular pressure during systolic contraction, correlates with the myocardial oxygen demand (tension-time index). Oxygen supply to the myocardium occurs during diastole and is related to the pressure gradient producing blood flow and to the duration of diastole. Oxygen supply can therefore be related to the area under the diastolic pressure curve (diastolic pressure-time index). The supply:demand ratio, i.e. DPTI:TTI should be greater than unity at all times as if it falls to less than one myocardial oxygenation is in jeopardy (Brazier *et al.*, 1974) (see Fig. 2.1 (Chapter 2)).

The rate pressure product (RPP), the product of heart rate and systolic pressure, is a simple non-invasive parameter which has been shown to correlate with myocardial work and therefore myocardial oxygen uptake (Nelson *et al.*, 1974). The anaesthetist, always remembering that a slow heart rate is more conducive to myocardial oxygen supply, should have a predetermined value of RPP which he will not allow the patient to exceed. Kaplan correlated the RPP with ischaemic changes on the electrocardiogram (Kaplan, 1979) and recommends that an RPP of 12 000 with a pulse rate not greater than 90 beats per minute should not be exceeded.

Knowledge of factors controlling myocardial oxygen balance must be utilized when anaesthetizing patients with cardiovascular disease. The importance of adequate premedication in producing a calm co-operative patient in the anaesthetic room has already been mentioned. Induction of anaesthesia must be smooth and unhurried in order to minimize changes in heart rate and blood pressure. Thiopentone sodium, narcotics, benzodiazepines and inhalation techniques are all in current usage. The author's current practice is to induce patients with midazolam, a new benzodiazepine drug, and morphine, starting with a dose of 10 mg of each drug and giving alternate increments of 5 mg until unconsciousness is produced. Patients with poor left ventricular function require even greater vigilance at induction and we have found etomidate, a rapidly acting intravenous hypnotic noted for its lack of cardiovascular effects, to be a useful alternative agent.

After loss of consciousness the patient is allowed to breath nitrous oxide and oxygen in a 50:50 ratio and muscle relaxation is produced. Although not absolutely essential for cardiac surgery muscle relaxation is generally thought to be advisable in order that:

(1) ventilation can be properly controlled; and
(2) the truncal rigidity associated with high doses of narcotic (especially fentanyl) is avoided.

The muscle relaxant most commonly used, despite its occasional tendency to induce a troublesome tachycardia, is pancuronium bromide. Tubocurarine which produces vasodilatation by ganglionic blockade and release of histamine is best reserved for hypertensive coronary artery patients. Two new muscle relaxants, both claiming greater cardiovascular stability than the older agents have recently become available. Atracurium bresylate (Tracrium) and vecuronium (Norcuron) are both short-acting non-depolarizing competitive neuromuscular blockers. They can be used in bolus form but are better used as intravenous infusions during bypass (Flynn, *et al.*, 1984). Atracurium has the added advantage that it is hydrolysed in the tissues in a predictable fashion and does not depend on hepatic or renal function for its inactivation.

Provided the patient has good left ventricular function a volatile anaesthetic agent, e.g. halothane or enflurane, can be added to the inspired gas mixture at this time. These agents will further deepen the anaesthetic level and reduce rises in heart rate or blood pressure stimulated by laryngoscopy and intubation. The pressor response associated with laryngoscopy can be further attenuated by topical administration of a 4% lignocaine spray to the larynx and trachea or by giving a further small dose of benzodiazepine prior to intubation (Denhinger *et al.*, 1974).

Maintenance of anaesthesia is best provided by infusion of drugs. Continuous intravenous infusion ensures that the blood level of drugs is maintained at a constant level and avoids the peaks and troughs of drug action associated with bolus administration. Haemodynamic disturbance is also much less likely with constant infusion. Knowledge of the pharmacokinetic profile of a drug is necessary for this type of administration and in general drugs with short half-lives are more suited.

3.4.1 Sleep

Etomidate and althesin, both short-acting anaesthetic induction agents, seemed ideal for this purpose. However etomidate infusions have recently been shown to produce adrenocortical suppression (Ledingham and Watt, 1983) and althesin has been withdrawn due to an unacceptably high incidence of anaphylactic reactions. Methohexitone, a short-acting barbiturate or a benzodiazepine, e.g. midazolam, would appear to be the drugs best suited to infusion for maintenance of sleep at the present time.

3.4.2 Analgesia

Morphine infusions are widely used to provide analgesia during both the intra- and postoperative periods but from a pharmacokinetic point of view one of the newer short-acting narcotics, e.g. fentanyl (sublimaze) or alfentanyl (rapifen) would appear to be a more logical choice. The main disadvantage of these drugs is their potency and liability to produce respiratory depression in the postoperative period.

3.4.3 Muscle relaxation

Vecuronium and atracurium can both be administered as infusions. Using a nerve stimulator attached to a recording device a constant display of myoneural function can be obtained and the infusion rate adjusted as necessary.

Patients require to be at the deepest level of anaesthesia at the commencement of surgery. The greatest degree of surgical stimulus is from the time of skin incision up to and including the median sternotomy. If the anaesthetic technique fails to control adequately pulse and blood pressure it will be necessary for the anaesthetist to administer vasodilators and possibly β-adrenergic blockers to regain the status quo.

Many drugs can cause vasodilatation but in practice we prefer to use drugs with specific vasodilator properties. Drugs which produce vasodilation and affect conscious level, e.g. phenothiazines, are best avoided.

Pre-bypass hypertension is best treated by the use of volatile anaesthetic agents or an infusion of nitroglycerin or a combination of both. The volatile anaesthetic agents are best used in patients known to have good left ventricular function as their hypotensive effect is largely due to direct myocardial depression although systemic vascular resistance is also decreased. In our practice all patients undergoing coronary artery surgery are commenced on an infusion of nitroglycerin at induction of anaesthesia at a dose of 50 $\mu g\ min^{-1}$. This allows for rapid administration of the drug should the necessity arise. The superiority of nitroglycerin to nitroprusside in the pre-bypass period has been demonstrated by Kaplan and Jones (1979). They showed that although both nitroglycerin and nitroprusside reduce myocardial oxygen demand the coronary perfusion pressure is better maintained by nitroglycerin. A decrease in coronary perfusion pressure in patients with obstructed coronary arteries may result in a coronary 'steal' syndrome where already ischaemic areas of myocardium are further compromised. Assuming that surgery has achieved full revascularization of the myocardium sodium nitroprusside is best reserved for the treatment of post-bypass hypertension.

We have also found nitroglycerin to be an extremely useful drug in patients undergoing valve replacement surgery. As well as controlling hypertension the drug can be used in the treatment of hypotension especially at the discontinuation of bypass. Not infrequently patients with a low systemic pressure and high left atrial pressure are dramatically improved by the administration of nitroglycerin. The left atrial pressure falls and the cardiac output and systemic pressure increase.

The administration of vasodilators results in an increase in heart rate. Small intravenous increments of a β-adrenergic blocking drug, e.g. oxprenolol, may be necessary to ensure that the predetermined limits of pressure and rate are not exceeded.

3.4.4 **Heparinization** (see Chapter 16)

Monitoring of the degree of anticoagulation and its reversal have been greatly simplified with the introduction of the activated clotting time (ACT). An initial dose of heparin (300 units kg^{-1}) is administered intravenously several minutes prior to bypass cannulation. The ACT should be maintained above 400 s for the duration of cannulation. Following decannulation protamine sulphate is administered until the ACT returns to control values (usually less than 140 s) (Dutton *et al.*, 1983).

3.4.5 Maintenance during bypass

During bypass the oxygenator takes over the role of the ventilator and ventilation can therefore be stopped. The lungs are held inflated at an airway pressure of about 1 kPa in order to prevent small airway closure and the development of absorption atelectasis during the non-ventilated period, although there is no evidence to support the usefulness of this manoeuvre.

Anaesthesia during this period can only be maintained by the intravascular administration of drugs. Using the infusion techniques described this presents no problem, although it may be necessary to increase infusion rates or give a small bolus dose of maintenance agents at the initiation of bypass due to the dilutional effect of the priming fluid. The rates of infusion can however be reduced again if the patient is being cooled as hypothermia will potentiate the effects of the circulating anaesthetic agents and muscle relaxants.

3.4.6 Perfusion pressure during bypass

The ideal perfusion pressure during bypass is unknown. While some centres disregard perfusion pressure completely arguing that hypothermia ensures end organ function and that flow is all important, other groups aggressively treat any fall in mean pressure below figures as high as 80 mmHg (10.7 kPa). The treatment of low perfusion pressures with vasopressors, thus probably worsening perfusion to certain regions, has always seemed an illogical practice and it is the author's practice to accept a low perfusion pressure in the certain knowledge that it will gradually rise during bypass. Urine production and cerebral function monitoring are certainly not affected at pressures down to 30 mmHg (4 kPa) though it is accepted that these may be crude indicators. The advocates of maintaining high perfusion pressure have as yet brought forward no convincing evidence of an altered incidence of postoperative organ dysfunction in their patients. Awareness and calculation of peripheral vascular resistance index levels would be a welcome improvement in haemodynamic management during perfusion.

3.4.7 Discontinuation of bypass

As the patient is gradually rewarmed to normothermia the dose of anaesthetic drugs again requires to be increased. Bypass should only be terminated once certain conditions are satisfied:

(1) The heart has been emptied of any residual air. (Positive pressure ventilation and a Valsalva manoeuvre during removal of the left ventricular vent cannula may assist with de-airing.)
(2) Ventilation of the lungs has recommenced. Volatile agents should not be used at this stage. The avoidance of nitrous oxide is probably wise post-bypass. Because of its solubility characteristics the gas is liable to diffuse from the blood into air-filled spaces. The consequences of this physical property could be extremely serious if air bubbles are present in the arterial circulation. Patients should be ventilated with 100% oxygen or oxygen-enriched air following bypass.
(3) Temperature $\geqslant$36.5°C.
(4) Acid–base status within normal limits.
(5) Potassium level within normal limits.
(6) Cardiac rhythm is stable.

Termination of bypass is really a practical application of Starling's Law. Preload is adjusted to provide an adequate cardiac output and systemic pressure. All of our patients come off bypass on a nitroglycerin infusion (50–200 $\mu g\ min^{-1}$) the dose being adjusted to provide a systemic pressure of 80–120 mmHg (10.7–16 kPa). This regime is used to provide:

(1) Optimal filling pressures in a dilated patient.
(2) Maximal coronary perfusion.
(3) More efficient rewarming.

The use of inotropic drugs following cardiac surgery has greatly decreased over the past few years. The introduction of modern cold cardioplegia techniques, a better understanding of the physiology involved, and improved surgical and anaesthetic techniques have all combined to improve myocardial performance post-bypass. Calcium chloride (1 g) can be a useful drug in the early post-bypass period if the heart is slow to recover from a residual cardioplegic effect.

A falling arterial and rising left atrial pressure despite the above regime may indicate that an infusion of inotrope is required. All inotropic drugs will increase myocardial oxygen consumption by increasing preload or afterload. The apparent improvement in myocardial performance on their introduction may be at the cost of disrupting the myocardial oxygen supply:demand ratio and the improvement may prove to be only transient. Dopamine, a noradrenaline precursor, is our first choice inotrope. An infusion of this drug will increase output by augmenting stroke volume and will have a lesser chronotropic effect than adrenaline or isoprenaline. Effective infusion rates of dopamine can vary from 2 to 20 $\mu g\,kg^{-1}\,min^{-1}$. If a primarily chronotropic effect is required then epicardial pacing wires are sutured to the heart or an isoprenaline infusion can be used although this will produce a much less-easily controlled rate than the pacemaker.

In the routine case however it is hypertension and not hypotension which is most commonly seen post-bypass. Post-bypass hypertension is due to increased peripheral vascular resistance thought to be produced by the release of vasoactive substances during bypass, e.g. angiotensin, serotonin. Drugs with a predominantly afterload reducing effect are most useful in treating this high vascular resistance. Sodium nitroprusside is our drug of choice. Infused at a rate of 1–8 $\mu g\,kg^{-1}\,min^{-1}$ it produces a rapid and easily controllable fall in peripheral resistance thus reducing myocardial work and oxygen demand (Campbell *et al.*, 1982). Specific blocking drugs for both angiotensin and serotonin activity are currently available. Captopril, an angiotensin converting enzyme inhibitor, which blocks the conversion of angiotensin I into angiotensin II, and ketanserin, a specific serotonin blocker, although not in routine use may have a part to play in the control of post-bypass hypertension.

3.5 POSTOPERATIVE CARE

The anaesthetist's responsibility for analgesia and ventilation of the patient should certainly continue until the time of removal of the endotracheal tube.

Transfer of the patient from the operating theatre to the intensive care unit requires certain provisions:

(1) Blood pressure and electrocardiogram require to be continuously monitored.

(2) Portable oxygen supply and a means of ventilating the patient, e.g. Ambu bag.
(3) Battery-driven infusion pumps to ensure that anaesthetic, inotropic, or vasodilator drugs continue to be infused during this critical period.
(4) A defibrillator.

All parameters, with the exception of the cerebral function monitor, mentioned in the monitoring section should continue to be monitored in the intensive care unit. Blood loss into calibrated drains is an additional measurement in the postoperative period.

Hypoxaemia or hypercarbia in the postoperative period will cause reduced myocardial efficiency and an increased tendency to arrhythmias. Both of these complications are less likely to occur if the patient is ventilated. The majority of our patients are routinely ventilated for a minimum period of six hours. This period allows:

(1) The effect of muscle relaxants, and analgesic-induced respiratory depression to wear off.
(2) Complete rewarming to take place. Despite the achievement of normothermia at the end of bypass an inevitable 'after drop' in temperature takes place.
(3) The identification and treatment of cardiac arrythmias.
(4) The identification and treatment of excessive bleeding.

Ventilator settings are adjusted depending on serial blood gas measurements with approximately normal results being regarded as optimal.

Pulmonary shunting is a not infrequent problem at this stage. A PaO_2 of less than 200 mmHg (26.7 kPa) at an F_IO_2 of 70% should be considered as significant shunting. The position of the endotracheal tube, the presence of bronchospasm or blood or air in the thoracic cavity should be checked and if found, treated. Interstitial pulmonary oedema or atelectasis are other possible causes of the shunting and are best dealt with by the introduction of positive end expiratory pressure (PEEP).

Postoperative analgesia should be by constant intravenous infusion. Morphine (1–4 mg h^{-1}) or fentanyl (50–150 μg h^{-1}) are regimes which produce an analgesed, co-operative patient capable of tolerating artificial ventilation and able to breathe spontaneously if disconnected from the ventilator. Small increments of midazolam (1–2 mg) or diazepam (1–5 mg) may be required if the patient is difficult to control.

Cardiac surgery has become a much more routine procedure in recent years. There is undoubtedly a tendency for numbers to be all important and for good academic research to be relegated to second place. This is unfortunate as much work requires to be done. New drugs and new equipment are constantly appearing which require detailed evaluation.

Perhaps the area most requiring research, however, is in the morbidity associated with cardiopulmonary bypass. The identification and aetiology of post-bypass neurological damage must lead to further improvement in bypass technique. Whether these syndromes are caused by microemboli or perfusion pressure inadequacy during bypass remains an intriguing question.

The present low mortality associated with cardiopulmonary bypass must not be allowed to mask the continuing morbidity. Research must be encouraged to ensure that cardiac surgery continues to advance and that patient safety is guaranteed.

REFERENCES

Brazier, J., Cooper, N. and Buckberg G. (1974) The adequacy of subendocardial oxygen delivery: The interaction of determinants of flow, arterial oxygen content and myocardial oxygen need. *Circulation*, **49**, 968–77.

Campbell, C. S., Wallwork, J., Taylor, K. M. and Wheatley, D. J. (1982) The haemodynamic effects of sodium nitroprusside following cardiopulmonary bypass: a clinical study. *J. Cardiovasc. Surg.*, **23**, 41–8.

Denhinger, J. K., Ellison, N. and Ominsky, A. J. (1974) Effects of intratracheal lignocaine on circulatory responses to tracheal intubation. *Anaesthesiology*, **41**, 409–12.

Dutton, D. A., Hothersall, A. P., McLaren, A. D., Taylor, K. M. and Turner, M. A. (1983) Protamine titration after cardiopulmonary bypass. *Anaesthesia*, **38**(3), 264–8.

Flynn, P. J., Hughes, R. and Walton, B. (1984) Use of atracurium in cardiac surgery involving cardiopulmonary by-pass with induced hypothermia. *Br. J. Anaesth.*, **56**, 967–72.

Harrison, D. C. and Alderman, E. L. (1976) Discontinuation of propranolol therapy: Cause of rebound pectoris and acute coronary events. Editorial, *Chest*, **69**, 1.

Hoffman, J. I. E. and Buckberg, G. D. (1975). Pathophysiology of subendocardial ischaemia. *Br. Med. J.* **1**, 76–9.

Kaplan, J. A. (1979) *Cardiac Anaesthesia*. Grune & Stratton, New York.

Kaplan, J. A. and Jones, E. L. (1979) Vasodilator therapy during coronary artery surgery: Comparison of nitroglycerin and nitroprusside. *J. Thorac. Cardiovasc. Surg.*, **77**, 301–9.

Ledingham, I. McA. and Watt, I. (1983) Influence of sedation on mortality in critically ill multiple trauma patients. *Lancet*, **i**, 1270.

Miner, J. A. and Conti, C. R. (1978) Topical nitroglycerin for ischaemic heart disease. *J. Am. Med. Assoc.*, **239**, 2166–7.

Nelson, R. R., Gobel, F. L., Jorgensen, C. R., Wang, K., Wang, Y. and Taylor, H. L. (1974) Haemodynamic predictors of myocardial oxygen consumption during static and dynamic exercise. *Circulation*, **50**, 1179–89.

Todd, J. G. and Nimmo, W. S. (1983) Effect of premedication on drug absorption and gastric emptying. *Br. J. Anaesth.*, **55**, 1189–93.

4

Anaesthetic techniques for cardiopulmonary bypass in children

DONALD C. MILLER

4.1 INTRODUCTION

It has been estimated that the incidence of congenital heart disease is of the order of 7 per 1000 (Carlgren, 1969) and that there is little variation in different populations. Acquired heart disease in infants and children is relatively rare and occurs in approximately 10% of all cases. The number of infants with severe heart defects is around 3:1000 and about half of all children with congenital heart defects will die in the first year of life without effective treatment.

If congenital heart disease is suspected in early life it is very important that a positive attitude is taken towards investigation and assessment of the actual defect so that if surgical intervention is indicated the patient is in the best condition to survive the operative procedure.

The number of operative procedures undertaken at our hospital is shown in Fig. 4.1. The apparent increase in numbers from 1977 to 1981 is probably related to the increasing rate of referral rather than any change in the incidence of disease in the population.

The actual classification of the various defects has been well documented (Young, 1980) but for the practising anaesthetist it is convenient to adopt a broad physiological classification as detailed.

I Intracardiac shunt with mixing of the two circulations.
II Decreased pulmonary blood flow.
III Increased pulmonary blood flow.
IV Obstruction to left or right ventricle.

It must be appreciated that some defects may occur which include several

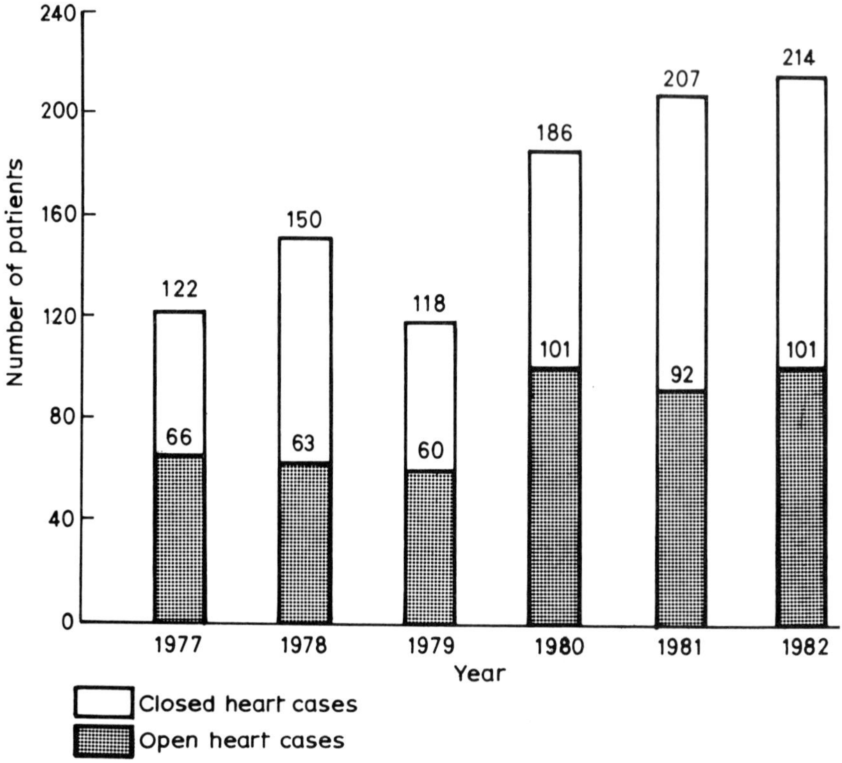

Fig. 4.1 Total number of paediatric cardiac surgical operations performed at the Royal Hospital for Sick Children, Glasgow (1977–82).

of the above categories and the surgical procedure is intended to improve the haemodynamic situation rather than the correction of every anatomical abnormality.

As modern techniques of anaesthesia and surgery incorporating bypass with hypothermia have improved results in the young infant so also has the enthusiasm for primary correction of the heart defect. The advantages of early correction of the defect over an early palliative procedure with late total correction will be dependent on the age and general condition of the infant and also the complexity of the lesion involved.

4.2 ANAESTHETIC CONSIDERATIONS

A major problem which confronts the anaesthetist involved in the field of paediatric cardiac surgery is the wide range of patients he is called upon to anaesthetize. The range includes many difficult operative procedures and a wide variation in patient age. The older child may be of almost adult size and outlook with the physiological and pharmacological problems of acquired heart disease. The youngest may be days or hours old with all the problems of the small sick neonate.

Psychological aspects must be considered in all children over two years of age. In the younger age group the principal fear is of separation from the mother and many hospitals now have facilities to allow one of the parents to live in with their child. A problem arises – is the presence of the parent in the induction room or intensive care unit in the best interests of the patient? Older children may have other fears; fear of anaesthesia, of pain and of mutilation (Pinkerton, 1981). The anaesthetist must remember these factors so that each individual child may be handled in a way which will minimize psychotrauma.

Undoubtedly, the major challenge at present is in the anaesthesia for the neonate with a major heart defect. The physiological differences between the neonate and the older child have been well documented (Hatch and Sumner, 1981; Smith, 1980) and it is important that those involved in cardiac anaesthesia for such infants are well acquainted with all aspects of anaesthesia for this age group.

Firstly, other non-cardiac congenital defects may occur in association with the cardiac lesion and there may be difficulties with endotracheal intubation and/or venous access. Temperature regulation is difficult for the neonate and hypothermia pre-operatively may lead to metabolic acidosis with increasing myocardial depression. Neonatal body systems are immature with decreased renal function and delayed liver metabolism which may be compromised further by the presence of congestive cardiac failure. Detoxification of many drugs such as the barbiturates, morphine and diazepam may be delayed and cumulation is likely unless careful consideration is given to the dosages used. Synthesis of vitamin K-dependent coagulation factors (II, VII, IX and X) by the liver is slow until the age of two months when normal adult values may be obtained.

The sensitivity of the neonate to the non-depolarizing muscle relaxants is well known (Bush and Stead, 1962) but is of minimal importance in these cases as most patients requiring surgery in the first month of life for cardiac abnormalities will require postoperative ventilation.

The nature of the cardiac defect must be a major consideration in the choice of the anaesthetic agents used. It is important to understand the nature of the haemodynamic problem so that the induction of anaesthesia will be speedy and safe. The use of myocardial depressant agents such as halothane may be acceptable in the older child with a simple ASD but may not be acceptable in the infant with cardiac failure. Inhalational agents will in general be unsatisfactory in the cyanosed child with poor pulmonary blood flow, while drugs which promote rapid vasodilatation and systemic hypotension may lead to increased right–left shunting and progressive hypoxaemia.

It is therefore important that the paediatric cardiac anaesthetist spends time pre-operatively to acquaint himself thoroughly with the child and all his problems before embarking upon an anaesthetic sequence which may be demanding and difficult.

4.2.1 Premedication

It is well recognized that in considering cardiac patients being prepared for heart surgery any distress pre-operatively may have serious consequences. Crying and struggling with breath holding may cause marked changes in intracardiac shunts and lead to hypoxaemia and metabolic acidosis. Prolonged starvation in a young infant may also produce distress and hypoglycaemia (Thomas, 1974). It is important that wherever possible, operative schedules are adhered to when dealing with this group of patients.

Some forty years ago Harmel and Lamont (1946) suggested that patients being prepared for heart surgery should be sufficiently depressed by premedicant agents that if undisturbed they would sleep. Older children who may have had previous operations and investigations should be consulted at the pre-operative visit to explain what is proposed and wherever possible techniques should be modified to take account of patient preference. In this group oral and/or intramuscular premedication may be employed depending on preference and the fitness of the patient. Diazepam 0.2 mg kg^{-1} or diazepam 0.1 mg kg^{-1} with droperidol 0.2 mg kg^{-1} (Fozard and Manford, 1977) or trimeprazine 1–2 mg kg^{-1} (Davies and Doughty, 1966) orally have all been used. Morphine 0.2 mg kg^{-1} or papaveretum 0.25 mg kg^{-1} with hyoscine or atropine have also been employed intramuscularly with success. Some authors advocate a combination of oral premedication followed by intramuscular agents given nearer the time of operation (Moffitt *et al.*, 1970; Abbott, 1981).

Small infants under 5 kg body weight or those who are ill with cardiac failure present a different problem and normally atropine 30 μg kg^{-1} is given intramuscularly one hour pre-operatively. It is important to give atropine either with the premedicant drugs or intravenously prior to induction if it is considered necessary to use ketamine as part of the anaesthetic sequence. Ketamine will produce a marked increase in tracheobronchial secretions unless a drying agent is used. This could have serious consequences in this type of patient.

4.2.2 Induction of anaesthesia

The choice of induction agents is dependent on the age and general condition of the patient. In older children with simple cardiac defects any agent which does not produce profound circulatory effects may be used. Thiopentone $5\,mg\,kg^{-1}$ intravenously is normally well tolerated by this group. If an inhalational induction is requested then nitrous oxide/oxygen with halothane or enflurane may produce satisfactory results.

Halothane however, is quite unsuitable for the smaller sick child in congestive cardiac failure because of its effects on the myocardium (Price, 1960). In addition, cyanotic children will not absorb inhalational agents because of low pulmonary blood flow. In some of these cases it may be possible to use a reduced dose of thiopentone $2\,mg\,kg^{-1}$ or morphine $0.2\,mg\,kg^{-1}$ followed by relaxant. However, probably the agent of choice in this difficult situation is ketamine $1–2\,mg\,kg^{-1}$ intravenously or $5\,mg\,kg^{-1}$ intramuscularly. Ketamine maintains the systemic blood pressure and heart rate and should therefore minimize change in right to left shunting. It is also useful in small infants since it may be given intramuscularly when venous access is very difficult. As hypoxaemia has been reported following ketamine administration it is important that the patient should receive oxygen immediately after induction (Coppel and Dundee, 1972; Zsigmond *et al.*, 1976).

The choice of muscle relaxant is more difficult. Wherever possible suxamethonium should be avoided and a non-depolarizing agent used such as d-tubocurarine or pancuronium. d-Tubocurarine may produce histamine release and in some individuals marked systemic hypotension. This may lead to increased right to left shunt with hypoxaemia and acidosis. Pancuronium has little effect on the systemic blood pressure but it may produce a marked tachycardia. This drug is not advised in patients with known ventricular hypertrophy and ventricular outflow obstruction. Vecuronium, a new muscle relaxant, requires further assessment but may prove useful for induction because of its minimal cardiovascular effects.

4.2.3 Intubation and cannulation techniques

After ventilation via mask with an appropriate mixture of oxygen and nitrous oxide an endotracheal tube is passed. It is important that in young children the diameter is such that there should be a slight leak around the tube. In infants up to 6 months of age a nasotracheal tube may be passed at this stage if postoperative ventilation is envisaged. This avoids the problem of changing tubes postoperatively when the child's condition may be less stable. Haemorrhage from the post-nasal space is not a major problem in these patients provided care is taken.

It must always be remembered that many cardiac patients have communications between the venous and arterial circulations. Great care must be taken with the injection of drugs, the insertion of cannulae, and the setting up of intravenous infusions to minimize the risk of air embolism.

4.2.4 Maintenance of anaesthesia

(a) Pre-bypass

The technique used to maintain anaesthesia will be dependent upon the size of the patient and the complexity of the operation involved. Other considerations will be the use of hypothermia and the extent to which postoperative ventilation is thought desirable. Usually after induction and insertion of the monitoring lines the patient is transferred to theatre and ventilated with a suitable ventilator fitted with a humidifier. An oxygen/nitrous oxide mixture is regulated to produce an adequate PaO_2. In cyanosed children the low PaO_2 is related to intracardiac shunting and will not be improved markedly by increasing the inspired oxygen concentration. The initial minute volume settings are determined after consultation with a nomogram but the ventilation of the patient is controlled throughout the operation by repeated blood gas analysis or in-line oxygen sensors if available.

In older children a narcotic technique may be used similar to that described by Lowenstein (1971) for adult patients using a total dose of morphine 1–2 mg kg^{-1}. A similar technique using fentanyl as the principal agent in a total dose of 5–20 μg kg^{-1} has also been described (Stanley and Webster, 1978). If a raised FIO_2 is required because of hypoxaemia then the technique may be modified by decreasing the narcotic dose and adding small increments of a volatile agent such as halothane or enflurane. Care must be taken to avoid myocardial depression and these agents are contraindicated in the presence of pre-operative cardiac failure. In the poor risk case the use of ketamine in small increments with a high inspired FIO_2 is a very suitable technique.

It should be remembered that retrolental fibroplasia is a risk in the premature low birth-weight infant. Currently, few of these patients present for bypass surgery although an increasing number present for closure of patent ductus arteriosus. Although the aetiology of retrolental fibroplasia is not completely understood it is important that in premature cases the PaO_2 should not exceed 80 mmHg (10.7 kPa).

The use of corticosteroid pretreatment to minimize oedema and stabilize membranes has been advocated and decamethonium 0.2 mg kg^{-1} or methylprednisolone sodium 30 mg kg^{-1} should be given intravenously pre-bypass or added to the pump prime.

(b) Bypass

After heparinization with 3 mg kg^{-1} heparin the arterial and venous cannulae are inserted. At this stage a further increment of relaxant and narcotic is usually given. If normothermic perfusion is envisaged then a further dose of anaesthetic agent such as thiopentone, ketamine or diazepam should be given to ensure adequate central depression. The withdrawal of nitrous oxide prior to starting bypass has been recommended to minimize possible gaseous micro-embolic effects (Bethune, 1976).

Once the patient is on full bypass, blood flow through the lungs is minimal and ventilation may be discontinued. At this point atelectasis will occur to some extent and is more severe if the pleural cavities have been opened. There has been much debate about how airway closure may be minimized. Ventilation with air, helium and oxygen/air mixtures have all been advocated. It would seem reasonable to maintain the lungs inflated at a constant pressure of 5–8 cmH_2O provided this does not interfere with the surgical field. In this regard, it is far more important to ensure that the lungs are fully expanded at the end of cardiopulmonary bypass by vigorous hand ventilation and that the surgeon is encouraged to empty all fluid from the pleural cavities.

Perfusion pressure during bypass is usually kept at 50–70 mmHg (6.7–9.3 kPa) to maintain adequate cerebral perfusion. On starting bypass the pressure will often be low but quickly reaches an acceptable level without interference. Later, particularly if hypothermia is employed, there will be a rise in perfusion pressure which may require intervention. Provided that anaesthesia is adequate, drugs with some α-receptor blocking effect may be tried, e.g. chlorpromazine 0.2 mg kg^{-1} or droperidol 0.2 mg kg^{-1}. If these measures fail phentolamine 0.1–0.2 mg kg^{-1}, phenoxybenzamine 1 mg kg^{-1} or sodium nitroprusside by infusion should control any undue rise in arterial pressure. It is wise to use sodium nitroprusside with care during hypothermia as degradation may be slower at low temperatures.

(c) Post-bypass

When the cardiac repair is complete the patient is rewarmed to 37°C and preparations made to wean him from the heart–lung machine. Ventilation of the lungs is restarted with 100% oxygen and the lungs actively expanded to exclude any gross collapse. The acid–base status and electrolyte results are checked to ensure normal potassium and calcium levels and that metabolic acidosis is not present. Filtered, warmed whole blood should be available immediately and also fresh frozen plasma thawed if appropriate.

Protamine sulphate is given to reverse the heparin as soon as the patient is off pump and the cannulae removed. The usual dose is in the range of 1–1.5 mg for each 1 mg of heparin given. As this drug may produce marked hypotension in sensitive individuals it must be given slowly. The wound is inspected for signs of clot and the activated clotting time repeated frequently to demonstrate adequate reversal. In the very young and in children who were cyanosed pre-operatively concentrated coagulation factors and platelet infusions may be required to produce adequate clotting.

If cardiac output is low in the immediate post-bypass period it is important to exclude acidosis and hypocalcaemia before resorting to inotropic agents. However, if myocardial support is indicated then dopamine, isoprenaline or adrenaline may be given by infusion via a central line. If excessive arterial hypertension occurs sodium nitroprusside is given by infusion. It is important that an accurate volumetric pump is used to control these infusions of potent vasoactive agents, thus ensuring safe administration.

On completion of the operation the patient is transferred to the intensive care ward and ventilated postoperatively until there is cardiovascular stability and minimal blood loss.

4.3 MONITORING TECHNIQUES FOR PAEDIATRIC CARDIAC SURGERY

One of the factors which has contributed to the successful management of children and infants during corrective cardiac surgery has been the improvement in monitoring techniques.

4.3.1 ECG

On arrival in the anaesthetic room prior to the induction of anaesthesia the patient is connected to an ECG monitor to give a lead II trace. With modern solid-state devices and disposable electrodes a reliable trace with minimal interference is possible. It must be realized however that in infants and small children who have a resilient myocardium it is possible to have normal ECG with little or no cardiac output and a good cardiac output but bizarre cardiac rhythm. In these patients the onset of bradycardia is the most consistent sign of impending disaster.

4.3.2 Blood pressure

The blood pressure may be accurately measured using an ultrasonic doppler detector (Arteriosonde 1010) or alternatively an automatic oscillotonometer (Dinamap). Both these devices have been shown to be accurate (Kalka, 1971; Friesen and Lichtor, 1981) provided the cuff size is appropriate. The problem with indirect measurement of the blood pressure in children is related to difficulty with standardization of cuff sizes (Park *et al.*, 1976). After induction of anaesthesia a 22 G cannula is inserted into the radial artery provided the collateral circulation of the hand is considered adequate.

4.3.3 CVP

One or more CVP lines are inserted using the Seldinger technique and a suitable placement unit. Either the right or left internal jugular vein may be used although damage to the thoracic duct may occur if the left is chosen. There may be marked differences in the size and position of the vein in children and both sides of the neck should be examined carefully before attempting to cannulate. It is recommended that before inserting the large placement needle that the position of the vein is verified using a small 23 G needle. Complications of the technique include carotid artery puncture and pneumothorax but provided the risks are appreciated and care taken it is a satisfactory method. It is also possible to use the femoral vein to place a catheter percutaneously in the IVC. In small children it is difficult to gain access to the SVC vein via the median cubital vein.

However, in acutely ill infants it is our policy to take the patient directly to the theatre and after induction of anaesthesia perform a cut-down in the median cubital fossa to gain arterial and venous access.

If it is anticipated that there may be a problem with left ventricular performance in the immediate postoperative period then a Swan–Ganz catheter may be inserted intra-operatively. It is also possible to leave a left atrial line *in situ*. The cardiac output may then be determined by the thermal dilution technique and the left atrial pressure constantly monitored.

4.3.4 Temperature

Temperature monitoring is especially important in the very young and in operative techniques involving hypothermia. Normally two probes are inserted, one in the nasopharynx or upper oesophagus which will approximate to core temperature, and the other in the rectum.

The temperature differences from the two probes will give some indication of the effectiveness of cooling and rewarming during the procedure. It is also important to measure the blood temperature from the bypass pump and the temperature at the warming blanket–patient interface.

Postoperatively the core–skin temperature gradient will give valuable information concerning the state of the peripheral circulation and cardiac output.

4.3.5 Urine output

Except in the simplest of cases, the bladder is catheterized immediately after induction of anaesthesia and the urine output carefully monitored. During bypass output may be variable depending on perfusion pressure and type of flow used. Postoperatively urine production should be of the rate 2 ml kg^{-1} h^{-1} and a fall in urine output may indicate either hypovolaemia and the need for fluids, or a developing myocardial problem.

4.3.6 Blood gas analysis and electrolytes

Arterial blood gases must be monitored carefully during surgery to ensure adequate ventilation and to check acid–base status. The electrolyte levels are also carefully observed as large changes in concentration may occur. It is important to ensure that hypocalcaemia does not occur in the immediate postoperative period.

4.3.7 Heparinization

The degreee of heparinization is controlled by measuring the activated clotting time (ACT). After initial baseline determinations measurements are made throughout the bypass procedure to ensure that this time is above 400 s. At the end of the procedure protamine is given and the activated clotting time should return to near the original value. If this does not happen despite adequate protamine then a clotting screen should be performed and appropriate factors given.

4.3.8 Cerebral perfusion

The adequacy of cerebral perfusion is difficult to assess particularly if hypothermia is employed. The size of the pupil is not reliable as reduced temperature, the use of narcotics and other drugs such as atropine and adrenaline will all have an effect. The electroencephalogram could produce useful information but it is very difficult to obtain reasonable traces in most operating threatres. The cerebral function monitor (CFM) will however give useful information as it shows an integrated measurement of cerebral activity. Certainly the fall in cerebral perfusion will be paralleled by a fall in activity on the monitor.

Figure 4.2 shows the effects of cooling on the level of CFM activity and also the loss of all demonstrable activity when perfusion is stopped at a temperature of 18°C. This patient subsequently made an uneventful recovery after intracardiac repair for transposition of the great vessels.

Figure 4.3 shows the effects on the cerebral function monitor trace of cardiac standstill which occurred on insertion of the venous lines prior to bypass. The level of cerebral activity fell toward zero until bypass commenced and cerebral perfusion was resumed.

4.4 CEREBRAL PROTECTION IN PAEDIATRIC CARDIAC SURGERY

Although the mortality figures for open heart surgery have fallen progressively over recent years there is still a significant morbidity in terms of cerebral

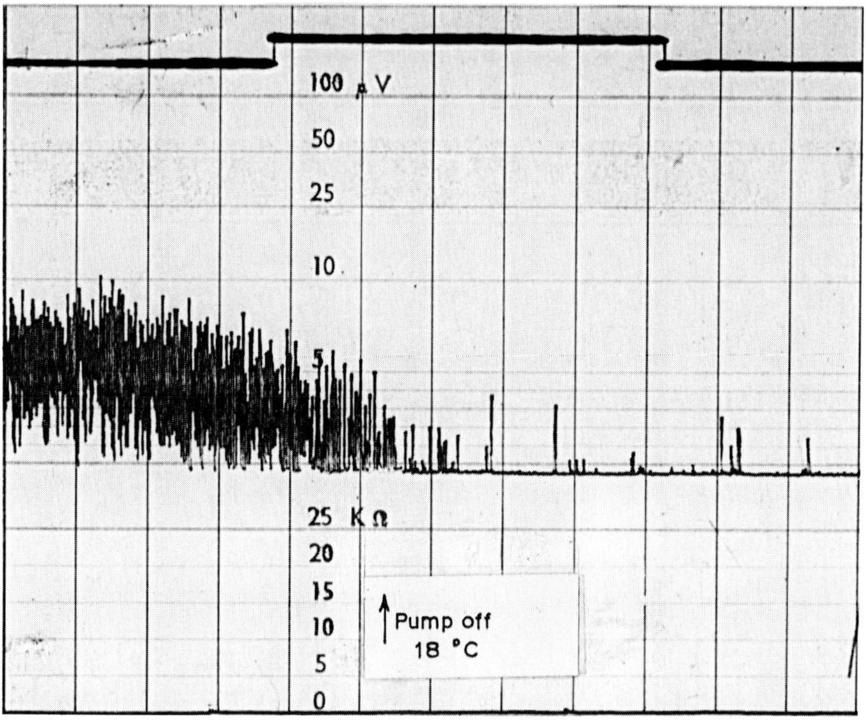

Fig. 4.2 Cerebral function monitor (CFM) trace. The upper portion indicates compressed and filtered signals of electrical cerebral activity at a rate of 30 cm h^{-1}. The lower portion indicates interference and electrical artefacts. The effects of cooling to 18°C and circulatory arrest are demonstrated.

damage. In children there is evidence of underachievement (Lincoln, 1982) and if cerebral damage is severe then subsequent development may be so retarded that the patient becomes a burden to his family and the community. Several of the factors involved in cerebral damage during cardiac surgery are outlined in Table 4.1.

Many of the causes of embolism are related to the surgery, the bypass circuit and oxygenator. However, if the anaesthetist is not meticulous in ensuring that all intravenous lines are free from air then air embolism may occur prior to bypass. As the pump circuit will contain some small gaseous microemboli it has been suggested that nitrous oxide should be withdrawn from the patient before commencing bypass.

Blood aggregates may be added to the patient's circulation with the transfusion of stored blood unless a suitable blood filter is employed. It is usual to filter all blood products given to the patient except of course platelet concentrations.

Table 4.1 Causes of cerebral dysfunction during open-heart surgery

Embolism	*Haemodynamic factors*
Gas (1) 'Surgical' – heart and pulmonary veins	Duration of bypass
(2) Pump oxygenator circuit	Cerebral metabolism – Temperature – Drugs
Foreign material	
Blood aggregates	Time of circulatory arrest
Fibrin	Perfusion pressure
Calcium	Cerebral circulation autoregulation
Denatured protein	Pulsatile flow or constant flow
Fats	

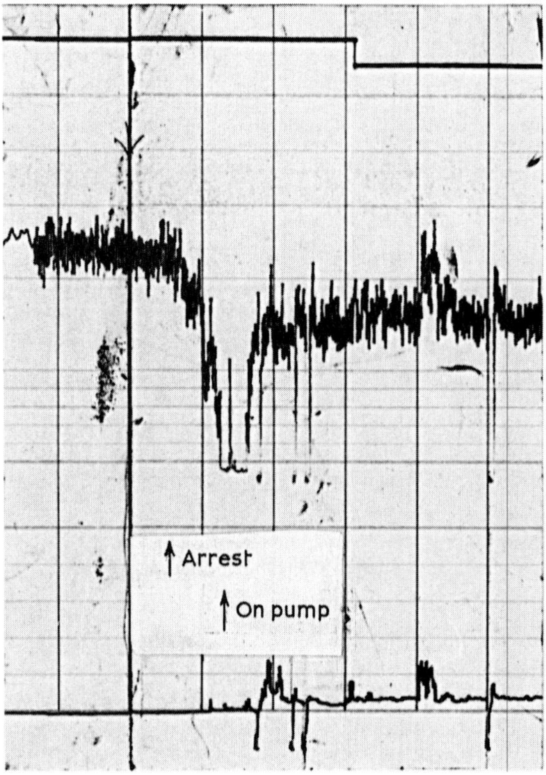

Fig. 4.3 Cerebal function monitor (CFM) trace. This trace demonstrates the effect of cardiac standstill on cannulation of the heart. The cerebral activity decreases to zero until bypass commences with cooling.

Great interest has been generated by the possibility of using drugs to protect the brain during bypass surgery particularly in children when deep hypothermia and circulatory arrest is planned. Barbiturates have been shown to be protective in a variety of situations both clinical (Aitkenhead, 1981) and in animals (Bleyart *et al.*, 1978). However, it seems likely that deep hypothermia and drugs which depress cerebral metabolism afford the same protection. The rationale in giving drugs in this type of case would be to protect areas of the brain which were not cooled adequately. The use of barbiturates in the postoperative period is more controversial but if a known cerebral insult has occurred such as embolism or period of inadequate perfusion it would seem reasonable to adopt a regime of barbiturates, controlled ventilation and cerebral pressure monitoring for the first 48 hours post-bypass.

The cerebral circulation in the young patient will be free of disease and therefore responsive to vasodilatation and constriction. The perfusion pressure is usually maintained within the range 50–70 mmHg (6.7–9.3 kPa). On commencement of bypass the pressure may be lower, particularly if the patient is vasodilated. Consideration must be given to cerebral perfusion when deciding what length of time a low perfusion pressure can be tolerated. Usually the pressure returns to an acceptable level with no intervention after one or two minutes.

When actively cooling with bypass for moderate to deep hypothermia it is important to endeavour to ensure that there is no cerebral vasoconstriction. As carbon dioxide is a potent vasodilator the $PaCO_2$ should be kept to 40–50 mmHg (5.3–6.7 kPa). There is evidence to suggest that pulsatile flow is also beneficial as constant flow may cause the cerebral microcirculation to constrict (Matsumoto *et al.*, 1971).

The use of drugs to reduce cerebral metabolism and perhaps enhance the protection produced by hypothermia is a technique of great interest to anaesthetists. Possibly with further development, new drugs will be produced which will ensure complete cerebral protection and minimize the need to use hypothermia with all its associated disadvantages.

REFERENCES

Abbott, T. R. (1981) Anaesthesia for cardiac surgery in children. *Paediatric Anaesthetics. Trends in Current Practice*, Butterworth, London.

Aitkenhead, A. R. (1981) Do barbiturates protect the brain. *Br. J. Anaesth.*, **53**, 1011–13.

Bethune, D. W. (1976) Organ damage after open-heart surgery. (Letter) *Lancet*, **ii**, 1410.

Bleyart, A. L., Nemolo, E. M., Safar, P. *et al.* (1978) Thiopentone amelioration of brain damage after global ischaemia in monkeys. *Anaesthesiolgy*, **49**, 390–8.

Bush, G. H. and Stead, A. L. (1962) The use of d-tubocurarine in neonatal anaesthesia. *Br. J. Anaesth.*, **34**, 721–8.

Carlgren, L. E. (1969) The incidence of congenital heart disease in Gottenberg. *Ass. Paed. Cardiol.*, Bulletin 5.

Coppel, D. and Dundee, J. W. (1972) Ketamine anaesthesia for catheterisation. *Anaesthesia*, **27**, 25–31.

Davies, D. R. and Doughty, A. (1966) Oral premedication in children with trimeprazine. *Br. J. Anaesth.*, **38**, 878–85.

Fozard, J. R. and Manford, M. L. M. (1977) A controlled clincial trial of oral droperidol and droperidol plus diazepam for premedication in children. *Br. J. Anaesth.*, **49**, 1147–51.

Friesen, R. H. and Lichtor, J. L. (1981) Indirect measurement of blood pressure in neonates and infants utilising an automatic normovasive oscillometric monitor. *Anaesth. Analg.*, **60**, 742–5.

Harmel, H. H. and Lamont, A. (1946) Anaesthesia in the surgical treatment of congenital pulmonary stenosis. *Anaesthesiology*, 7, 477–98.

Hatch, D. J. and Sumner, E. (1981) Neonatal Anaesthesia. *Current Topics in Anaesthetics* Series. Arnold, London.

Kalka, O. H. (1971) Direct and indirect blood pressure measurements in newborn infants. *Am. J. Dis. Child.*, **122**, 425.

Lincoln, C. (1982) Psychological sequelae following cardiac surgery in infancy with and without circulatory arrest. *Br. Heart J.* **47**, 194.

Lowenstein, E. (1971) Morphine anaesthesia: a perspective. *Anaesthesiology*, **35**, 563–5.

Matsumoto, T., Wolferth, C. C. and Pertman, M. H. (1971) Effects of pulsatile and non-pulsatile perfusion upon cerebral and conjunctival microcirculation in dogs. *Am. Surg.*, **37**, 61.

Moffitt, E. A. McGoon, D. C. and Rutter, D. G. (1970) The diagnosis and correction of congenital cardiac defects. *Anaesthesiology*, **33**, 144–60.

Park, M. K., Kawabori, I. and Guntheroth, W. G. (1976) Need for an improved standard for blood pressure cuff size. *Clin. Paediatr.*, **15**, 784.

Pinkerton, P. (1981) Preventing psychotrauma in childhood anaesthesia. *Paediatric Anaesthetics. Trends in Current Practice.* Butterworth, London.

Price, H. L. (1960) General anaesthesia and circulatory homeostasis. *Physiol. Rev.*, **40**, 187.

Smith, R. M. (1980) *Anaesthesia for Infants and Children.* Mosby Co., St Louis.

Stanley, T. H. and Webster, L. R. (1978) Anaesthetic requirements and cardiovascular effects of fentanyl-oxygen, fentanyl, diazepam oxygen anaesthesia in man. *Anaesth. Analg.*, 57, 411–15.

Thomas, D. K. M. (1974) Hypoglycaemia in children before operation – its incidence and prevention. *Br. J. Anaesth.*, **46**, 66–8.

Young, D. (1980) Pathophysiology of congenital heart disease. *Int. Anesth. Clin.*, **18**, 5–25.

Zsigmond, E. K., Mabuku, A., Kothay, S. P. and Jallad, M. (1976) Arterial hypoxaemia caused by intravenous ketamine. *Anaesth. Analg.*, 55, 311–14.

5
Cannulation for cardiopulmonary bypass

K. G. DAVIDSON

5.1 INTRODUCTION

The techniques of cannulation for cardiopulmonary bypass have developed gradually over the last 20 years as surgeons have identified the various manoeuvres which enable them to place a patient on cardiopulmonary bypass with greater speed and safety. The techniques used are by no means standardized and considerable differences exist between different cardiac surgical units, between different surgeons in the same unit, and between different operations performed by the same surgeon. This chapter will describe some of the more commonly used techniques for arterial and venous cannulation in different situations, including closely related manoeuvres such as cardiac decompression. No attempt will be made to describe all possible cannulation techniques, merely some of the more popular ones.

5.2 PREPARATION FOR CANNULATION

Those incisions employed for cardiac surgical procedures will be described, and the implications for cannulation outlined.

5.2.1 Median sternotomy

This is the preferred incision of the vast majority of cardiac surgeons today for most cardiopulmonary bypass surgery. The sternal halves are held open by a retractor, the pericardium opened from the diaphragm to the aorta and adequate exposure of the ascending aorta obtained by dissecting off the thymus gland. The right atrium is exposed by retracting the right edge of the pericardium, often by suturing it to the right blade of the retractor or the wound edge.

5.2.2 Right thoracotomy

An anterolateral thoracotomy at about the level of the right 5th rib gives quite good access to the atria and is favoured by some surgeons for mitral valve replacement, particularly in the presence of a previous median sternotomy. Access to the ascending aorta from this approach can be difficult and access to the left ventricle impossible without continuing the incision across the sternum. Cardiopulmonary bypass can be set up from the right atrium to ascending aorta without difficulty in the majority of cases.

5.2.3 Left thoracotomy

A left anterolateral thoracotomy at about the level of the 5th rib is rarely used for cardiopulmonary bypass surgery. If partial left heart bypass is required during surgery on the descending thoracic aorta, left atrial cannulation may be carried out, the arterial return being placed either into the aorta or the femoral artery. A left thoracotomy with cardiopulmonary bypass has also been described for dealing with left-sided accessory conduction pathways and for redo coronary surgery where only the circumflex system is involved.

5.2.4 Bilateral transverse thoracotomy

This was a popular incision for cardiopulmonary bypass in the 1960s, but was abandoned in favour of median sternotomy largely because of the much improved access which the latter approach gave to the ascending aorta for aortic valve replacement and coronary surgery. Median sternotomy also proved a more rapid incision when emergency cannulation for cardiopulmonary bypass was required.

5.3 CANNULATION TECHNIQUE

It is essential to ensure that the patient is fully heparinized prior to the insertion of any bypass cannulae into either the venous or arterial side. Responsibility for this step may be taken by the anaesthetist, in which case the heparin should be inserted through a correctly sited central venous line, or alternatively by the surgeon who can inject the anticoagulant directly into the right atrium. The dose of heparin required is worked out according to the patient's weight (usually 3 mg per kg body weight). Some centres also add heparin to the priming fluid in the cardiopulmonary bypass circuit. When the patient has been heparinized, the activated clotting time (ACT) should ideally be checked and an ACT >450 s confirmed.

5.3.1 Ascending aorta cannulation

The ascending aorta is the site most often used for the arterial return in routine cardiopulmonary bypass operations. Access to it is easy, cannulation is safe, and the incidence of complications relatively low. It is helpful to reduce the movement of the aorta during cannulation, either by traction on a tape passed round the aorta, or by steadying the aortic adventitia with forceps. The exact cannulation site on the ascending aorta must be chosen with care, bearing in mind several factors: (a) *the type of operation planned* – high cannulation is required if multiple grafts are to be attached to the ascending aorta; more room on the ascending aorta is also required for aortic valve replacement than for mitral: (b) *the type of arterial return cannula chosen* – there are many commercially available of different design and with appropriate size ranges (Fig. 5.1). Most are tapered so that the part inserted into the aorta is 5–8 mm in diameter for adults. It may be a straight cannula designed to sit in the middle of the lumen of the aorta, a cannula with a right-angled bend near the tip designed to point towards the aortic arch, or even a long cannula designed to be fed some distance round the arch of the aorta: (c) *the quality of the wall of the aorta* – whichever area of the aorta is selected for cannulation it should be carefully palpated to ensure that it is not unduly atheromatous.

(a) Purse string sutures

The point on the aortic wall selected for cannulation is encircled with one, or more commonly two concentric purse string sutures leaving an area within the purse string large enough to accept the cannula with a margin of aortic wall around it. The purse string sutures will often be in the shape of a circle or diamond and should take an adequate bite of aortic wall to retain their grip but should if possible not go through into the lumen. Tourniquets are applied to the purse string sutures to give haemostasis and secure fixation when the cannula is *in situ*. Having ensured that the patient is fully heparinized, it is best to cannulate the aorta at a time when the patient's systolic blood pressure is at a fairly normal level. If the patient is hypertensive, bleeding can occur alongside the cannula despite the purse strings, and may produce an unsightly, though not usually dangerous, subadventitial haematoma. If the patient is severely hypotensive there is little resistance from the wall of the flaccid aorta and cannulation can be difficult. The exact technique used to introduce the cannula varies considerably according to the individual preferences of the surgeon. The tidier the technique the better. Considerable efforts must be made to develop a technique which will avoid spraying the surgeon, the assistants, the scrub nurse and any onlooker who happens to get too close, with large quantities of arterial blood. The principles are obvious – an

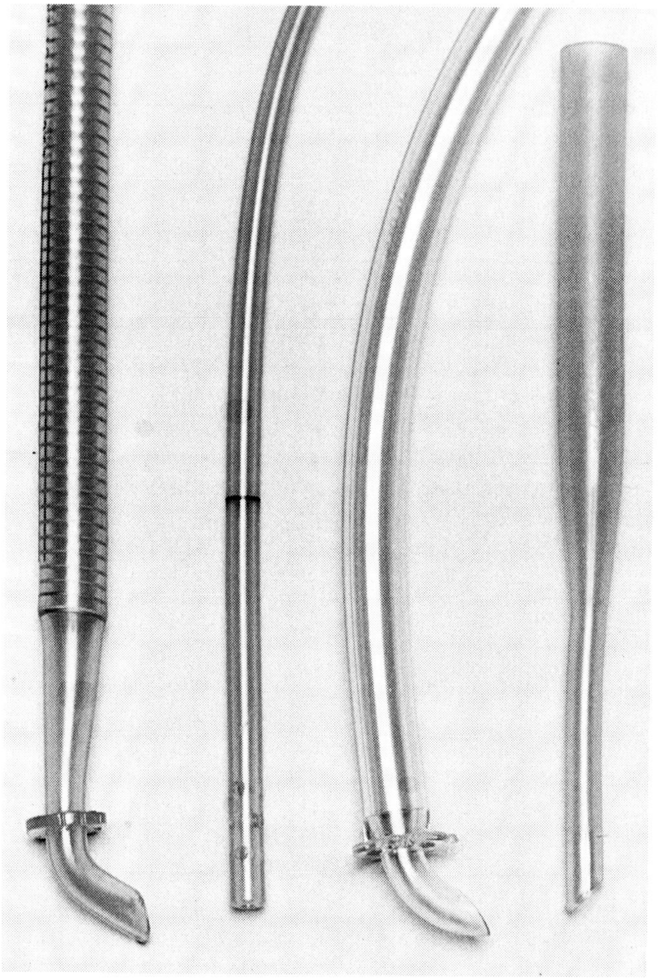

Fig. 5.1 Four commonly used arterial return cannulae.

incision about the size of the tip of the selected cannula is made with a scalpel within the purse string. The resulting hole must be occluded either with a finger, by approximating the edges with tissue forceps, by the application of a clamp partially to occlude the aorta, or by the rapid introduction of the tip of the cannula. If a clamp is utilized it may be applied prior to making the incision, but some surgeons dislike applying a clamp to this part of the aorta unless it is necessary, because of the risk of damage to the aortic wall. When the cannula has been introduced, the purse string sutures are tightened using the rubber tourniquets and haemostasis secured. Blood is then allowed to flow back up the arterial cannula prior to connecting it to the arterial line of the bypass circuit, ensuring that all air is evacuated from the line. The position of the tip of the arterial cannula in the aorta should be checked by palpation at this stage to ensure that it is pointing in an appropriate direction, in particular not directed preferentially towards any of the head and neck vessels and not abutting directly onto the wall of the aorta.

(b) Problems associated with cannulation of ascending aorta

The cannula will not enter the aortic lumen

If after 2 or 3 attempts the cannula will not pass through the incision in the aortic wall into the lumen, a side clamp should be applied to the aorta at the cannulation site and the incision inspected. Sometimes a flap of adventitia requires to be trimmed off, or occasionally the incision requires to be enlarged. Care should be taken to ensure that there is not an atheromatous plaque preventing cannulation, as cannulation through such a plaque may produce aortic dissection or embolism. If aortic dissection occurs (incidence <1 in 500 cases), immediate institution of femoral arterial return and ascending aortic repair or replacement must be attempted.

The cannula goes into the aorta but bleeding persists once the tourniquets have been tightened

There is no point in over-tightening the tourniquets as this may further damage the aortic wall. The assistant should control the bleeding by direct pressure or by altering the position of the cannula; complete the venous cannulation and go onto cardiopulmonary bypass. If there is still significant leakage around the cannula when on full flow, place an additional purse string suture with a tourniquet around the cannula.

If excessive bleeding occurs, as for example when the aorta tears beyond the purse string suture, or the purse string sutures break, it may be better to remove the cannula, control the tear by digital pressure and apply a clamp to regain control. It may be possible to retrieve the situation merely by the insertion of new purse string sutures, but sometimes the incision has to be closed and an alternative site on the ascending aorta selected.

5.3.2. Femoral artery cannulation

In the early days of cardiopulmonary bypass the femoral artery was the cannulation site of choice for many surgeons. Most surgeons have now changed to using the ascending aorta whenever possible and reserving the femoral, or even the external iliac artery above the inguinal ligament, for situations where the ascending aorta cannot be used safely. Thus, the femoral artery is the cannulation site of choice for most operations involving aneurysms of the ascending aorta, ascending aortic dissections, most patients with tamponade requiring cardiopulmonary bypass and in some other emergency situations where access to ascending aorta cannot safely be obtained or obtained sufficiently rapidly (e.g. in redo surgery).

(a) Exposure

The common femoral artery is easily exposed in the groin, either under local or general anaesthesia. The superficial femoral artery is usually too small to accept an adequate cannula and it is preferable to use the common femoral artery. If it is small or atheromatous, the external iliac artery may be used, with an extraperitoneal approach above the inguinal ligament. In most patients the common femoral artery is suitable and tapes should be passed round it above and below the selected cannulation point. The patient is then heparinized, proximal and distal clamps applied to the artery and a large enough incision made in the artery to accept the cannula. The size of cannula should be the largest one which will fit easily into the artery. The proximal clamp is released and the cannula inserted for a short distance into the external iliac artery. The cotton tape with a rubber tourniquet is then carefully tightened just enough to prevent bleeding around the cannula. The cannula is joined up to the arterial line of the cardiopulmonary bypass circuit in the usual way, taking care to expel all air. The cannula and pump tubing are then securely anchored to the groin to prevent displacement.

(b) Problems associated with femoral artery cannulation

When the artery is first exposed it should be palpated carefully to ensure that it is of an adequate lumen to accept an appropriate cannula. If it is very atheromatous, it is probably wiser not to attempt cannulation at this site, in which case the other femoral artery may be exposed in the hope that it will be better. If that fails, the external iliac artery is another alternative. Occasionally when cannulation has been successful, the flow through the cannula appears limited and the arterial line pressure is very high. This may be due to atheromatous obstruction in the common or external iliac, or the cannula may not be lying correctly in the lumen of the artery. If repositioning of the cannula is unsuccessful, the other femoral or iliac artery will have to be approached. The most frequent problems with femoral artery cannulation are related to damage done to the artery by too large a cannula tearing the arteriotomy, or by clamps or tourniquets damaging the intima. Careful repair of the femoral artery at the end of the procedure is required and if there is doubt about the adequacy of repair, then a patch graft or even an interposition of saphenous vein may be required. Retrograde dissection due to the introduction of the cannula into a false plane in the wall of the artery is potentially disastrous. Bypass must be stopped immediately, the artery explored and repaired, and alternative arterial access found.

5.3.3 Venous cannulation

Preparation for cardiopulmonary bypass includes ensuring adequate access for venous cannulation. This usually means exposing enough of the right atrium to insert purse string sutures and either one or two cannulae. As indicated previously, adequate heparinization must be achieved prior to the insertion of the cannulae. The right atrium is partially concealed at median sternotomy under the right half of the sternum and varies considerably in size and position. Adequate exposure is almost always achieved by opening the sternal spreader sufficiently and keeping the edge of the pericardium out of the way. Handling the atrium during cannulation often produces supraventricular arrhythmias which are usually transient, but can occasionally persist and produce quite dramatic hypotension – it may then be necessary to cardiovert the patient back into a more satisfactory rhythm or, if cannulation is almost complete, it may be simpler to commence cardiopulmonary bypass.

(a) Choice of venous cannulae

There is a wide range of venous cannulae available and choice depends on the individual preference of the surgeon and the exact type of operation planned (Fig. 5.2). The priority is to ensure adequate venous drainage throughout the entire procedure. This can be achieved in several ways.

(i) Cannulation of both vena cavae
This is one of the more commonly used cannulation systems and requires the insertion of 2 cannulae, 7–10 mm in diameter through purse string sutures in the right atrial wall into either vena cava. The cannulae may be straight or right angled, and may or may not be crossed within the atrial cavity. The cannula is advanced into the vena cava so that if the surgeon wishes, tapes with tourniquets can be passed round the cavae, preventing venous blood returning to the right atrium via the cavae. This cannulation system is mandatory for operations on the right side of the heart, as it allows the right atrium or right ventricle to be opened without air entering the venous side of the bypass circuit and producing an air-lock.

(ii) A two-stage single cannula
This is a relatively recent development, whereby a single cannula provides drainage of the inferior vena cava and the right atrium. To achieve this the cannula is constructed in two 'stages' – a 10 cm long distal portion about 1 cm diameter and a much wider proximal section ending in an open basket designed to sit in mid-cavity of the right atrium when the distal portion of the cannula is in the inferior vena cava. This provides good venous drainage and

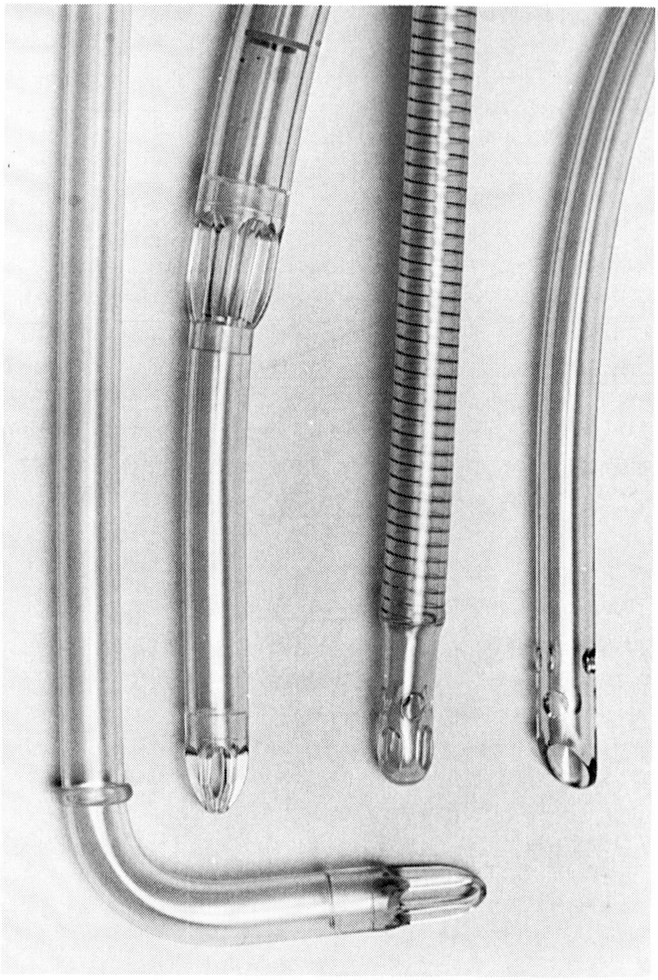

Fig. 5.2 Four commonly used venous cannulae. One is an example of the single 2-stage venous cannula, with right atrial basket, and internal tube passing to the IVC.

can be used for most procedures for valvular and coronary disease, though it is obviously not suitable for situations where the right atrium has to be opened, and may be less efficient when the heart is distorted to gain access to the posterior surface.

(b) Venous cannulae insertion technique

The technique of insertion of the cannula depends to some extent on the type of cannula selected and its size. If one cannula of the two-stage type is chosen, then it usually can be passed through the atrial appendage. A purse string suture is placed round the base of the atrial appendage, a clamp applied and an incision large enough to admit the cannula made in the tip of the appendage. If a two-cannula system is selected, then two purse string sutures a reasonable distance apart are required. These may be sited close to the cavo-atrial junctions or in more easily accessible parts of the atrium depending on surgical preference. Access to the tricuspid valve, or to congenital defects within the right atrium will obviously dictate positioning of atrial cannulation sites.

The right atrial wall is trabeculated and this may hinder the insertion of a cannula. There are two main methods for dealing with this – a side clamp may be applied to the atrial wall at the cannulation site, the atrium opened and the trabeculae divided; or an appropriately sized incision may be made within the purse string suture and a large artery forceps passed into the atrial cavity to ensure that there is no hindrance to the insertion of the cannula. When the cannula has been inserted into the appropriate position, the purse string suture is either tightened with a tourniquet or tied around the cannula to anchor it in place, to give haemostasis and to prevent air entering the atrium.

(c) **Problems with venous cannulation**

When the right atrial pressure is very high in situations such as tricuspid valve disease and massive pulmonary embolism, considerable bleeding can occur during venous cannulation, even from the needle holes made by the purse string suture. In this situation it may be best to apply a clamp to the base of the atrial appendage, then insert the purse string, and use either a single two-stage cannula or go on bypass with one caval cannula *in situ*, the second one being inserted once the patient has been established on cardiopulmonary bypass and the right atrial pressure substantially reduced. Sometimes when an attempt is made to insert a cannula into the inferior vena cava it will fail repeatedly to enter the cava. This may be due to a valve on the inferior cava and undue force must not be used. A tear at the cavo-atrial junction can be extremely difficult to repair. It is better to remove the cannula from the atrial purse string, insert the index finger and palpate the inside of the atrium to check whether there is any hindrance to the passage of the cannula. It is usually possible to manipulate the tip of the cannula past a valve into the cava without great difficulty. If a superior caval cannula is being used, it should be directed carefully away from the vena azygos as the tip of the cannula sometimes lodges at the cavo-azygos junction, thus hindering venous return.

5.3.4 Femoral venous cannulation

As with arterial cannulation there are some situations where the right atrium cannot be approached safely for cardiopulmonary bypass. This applies particularly to patients with tamponade, as for example from a dissecting aneurysm of the ascending aorta which has ruptured into the pericardium. Even in this situation however, it is sometimes possible to cannulate the right atrial appendage and establish bypass from the atrium to the femoral artery. Femoral venous cannulation is therefore rarely required, though it may be used when external cardiac massage is required to keep the patient alive until femoro-femoral bypass can be established. The femoral vein is exposed in much the same way as the femoral artery, usually in the region of the saphenofemoral junction. Improved venous drainage is obtained if the femoral cannula can be passed right up through the venous system to the high inferior vena cava and accordingly a cannula of suitable diameter and length must be selected. If it will not advance beyond the external iliac vein, then it is unlikely to produce satisfactory venous drainage. In this situation it may be possible to go on to partial bypass, open the chest and establish right atrial drainage so as to achieve a satisfactory venous return. Occasionally special situations arise where even this cannot be accomplished – patients who have developed false aneurysms of the ascending aorta present a particular problem. Good bypass must be established without opening the chest at all so that the patient can be cooled to a point where the circulation can be stopped and the chest opened. In this situation venous drainage may be taken from femoral and internal jugular veins to give adequate cardiopulmonary bypass and cooling.

5.4 DECOMPRESSION OF THE HEART DURING CARDIOPULMONARY BYPASS

One of the requirements for satisfactory operating conditions during cardiac surgery with cardioplegia is that a minimal amount of blood flows through the heart while the critical parts of the operation are being carried out. The whole cardiopulmonary bypass circuit must be correct in order to achieve this – otherwise a heart which is supposed to be cold, empty and asystolic, will soon be half full, warm and irreversibly damaged. One of the main elements in maintaining satisfactory perfusion is to provide adequate venous drainage under all circumstances obtaining during the operation. One way of achieving this is to use total cardiopulmonary bypass with cannulae in both vena cavae and tapes tightened around the intracaval portions of the cannulae. When the aorta is cross clamped in this situation, only a small amount of non-coronary collateral blood flow from the mediastinum will enter the heart. Even when the same cannulation technique is used without applying caval tapes, it is usual for the right side of the heart to be completely empty. Any blood which does return to the heart will have the effect of rewarming it to some extent, even though the temperature of the circulating perfusion fluid is reduced to 25–30°C. If hypothermia of this degree is used, then it is considered safe to reduce the pump flow rate from the commonly used figure of around 2.4 l m^{-2} min^{-1} down to about 1.5–1.8 l m^{-2} min^{-1}. The single two-stage cannula cannot be used if the right side of the heart requires to be opened, but it is used routinely by many surgeons for coronary and valve surgery. Care must be taken with this type of cannulation when there is considerable displacement of the heart, as may occur in gaining access to the circumflex coronary system or to a less than easily accessible mitral valve.

In addition to providing good venous drainage through the venous return cannulae, many surgeons also use a suction catheter or vent to assist in the complete evacuation of blood from the heart during cardiopulmonary bypass (Fig. 5.3). There are several methods of achieving this.

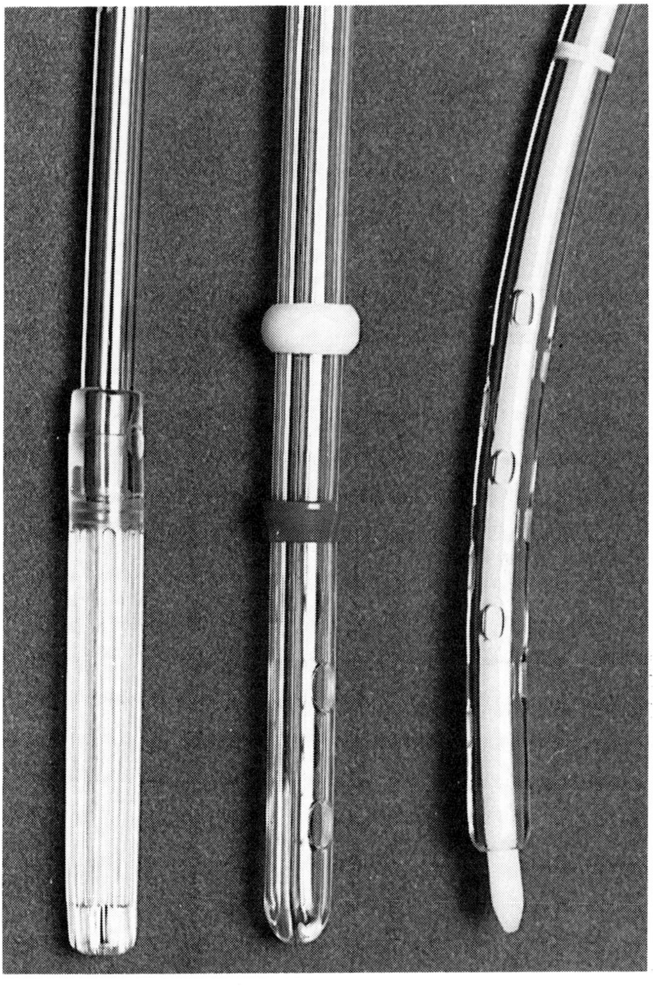

Fig. 5.3 Three commonly used vent catheters for left heart drainage.

5.4.1 Apex of left ventricle

In this method a purse string suture, often with teflon buttresses, is placed at the apex of the left ventricle, avoiding the coronary arteries, and a suction catheter is inserted into the cavity of the left ventricle through the suture. It is a simple and quite satisfactory method but is decreasing in popularity, particularly for coronary surgery where surgeons do not wish to produce any damage, however slight, to the muscle of the left ventricle. There is also a small morbidity associated with this type of decompression in that postoperative bleeding can occur through the suture at the apex and the development of a small aneurysm may occur rarely as a late complication. One of the advantages of an apical vent for mitral or aortic valve replacement is that the resulting small incision at the apex can be used as a method of extracting air from the ventricle at the end of the operation – care must also be taken to ensure that air is not sucked into the ventricle if the heart is allowed to beat with a vent *in situ*.

5.4.2 Right superior pulmonary vein

A small suction catheter may be inserted through a purse string suture in the right superior pulmonary vein just at its junction with the left atrium. A catheter with an introducer may be used so that the tube can be guided through the mitral valve into the left ventricle in operations where the left atrium is not going to be opened. This type of decompression has the advantage that it does not require an incision in cardiac muscle and the incision in the pulmonary vein can be used to evacuate air from the left side of the heart. Once again bleeding from the incision can be a problem and care must be taken not to narrow the pulmonary vein which can produce major problems of venous congestion in the upper and middle lobes of the right lung.

5.4.3 Left atrial appendage

This is not a particularly popular site for a suction catheter in adults, but it is possible to put a purse string suture in the apex of the left atrial appendage and to pass a catheter through this into the atrium.

5.4.4 Pulmonary artery

With this method a purse string suture is inserted in the main pulmonary artery, 2–3 cm above the pulmonary valve, and a suction catheter is passed through an incision within the purse string towards the bifurcation of the pulmonary artery. It achieves much the same objective as direct decompression of the left side of the heart, but again does not require an incision in cardiac muscle. The incidence of complications is low, though as always considerable care has to be taken in repairing the pulmonary artery and also in evacuating all air from the left side of the heart.

Which, if any, of the above techniques of cardiac compression is chosen is largely a matter of individual preference. The two most popular methods at present are probably the vent in the right superior pulmonary vein and the pulmonary artery. If the left ventricle is actually going to be opened, as for example with resection of a left ventricular aneurysm, decompression by another route is not required. Many surgeons however do not use a left ventricular decompression device routinely relying instead on good venous drainage with a reduced flow rate to keep the heart cold and empty.

5.5 CANNULATION IN EMERGENCY SITUATIONS

5.5.1 Cardiac arrest at induction of anaesthesia

With careful anaesthesia this is a relatively rare event but may still occur. Any patient who is haemodynamically unstable or liable to arrhythmias is better anaesthetized on the operating table in theatre, with continuous monitoring of ECG and arterial pressure. If cardiac arrest occurs at induction, and routine resuscitatory methods are not immediately effective in restoring circulation, there are two main alternatives. (a) External cardiac massage and ventilation with 100% oxygen are maintained while the femoral artery and vein are exposed. The patient is then heparinized, the artery and vein cannulated, and partial cardiopulmonary bypass commenced. By this method it is usually possible to maintain an adequate flow so that cardiac massage can be stopped and the chest opened. Better venous drainage can then be obtained by switching to standard atrial cannulation. (b) Continue external cardiac massage and ventilation with oxygen while the patient's chest is cleaned and draped. The skin, sternum and pericardium are then rapidly opened and internal cardiac massage started. It may be possible at this point to get the heart beating again by either cardioversion or drug treatment, but it is often better to continue internal cardiac massage while the patient is heparinized and an assistant cannulates the ascending aorta and right atrium for bypass.

5.5.2 Damage to the heart or great vessels while opening the chest

It is very rare for patients having their first heart operation to sustain any damage to the heart while the chest is being opened. The same does not apply to patients who have had previous heart operations, particularly previous median sternotomies. It is not unusual to find right ventricle, right atrium, or ascending aorta firmly adherent to the posterior table of the sternum, particularly as some surgeons do not close the pericardium after cardiac operations. In this situation if an attempt is made to split the sternum using an electric or compressed air saw with the blade oscillating in a vertical direction, then it may be very difficult to avoid damaging the heart or aorta. Even when using a saw with a blade which oscillates horizontally it is sometimes impossible to avoid damaging the underlying structures. If the bleeding is copious it should be controlled as much as possible by pressure over the sternum, the patient heparinized, the femoral artery and vein exposed and femoro-femoral bypass established. When the heart has been decompressed in this way it may be possible to open the sternum and control the situation at this stage. If the aorta is the source of the bleeding another alternative is to continue on partial bypass with cooling until the patient's temperature is 25–28°C. The patient's circulation is then allowed to drain into the pump reservoir and the pump flow is drastically reduced. The sternum is opened, the aorta cross clamped above the area of damage and normal flow resumed. The blood loss during such manoeuvres can be quite considerable, but of course as soon as the patient is heparinized, the discard suckers can be changed for the suckers which return the blood to the cardiotomy reservoir.

5.6 PERFUSION PROBLEMS DURING CARDIOPULMONARY BYPASS

5.6.1 High arterial line pressure

This is usually due to minor displacement of the tip of the cannula and it should be repositioned. Rarely it may indicate acute dissection of the aorta or femoral artery at the cannulation site, the cannula being in the false lumen.

5.6.2 Air in the arterial line

This disaster should ideally never occur. The pump must be stopped immediately, the source found and the air evacuated before starting the pump again. Air introduced into the patient's circulation (massive air embolism) requires immediate stopping of the arterial pump, full head-down position, aspiration of air from the heart and aorta, core cooling to 20–25°C and the introduction of steroid or barbiturate cerebral protective agents. Hyperbaric oxygen therapy has also been used with some success in massive air embolism cases.

5.6.3 Poor venous return

If there is no extracardiac obstruction to the tubing, the usual reason for poor venous return is malpositioning of the venous cannula or cannulae. Careful positioning at the time of insertion should prevent this complication.

5.6.4 Air-lock in venous line

Moderate amounts of air will pass down the venous line to the oxygenator without difficulty. Large amounts will stop the venous return by producing an air lock and this requires immediate action: (1) the source of entry of the air must be closed; (2) the air must be rapidly evacuated from the line and drainage re-established. This is often easily achieved by elevating the venous line a few inches at a time until the air reaches the oxygenator.

Safety aspects of air embolism are discussed further in Chapter 21.

6
Adequacy of perfusion – general review

B. SETHIA and D. J. WHEATLEY

6.1 INTRODUCTION

During cardiopulmonary bypass, the maintenance of the circulation is controlled directly by the perfusion team. It is therefore of vital importance that one appreciates what constitutes adequate cardiopulmonary bypass. The ultimate aim in cardiopulmonary bypass practice is the maintenance of adequate tissue perfusion and energy supply demand equality during the performance of cardiac surgical procedures at a time when many of the patient's normal physiological mechanisms are impaired. Adequacy of perfusion must also be defined in terms of the ultimate ability to ensure full return of pre-operative function to all organ systems of the patient after the operation. In this chapter the rationale for the conduct of cardiopulmonary bypass and methods for assessing its adequacy will be discussed.

Currently in the USA, over 100 000 open heart operations are performed annually. The reported results for coronary surgery, well exemplified by the 2.3% overall operative mortality reported for the Collaborative Study in Coronary Artery Surgery (Kennedy *et al.*, 1980), attest to the adequacy of perfusion in most cardiopulmonary bypass procedures. From this it might be deduced that cardiopulmonary bypass techniques are already adequate. However, review of the history of the development of cardiopulmonary bypass techniques soon dispels this assumption. It is evident that current methods of assessing the adequacy of cardiopulmonary bypass, based almost entirely on clinical experience, may be totally inadequate. The fact that the major haemodynamic variables are under human control emphasizes the need for constant vigilance in the conduct of extracorporeal circulation. That fatal accidents may ocur as often as one in every 1000–1500 perfusions (Wheeldon *et al.*, 1981) further indicates the need for review of the adequacy of cardiopulmonary bypass.

Perfusion attained with current cardiopulmonary bypass techniques does not often simulate accurately 'normal' physiological perfusion – restraints inherent in current technology preclude this. During the period of cardiopulmonary bypass there may be alterations in blood volume, total systemic blood flow, arterial and venous tone, arterial and venous blood pressure, pulsatility, blood viscosity, haematocrit and temperature. In addition, factors, such as microemboli or tissue oedema, may progressively impair the adequacy of perfusion.

The protective effects of anaesthesia, hypothermia and altered perfusate viscosity, as well as the limited time during which artificial perfusion is required, may make accurate simulation of normal perfusion unnecessary. Indeed, there are on occasions surgical circumstances when normal perfusion is undesirable. However, perfusion of the body during cardiopulmonary bypass must always be considered inadequate when there is a significant discrepancy between energy supply to tissue capillary beds and the energy demands of these tissues necessary for full functional recovery upon restoration of the natural circulation.

The following discussion is primarily directed toward the conduct of short-term cardiopulmonary bypass as required for cardiac surgery. In the conduct of cardiopulmonary bypass over several days, further parameters – particularly those relating to long-term gas exchange and blood trauma – assume a relatively greater importance, though assessment of the adequacy of perfusion is otherwise similar (see Chapter 13).

6.2 GENERAL CONSIDERATIONS OF THE ADEQUACY OF PERFUSION

The perfusion team must keep in mind the possibility of particular technical aspects of cardiopulmonary bypass which may result in local or regional inadequacy of perfusion. Although these are easy to understand, in clinical practice they may well be overlooked unless the team has a specific awareness of these problems.

Local inadequacy of perfusion is the consequence of an obstruction to the arterial supply or venous drainage of a particular region of the body. Femoral arterial cannulation for cardiopulmonary bypass may result in poor perfusion in the ipsilateral leg which is dependent on collateral flow during the bypass procedure. This rarely amounts to inadequate perfusion if judged by functional recovery. More serious, however, is the possibility of accidental selective perfusion of the brachiocephalic trunk, the common carotid artery, or the left subclavian artery by an inappropriately placed aortic cannula – care in selection of the site for cannulation and in directing the cannula tip is essential to prevent this problem.

Venous obstruction may be caused by unsatisfactory placement of a superior vena caval cannula, which may obstruct the innominate vein. In addition, venous obstruction may occur when the venous cannulae have an inadequate internal diameter (a commoner problem with neonates and small children). Failure to cannulate a large persistent left superior vena cava may similarly impair cerebral venous drainage. Attention to venous pressures and systemic arterial pressure during perfusion, observation of the clinical appearance of the upper extremity, as well as attention to the pump flow rates and line pressures, will help to identify such surgical mishaps.

Pre-existing arterial atherosclerosis may cause little obstruction to flow at normal pressure, but serious flow reduction may occur with reduction of blood pressure on cardiopulmonary bypass. Thus, it is possible that carotid atherosclerosis may result in cerebral injury due to inadequate perfusion in what would otherwise appear to be satisfactory cardiopulmonary bypass conditions. At present there is little information on patients with carotid artery stenosis to determine whether adequate cerebral blood flow during cardiopulmonary bypass can be achieved through increasing the aortic pressure or systemic flow rate (Ellis *et al.*, 1980).

Inadequate perfusion may be exacerbated by anatomical factors, which may result in an excessive 'run off' from the systemic circulation, as may occur with an uncontrolled ductus arteriosus, large aortopulmonary collateral vessels, or even severe aortic regurgitation where the possibility of ventricular distension further compounds inadequate myocardial perfusion.

6.3 SPECIFIC ASPECTS OF PERFUSION

It is not currently possible to produce a dogmatic 'recipe' for the conduct of adequate cardiopulmonary bypass. Of the many major factors, those for individual consideration are:

(1) Perfusate – this is discussed in detail in Chapter 14 but the specific aspects of haematocrit and blood viscosity have particular relevance to the adequacy of perfusion.
(2) Pressure and systemic flow rate – particularly with regard to perfusion of the cerebral circulation and other vital organs.
(3) Pulsatility.
(4) Temperature.

Factors, such as microemboli, the relevance of filtration and the influence of anaesthesia, have an important bearing on adequacy of perfusion and are discussed elsewhere (Chapters 3, 4, 18 and 19). Other concomitants of current cardiopulmonary bypass techniques, whilst not strictly producing inadequate perfusion, nevertheless emphasize the inadequacies of current artificial perfusion. These include activation of the complement system, suppression of immunity, reduction in platelets and sequestration of tissue fluid (Hammerschmidt *et al.*, 1981; Parker-Williams, 1972; Rosenkranz *et al.*, 1980).

Particular attention should be paid to the opinion that the most important manifestations of inadequate perfusion are those of central nervous system dysfunction. Cerebral morbidity remains unacceptably high even in current practice. It is clear that risk factors for perioperative neurological dysfunction may include age and past history of cerebrovascular accidents (Branthwaite, 1973). A pre-operative history of transient ischaemic episodes does not increase the likelihood of permanent post-operative neurological impairment (Sotaniemi, 1980). It is possible, however, that the type and duration of cardiac disease may determine the risk of post-operative neurological dysfunction (Lee *et al.*, 1971).

Evaluation of the adequacy of cerebral perfusion during cardiopulmonary bypass remains unsatisfactory in the absence of adequate intra-operative assessment of cerebral function. Although the electroencephalogram (Salerno *et al.*, 1978) and cerebral function monitor (Branthwaite, 1973) are commonly employed in monitoring the adequacy of cerebral function, the effects of hypothermia, haemodilution and anaesthesia impose limitations on the accuracy of electrophysiological assessment during cardiopulmonary bypass. Determination of arterial-jugular venous oxygenation differences (Wollman *et al.*, 1966) is inaccurate for the same reasons. Use of biochemical markers of brain cell injury may prove more sensitive (Taylor *et al.*, 1980; Taylor, 1982).

6.3.1 Perfusate

In most units it is now customary to use a clear fluid prime for adult cardiac surgery, so that the haematocrit during perfusion is around 25%. This practice is supported by studies of haemodynamics during open heart surgery (Nadjmabadi *et al.*, 1978). Despite the practical advantage of avoiding homologous blood primes, from the point of view of perfusion, it is important to consider the oxygen-carrying capacity of the perfusate and its viscosity. During hypothermia, the consequent increases in blood viscosity and in vasoconstriction are counteracted by haemodilution (Ream, 1982). Haemodilution has also been shown to oppose the adverse effect of hypothermia and pump oxygenation on blood flow, oxygen delivery and renal function (Utley *et al.*, 1981). Disadvantages of haemodilution, e.g. decreased oxygen carrying capacity, decreased plasma colloid oncotic pressure and elevated interstitial water content (English *et al.*, 1971; Rosenkranz *et al.*, 1980), are counteracted by the benefits of hypothermia (Utley *et al.*, 1981; Lilleaasen and Stokke, 1978). Haemodilution becomes even more important in children with cyanotic congenital heart disease, where it indeed may be important to reduce the increased viscosity which accompanies the secondary polycythaemia. In summary, there is now considerable evidence to substantiate the benefits of haemodilution with resultant haematocrit figures in the range of 20–25% in combination with a degree of hypothermia (Nadjmabadi *et al.*, 1978; Ream, 1982).

6.3.2 Pressure and flow

A fall in systemic vascular resistance with corresponding fall in perfusion pressure is a common occurrence at the outset of cardiopulmonary bypass in spite of rapid achievement of maximally attainable flow rates. There is thereafter a progressive increase in vascular resistance during surgery, and this vasoconstriction is exacerbated by hypothermia. Nevertheless, the initial problem facing the perfusionist, surgeon or anaesthetist, is in deciding what represents an adequate perfusion pressure. As with most of the parameters of perfusion, most studies have centred on central nervous system effects.

Ellis *et al.* (1980) produced evidence in 30 adult patients undergoing aortocoronary bypass grafting to support the validity of reduction of flow rate below 40 ml kg^{-1} and arterial pressure below 60 mmHg (8 kPa) in combination with systemic hypothermia at 28°C. Satisfactory cardiopulmonary bypass was achieved with minimal rewarming of the myocardium via non-coronary collateral circulation. Furthermore, late cerebral dysfunction was not observed. Kollka and Hilberman (1980) have demonstrated in 204 patients undergoing open heart surgery, that a mean arterial pressure in the region of 50 mmHg (6.7 kPa) produced no increase in long-term neuropsychological dysfunction and suggested that pressure *per se* is not the major determinant of postoperative neurological and neuropsychological dysfunction. They used moderate hypothermia with a core temperature of 30°C. It is of interest that this group, in common with many others, are reluctant to allow mean arterial pressures to fall below 30 mmHg (4 kPa) and use vasopressor drugs to increase the unusually low pressures when they occur.

Stockard *et al.* (1974) have advocated a minimum cerebral perfusion pressure of 50 mmHg (6.7 kPa) during cardiopulmonary bypass. In a study of 100 patients Tufo *et al.* (1970) detected postoperative neurological abnormalities in 44% and found a threefold increase in cerebral damage if the mean perfusion pressure fell below 40 mmHg (5.3 kPa) compared with 60 mmHg (8 kPa). It is of relevance to note that hypothermia was only employed in 38% of patients in this series.

Selkoe and Myers (1979) demonstrated a highly reproducible threshold for the development of ischaemic brain injury at a mean arterial blood pressure of 25 mmHg (3.3 kPa) in 12 out of 13 monkeys. Mean blood pressures of 35–40 mmHg (4.7–5.3 kPa) were sustained for up to three hours without evidence of neurological or cardiovascular sequelae. Pentobarbital anaesthesia, which may provide some degree of cerebral protection, was used in this series of experiments, and in clinical practice it is becoming not unusual to employ this type of agent with this rationale.

It is clear that total body hypothermia does confer some degree of cerebral protection against periods of hypotension. In the extreme form, the use of profound hypothermia in paediatric cardiac surgery permits circulatory arrest for periods of up to 60 minutes without major clinical evidence of long-term cerebral injury. Wright *et al.* (1979) discovered impairment of neuropsychological function in children undergoing profound hypothermia compared to similar children subjected to standard cardiopulmonary bypass. However Tharion *et al.*, (1982) in a review of 550 operations noted a residual neurological deficit in only 4.5% of survivors after profound hypothermia with circulatory arrest. Most clinical reports of cardiopulmonary bypass with low pressure are also using low flow techniques, and indeed the low pressure is usually the consequence of the low flow. Furthermore, in the profound hypothermia group with circulatory arrest, the low pressure is a concomitant of total absence of systemic flow. Evidently further studies are required to elucidate the status of this particular technique for protection of cerebral function.

It is likely that autoregulation of cerebral blood flow is maintained during hypothermic cardiopulmonary bypass, certainly at mean arterial pressures in excess of 60 mmHg (8 kPa) and possibly even lower. There appears to be no reduction in perfusion of the cerebral microcirculation when flow is reduced over a wide range. Indeed, it is likely that the brain is more resistant to periods of low perfusion pressure than was previously recognized (Taylor, 1982). In a clinical study using non-pulsatile flow, Fox *et al.* (1982) deduced that most of the cerebral microcirculation was perfused at a flow rate of 1.2 $l\,min^{-1}\,m^{-2}$ at 20°C, though direct measurement of cerebral blood flow was not performed. For most cardiac surgical procedures it is a major advantage to have low flow and low pressure in the systemic circulation, as this is associated with a reduction of blood trauma from the pump–oxygenator system. In addition, the decreased coronary collateral flow obtained using flow rates below 2.2 $l\,min^{-1}\,m^{-2}$ (Conti *et al.*, 1978) contributes significantly towards the preservation of myocardial hypothermia.

6.3.3 The pulsatile nature of flow (see Chapter 7)

The controversy over the relative merits of pulsatile and non-pulsatile cardiopulmonary bypass reflects our ignorance regarding the optimal haemodynamics for cardiopulmonary bypass. In a study of 27 rhesus monkeys using non-pulsatile bypass and normothermia, Lees *et al.* (1971) demonstrated a 50% decrease in total systemic vascular resistance, an increase in the percentage of blood flow to the alimentary tract and a decrease in systemic flow to the cerebral hemispheres, heart and peripheral organs.

These observations were confirmed by Rudy *et al.* (1973) but this group also noticed the absence in reduction of cerebral blood flow when the haematocrit was reduced to 25%. Halley *et al.* (1959) in a study on 58 dogs also noted the constancy of cerebral blood flow and cerebral vascular resistance during extracorporeal circulation.

Early data (Wesolowski *et al.* 1955) suggested that there was no significant difference in renal function with pulsatile and non-pulsatile perfusion. Boucher *et al.* (1974) demonstrated in monkeys that pulse pressure did not affect organ blood flow or systemic vascular resistance during cardiopulmonary bypass. However, more recent work suggests that pulsatile flow may confer benefit in terms of microcellular oxygenation and improved organ function during cardiopulmonary bypass (Dunn *et al.*, 1974; Mavroudis, 1978). This concurs with the theoretical concepts advanced by Shepard *et al.* (1966) which emphasizes the importance of an energy gradient in the production of pulsatile blood flow. Taylor *et al.* (1978, 1982) have demonstrated an attenuation of hormonal changes during pulsatile perfusion and a reduction in mortality and in the incidence of deaths attributable to post-perfusion low cardiac output. Nevertheless, other evidence declaims the value of pulsatile perfusion during hypothermia (Singh *et al.*, 1980) and has suggested that the importance of pulse pressure is minimal (Edmunds, 1982). The observation (Taylor *et al.*, 1980) of a greater increase in brain-specific creatine kinase isoenzyme in the cerebrospinal fluid of dogs during pulseless cardiopulmonary bypass, and of increased urine and serum amylase values (Moores *et al.*, 1977) in patients undergoing pulseless cardiopulmonary bypass suggests that pulseless perfusion may be detrimental despite the absence of overt clinical impairment. Non-pulsatile coronary perfusion in patients with coronary artery disease may result in some degree of myocardial injury on account of a reduction in subendocardial blood flow (Pappas *et al.*, 1975). Further studies are required in order to delineate the most effective forms of pulsatile perfusion for routine clinical practice. The simplicity of the currently available pulsatile roller-pump systems and the absence of any demonstrable adverse effects from pulsatile flow makes pulsatility even on basic physiological principles a reasonable adjunct to cardiopulmonary bypass.

6.3.4 Temperature

Considerable research has been directed toward the protective role of hypothermia during cardiopulmonary bypass. Despite early suggestions (Bjork and Hultquist, 1960) that profound hypothermia might induce brain damage in children after open heart surgery, subsequent clinical work has confirmed the efficacy of the technique. Assessment of cerebral perfusion during profound hypothermia remains an unsolved problem. Weiss *et al.*

(1975) demonstrated that there was no correlation between the electroencephalogram and late function. The extent of the metabolic insult could not be inferred from electroencephalographic data. It seems likely that the problems associated with profound hypothermia are related to uneven brain cooling and rewarming. This has been demonstrated experimentally in baboons by Aoyagi *et al.* (1974). They noted paradoxical alterations in the cerebral microcirculation leading to regional ischaemia, especially during rewarming from 18°C. These alterations were postulated as causes of focal or generalized cerebral damage.

Much of the present information regarding low flow, low pressure perfusion has been gained in combination with a degree of hypothermia. It would seem wise in the current state of knowledge to recommend a degree of hypothermia in all but the very shortest of cardiopulmonary bypass procedures, and it is our current practice to recommend a systemic blood temperature between 20°C and 28°C for adult cardiopulmonary bypass procedures.

It should be emphasized that no single parameter should be considered in isolation during the conduct of cardiopulmonary bypass. As already mentioned, we recommend cardiopulmonary bypass using a clear fluid prime so that the resultant haematocrit is 20–25%. Pump flow rate is maintained around $2.4\,l\,min^{-1}\,m^{-2}$ at the commencement and completion of cardiopulmonary bypass when systemic temperature is near normal. We often employ a lower flow rate, commonly $1.6\,l\,min^{-1}\,m^{-2}$, at a systemic core temperature of 28°C and we maintain the mean arterial pressure between 40–60 mmHg (5.3–8 kPa) during cardiopulmonary bypass using pulsatile flow for all cases. The complexity of the surgery determines the precise setting of each of these variables.

6.4 MONITORING OF THE ADEQUACY OF CARDIOPULMONARY BYPASS

Monitoring of the adequacy of cardiopulmonary bypass is most commonly achieved by a combination of clinical assessment of the patient, together with assessment of specific organ function. In practice, clinical assessment of organ perfusion is limited to observations on the perfusion of the upper extremities. Thus, for instance, an imbalance in cerebral perfusion may be indicated by inequality of the pupillary response to light. We have already alluded to the value of observing changes such as cyanosis or venous engorgement, suggestive of inadequate oxygenation or superior vena caval obstruction respectively. More objective assessment of the adequacy of cardiopulmonary bypass may be achieved as follows, though as the discussion indicates meaningful data are extremely limited.

6.4.1 Cerebral function

Many attempts have been made to use intra-operative electroencephalography or cerebral function monitoring as a parameter of the adequacy of cardiopulmonary bypass in relation to cerebral perfusion. Although these diagnostic aids may be of value in assessing cerebral function (Branthwaite, 1973), the validity of such records remains unproven at the lower extremes of flow, perfusion pressure and temperature. The effects of hypothermia, haemodilution and anaesthesia impose severe limitations on the accuracy of cerebral assessment during cardiopulmonary bypass (Salerno *et al.*, 1978). As yet there are no entirely satisfactory non-invasive techniques for assessment of cerebral function during cardiopulmonary bypass.

6.4.2 Renal function

Further assessment of the adequacy of perfusion during cardiopulmonary bypass may be afforded by the observation of urine output during the procedure, but poor urine output is frequently observed with the low flow and pressure techniques employed in cardiopulmonary bypass. A reduced urine output during cardiopulmonary bypass does not necessarily reflect inadequate renal perfusion or imply subsquent renal dysfunction.

6.4.3 Metabolic indices

Mixed venous oxygen pressures ($P\mathrm{vO_2}$) are also useful variables in evaluation of the adequacy of perfusion at the termination of cardiopulmonary bypass, as they reflect mean oxygen levels in the tissues being perfused. A mixed ($P\mathrm{vO_2}$) of 30 mmHg (4 kPa) or more is consistent in general with normal convalescence (Kirklin and Kirklin, 1981). These estimates can of course be continued into the post-operative period and, when correlated with cardiac index, give reliable information about the adequacy of cardiac performance (Parr *et al.*, 1975). Further investigations in the peri-operative period include measurement of the indices of renal and hepatic function, together with assay of cardiac specific enzymes and other enzymes, such as lactate dehydrogenase, released during cell injury (Welbourn *et al.*, 1966). The problem with these biochemical assessments of enzyme release is that they are not applicable for evaluation of any acute changes in a specific cardiopulmonary bypass procedure, but they do give information which may be of some value retrospectively.

Despite the relative paucity of biochemical estimations for evaluation of cardiopulmonary bypass, recent findings indicate that more specific assays for assessment of the adequacy of cardiopulmonary bypass may soon be available. In experiments on dogs, new assessment techniques for the measurement of cerebral injury have been based upon the direct measurement of biochemical markers in the cerebrospinal fluid (CSF) (Taylor *et al.*, 1980). It is clear that CSF sampling during cardiopulmonary bypass is unlikely to become routine clinical practice, but development of serum markers of brain cell injury may well improve the quality of open heart surgery. Of some interest are the observations by Aberg *et al.* (1982) which showed a significant increase in cerebrospinal fluid adenylate kinase in 18 out of 36 patients undergoing open heart surgery. This increase correlated with the post-operative change in intellectual function. Further studies are required in order to ascertain whether intra-operative enzyme studies correlate with post-operative neuropsychological assessment in a reproducible manner. It will, of course, be essential to obtain enzyme assays which are rapidly obtainable in the operating room if the conduct of cardiopulmonary bypass is to be altered during the performance of open heart surgery. Nevertheless, a clearer rationale for the conduct of cardiopulmonary bypass may be achieved through validation of serum markers of organ injury.

Another means of assessing the adequacy of tissue perfusion is the measurement of skeletal muscle surface pH which is thought to correlate with the onset of anaerobic metabolism (Couch *et al.*, 1971, Gazzaniga *et al.*, 1972). Although both the variables correlate well with the onset of decreased tissue perfusion (Gazzaniga *et al.*, 1972) they have not yet found a place in clinical practice.

6.5 OTHER CONCOMITANTS OF CARDIOPULMONARY BYPASS WHICH MAY AFFECT ITS ADEQUACY

Recent studies suggest that cerebral damage during cardiopulmonary bypass results from a combination of embolic and perfusion injuries (Taylor, 1982). Massive arterial air embolism may occur with modern rigid shell bubble oxygenators if an alarm system is not employed (Stoney *et al.*, 1980). Prevention of intra-operative air embolism is aided by meticulous evacuation of air from within the heart prior to discontinuation of cardiopulmonary bypass (Lawrence *et al.*, 1971).

Appreciation of the role of microembolism in the genesis of cerebral dysfunction has resulted in greater use of arterial line filters. The importance of filters was confirmed by Hallenbeck *et al.* (1979) who demonstrated preservation of neuronal function during cardiopulmonary bypass using dacron-wool filtration. Allardyce *et al.* (1966) also emphasized the importance of microembolism in the pathogenesis of organ dysfunction caused by prolonged use of pump oxygenation. Sotaniemi (1980) noted a lower instance of neurological dysfunction in patients following the use of a membrane oxygenator. More recently, interest has centred upon the importance of accurate control of heparinization combined with the use of agents such as prostacyclin in the reduction of cerebral microembolism (Faichney *et al.*, 1982). Evidence is also beginning to appear, indicating that microaggregates release potentially pathological vasoactive substances, e.g. histamine, serotonin, which may induce local vasoconstriction (Hosking *et al.*, 1984). In addition, the whole area of complement activation, white cell activation and release of free radical species is emerging as a most important aspect of perfusion pathophysiology (Fleming *et al.*, 1985).

In this review we have seen that the conduct of cardiopulmonary bypass is based more upon clinical experience than upon sound experimental data. In the same way, assessment of the adequacy of cardiopulmonary bypass will remain deficient until more sensitive and specific assays of cellular dysfunction are developed. Therein lies the challenge to the perfusionist, the anaesthetist and the surgeon.

REFERENCES

Aberg, T., Tyden, H., Ronquist, G., Ahlund, P. and Bergstrom, K. (1982) Release of adenylate kinase into the cerebrospinal fluid during open heart surgery and its relation to postoperative intellectual function. *Lancet*, **i**, 1139–41.

Allardyce, D. B., Yoshida, S. H. and Ashmore, P. O (1966) The importance of microembolism in the pathogenesis of organ dysfunction caused by prolonged use of the pump oxygenator. *J. Thorac. Cardiovasc. Surg.*, **52**, 706–15.

Aoyagi, M., Flasterstein, A. H., Barnette, J., VonKoch, L., Ross, J. N. and Kennedy, J. H. (1974) Cerebral effects of profound hypothermia (18°C) and circulatory arrest. *Circulation* (Suppl. 1), **51**, 52–60.

Bjork, V. O. and Hultquist, G. (1960) Brain damage in children after deep hypothermia for open heart surgery. *Thorax*, **15**, 284–91.

Boucher, J. K., Rudy, L. W. and Edmunds, L. M. (1974) Organ blood flow during pulsatile cardiopulmonary bypass. *J. Appl. Physiol.*, **36**, 86–90.

Branthwaite, M. A. (1973) Detection of neurological damage during open heart surgery. *Thorax*, **28**, 464–72.

Conti, V. R., Bertranou, E. G., Blackstone, E. H., Kirklin, J. W. and Digerness, S. B. (1978) Cold cardioplegia versus hypothermia for myocardial protection. *J. Thorac. Cardiovasc. Surg.*, **76**, 577–89.

Couch, N. P., Dmochowski, J. R., Van de Water, J. M., Harken, D. E. and Moore, F. D. (1971). Muscle surface pH as an index of peripheral perfusion in man. *Ann. Surg.*, **173**, 173–83.

Dunn, J., Kirsh, M. M., Harness, J., Carswell, M., Straker, J. and Sloan, H. (1974) Haemodynamic, metabolic and haematologic effects of pulsatile cardiopulmonary bypass. *J. Thorac. Cardiovasc. Surg.*, **68**, 138–47.

Edmunds, L. H. (1982) Pulseless cardiopulmonary bypass. *J. Thorac. Cardiovasc. Surg.*, **84**, 800–4.

Ellis, R. J., Wisniewski, A. W., Potts, R., Calhoun, C., Loucks, C. and Wells, M. R. (1980) Reduction of flow rate and arterial pressure at moderate hypothermia does not result in cerebral dysfunction. *J. Thorac. Cardiovasc. Surg.*, **74**, 173–80.

English, T. A. H., Digerness, S. and Kirklin, J. W. (1971) Changes in colloid osmotic pressure during and shortly after open intracardiac operation. *J. Thorac. Cardiovasc. Surg.*, **61**, 338–41.

Faichney, A., Davidson, K. G., Wheatley, D. J., Davidson, J. F. and Walker, I. D. (1982) Prostacyclin in cardiopulmonary bypass operations. *J. Thorac. Cardiovasc. Surg.*, **84**, 601–8.

Fleming, J., Royston, D., Westaby, S., Braude, S. and Taylor, K. M. (1985) Liberation of free radical species during cardiopulmonary bypass in man. *Thorax*, **40**, 240.

Fox, L. S., Blackstone, E. H., Kirklin, J. W., Stewart, R. W. and Samuelson, P. N. (1982) Relationship of whole body oxygen consumption to perfusion flow rate during hypothermic cardiopulmonary bypass. *J. Thorac. Cardiovasc. Surg.*, **83**, 239–48.

Gazzaniga, A. B., Byrd, C. L., Stewart, D. R. and Gross, R. E. (1972) Effects of dexamethasone and chlorpromazine on skeletal muscle surface hydrogen ion concentration during cardiopulmonary bypass. *Ann. Surg.*, **176**, 757–60.

Hallenbeck, J. M., Furlow, T. W. Jr, Ruel, T. A. and Greenbaum, L. J. Jr (1979) Extracorporeal glass-wool filtration of whole blood enhances post ischaemic recovery of the cortical sensory evoked response. *Stroke*, **10**, 158–64.

Halley, M. M., Reemtsma, K. and Creech, O. Jr (1959) Haemodynamics and metabolism of individual organs during extracorporeal circulation. *Surgery*, **46**, 1128–34.

Hammerschmidt, D. E., Stroncek, D. F., Bowers, T. K., Lammi-Keefe, C. J., Kurth, D. M., Ozalins, A., Nicoloff, D. M., Lillehei, R. C, Craddock, P. R. and Jacob, H. S. (1981) Complement activation and neutropenia occurring during cardiopulmonary bypass. *J. Thorac. Cardiovasc. Surg.*, **81**, 370–7.

Hosking, S., Man, W. and Taylor, K. M. (1984) Histamine release during cardiopulmonary bypass. In *Proc. Int. Symp., Frontiers of Histamine Research*, Paris.

Kennedy, J. W., Kaiser, G. C., Fisher, L. D., Maynard, C., Fritz, J. K., Myers, W., Mudd, J. G., Ryan, J. J. and Coggin, J. (1980) Multivariate discriminate analysis of the clinical and angiographic predictors of operative mortality from the Collaborative Study in Coronary Artery Surgery. *J. Thorac. Cardiovasc. Surg.*, **80**, 876–87.

Kirklin, J. K. and Kirklin, J. W. (1981) Management of the cardiovascular system after cardiac surgery. *Ann. Thorac. Surg.*, **32**, 311–19.

Kollka, R. and Hilberman, M. (1980) Neurological dysfunction following cardiac operation with low flow, low pressure cardiopulmonary bypass. *J. Thorac. Cardiovasc. Surg.*, **79**, 432–7.

Lawrence, G. H., McKay, H. A. and Sherensky, R. T. (1971) Effective measures in the prevention of intraoperative aeroembolus. *J. Thorac. Cardiovasc. Surg.*, **62**, 731–5.

Lee, W. H., Brady, M. P., Rowe, J. M. and Miller J. W. C. Jr (1971) Effects of extracorporeal circulation upon behaviour, personality and brain function. *Ann. Surg.*, **173**, 1013–23.

Lees, M. H., Kerr, R. H., Hill, T. D., Morgan, C. L., Ochsner, A. J., Thomas, C. and van Fleet, D. L. (1971) Distribution of systemic blood flow of the rhesus monkey during cardiopulmonary bypass. *J. Thorac. Cardiovasc. Surg.*, **61**, 570–86.

Lilleaasen, P. and Stokke, O. (1978) Moderate and extreme haemodilution in open heart surgery: fluid balance and acid–base studies. *Ann. Thorac. Surg.*, **25**, 127–33.

Mavroudis, C. (1978) To pulse or not to pulse. *Ann. Thorac. Surg.*, **25**, 259–71.

Moores, W. Y., Gago, O., Morris, J. D. and Peck, C. C. (1977) Serum and urinary amylase levels following pulsatile and continuous cardiopulmonary bypass. *J. Thorac. Cardiovasc. Surg.*, **74**, 73–6.

Nadjmabadi, M. M., Rastan, H., Saidi, M. T. *et al.* (1978) Haemodynamic effects of acute intraoperative haemodilution in open heart surgery. *Anaesthesist*, **27**, 364–9.

Pappas, G., Winter, S. D., Kopvriva, C. J. and Steele, P. P. (1975) Improvement of myocardial and other vital organ functions and metabolism with a simple method of pulsatile flow (IABP) during clinical cardiopulmonary bypass. *Surgery*, **77**, 34–44.

Parker-Williams, E. J. (1972) Platelets in prostheses and pumps. *Clin. Haematol.*, **1**, 413–19.

Parr, C. V. S., Blackstone, E. H. and Kirklin, J. W. (1975) Cardiac performance and mortality early after intracardiac surgery in infants and young children. *Circulation*, **51**, 867–74.

Ream, A. K. (1982) Cardiopulmonary bypass in *Acute Cardiovascular Management. Anaesthesia and Intensive Care* (eds. Allen K. Ream and Richard P. Fogdall), J. P. Lippincott & Co., Philadelphia, pp. 420–55.

Rosenkranz, E. R., Utley, J. R., Menninger, F. J., Dembitsky, W. P., Hargens, A. C. and Peters, R. M. (1980) Interstitial fluid pressure changes during cardiopulmonary bypass. *Ann. Thorac. Surg.*, **30**, 536–42.

Rudy, L. W., Heymann, M. A. and Edmunds, L. H. (1973) Distribution of systemic blood flow during cardiopulmonary bypass. *J. Appl. Physiol.*, **34**, 194–200.

Salerno, T. A., Lince, D. P., White, D. N., Lynn, R. B. and Charrette, E. J. P. (1978) Monitoring of electroencephalogram during open heart surgery. *J. Thorac. Cardiovasc. Surg.*, **76**, 97–100.

Selkoe, D. J. and Myers, R. E. (1979) Neurological and cardiovascular effects of hypotension in the monkey. *Stroke*, **10**, 147–57.

Shepard, R. C., Simpson, D. C. and Sharp, J. F. (1966) Energy equivalent pressure. *Arch. Surg.*, **93**, 730–40.

Singh, R. K. K., Barratt-Boyes, B. G. and Harris, E. A. (1980) Does pulsatile flow improve perfusion during hypothermic cardiopulmonary bypass? *J. Thorac. Cardiovasc. Surg.*, **79**, 827–32.

Sotaniemi, K. A. (1980) Brain damage and neurological outcome after open heart surgery. *J. Neurol. Neurosurg. Psychiat.* **43**, 127–35.

Stockard, J. J., Bickford, R. O., Myers, R. R., Aung, M. M., Dilley, R. B. and Schauble, J. F. (1974) Hypotension induced changes in cerebral function during cardiac surgery. *Stroke*, **5**, 730–46.

Stoney, W. S., Alford, W. C. J., Burrus, G. R., Glassford, D. M. and Thomas, C. S. (1980) Air embolism and other accidents using pump oxygenators. *Ann. Thorac. Surg.*, **29**, 336–40.

Taylor, K. M. (1982) Brain damage during open heart surgery. *Thorax*, **37**, 873–6.

Taylor, K. M., Bain, W. H., Davidson, K. G. and Turner, M. A. (1982) Comparative clinical study of pulsatile and nonpulsatile perfusion in 350 consecutive patients. *Thorax*, **37**, 324–30.

Taylor, K. M., Devlin, B. J., Mittra, S. M., Gillan, J. G., Brannan, J. J. and McKenna, J. M. (1980) Assessment of cerebral damage during open heart surgery. A new experimental model. *Scand. J. Thorac. Cardiovasc. Surg.*, **14**, 197–203.

Taylor, K. M., Wright, G. S., Reid, J. M., Bain, W. H., Caves, P. K., Walker, M. I. and Grant, J. K. (1978) Comparative studies of pulsatile and nonpulsatile flow during cardiopulmonary bypass. II. The effects on adrenal secretion of cortisol. *J. Thorac. Cardiovasc. Surg.*, **75**, 574–8.

Tharion, J., Johnson, D. C., Celermajer, J. M., Hawkes, R. M., Cartmill, T. B. and

Overton, J. M. (1982) Profound hypothermia with circulatory arrest. *J. Thorac. Cardiovasc. Surg.*, **84**, 66–72.
Tufo, H. M., Ostfeld, A. M. and Shekelle, R. (1970) Central nervous system dysfunction following open heart surgery. *J. Am. Med. Assoc.*, **212**, 1333–40.
Utley, J. A., Wachtel, C., Cain, R. J., Spaw, E. A., Collins, J. C. and Stephens, D. M. (1981) Effects of hypothermia, haemodilution and pump oxygenation on organ water content, blood flow and oxygen delivery and renal function. *Ann. Thorac. Surg.*, **31**, 121–33.
Weiss, M., Weiss, J., Cotton, J., Nicolas, F. and Binet, J. P. (1975) A study of the electroencephalogram during surgery with deep hypothermia and circulation arrest in infancy. *J. Thorac. Cardiovasc. Surg.*, **70**, 316–29.
Welbourn, N. E. Melrose, D. and Moss, D. W. (1966) Change in serum enzyme levels accompanying cardiac surgery with extracorporeal circulation. *J. Clin. Pathol.*, **19**, 220–32.
Wesolowski, S. A., Sauvage, L. R. and Pinc, R. D. (1955) Extracorporeal circulation: the role of the pulse in maintenance of the systemic circulation during heart lung bypass. *Surgery*, **37**, 663–82.
Wheeldon, D. R., Gill, R. D., Bethune, D. W. and English, T. A. H. (1981) How safe is cardiopulmonary bypass? *Thorax*, **36**, 79–80.
Wollman, H., Stephen, G. W., Clement, A. J. and Davidson, G. K. (1966) Cerebral blood flow in man during extracorporeal circulation. *J. Thorac. Cardiovasc. Surg.*, **52**, 558–64.
Wright, J. S., Hicks, R. O. and Norman, D. C. (1979) Deep hypothermia arrest: observations on later development in children. *J. Thorac. Cardiovasc. Surg.*, **77**, 466–8.

7
Pulsatile perfusion

K. M. TAYLOR

7.1 INTRODUCTION

When total cardiopulmonary bypass was employed clinically in the early 1950s, pioneering workers had, in many instances, attempted to develop pulsatile systems which would reproduce the pulsatile flow produced by the normal heart. The technological complexity of such systems did, however, prove at that time to be an insurmountable barrier and the use of short periods of non-pulsatile perfusion during cardiopulmonary bypass were found to be compatible with patient survival. Confidence increased and non-pulsatile perfusion became established as the routine mode of perfusion, the early non-pulsatile roller pump systems proving exceedingly reliable and safe in clinical use. For many years thereafter little attention was paid to the subject of pulsatile perfusion. Studies continued to appear however, demonstrating in terms of haemodynamics and metabolism that non-pulsatile perfusion appeared at least potentially to carry a detrimental effect on cell metabolism and organ function. These pathological effects were either preventable or at least diminished by the substitution of pulsatile flow. A few investigators continued to develop their own pulsatile pump systems for clinical use, although none progressed into commercial production and routine clinical application, probably due to excess of complexity and dubious reliability.

The emphasis in this intermediate phase was on the development of surgical techniques and it is only in the past few years that attention has been focused again on the topic of pulsatile perfusion. In view of the considerable expansion in industrial technology in recent years, the ultimate development of pumps able to deliver adjustable and reliable pulsatile flow might have been anticipated. In the past few years, such systems have indeed been developed and have been introduced into commercial production and clinical usage. The introduction of pulsatile perfusion systems after the long period of acceptance and proven reliability of non-pulsatile systems has led, not surprisingly, to some degree of resistance towards the incorporation of pulsatile perfusion systems into routine clinical practice. Many have expressed the opinion that pulsatile perfusion may introduce greater complexity for only a marginal benefit, although few would argue that pulsatile flow is not inherently more physiological. This problem of clinical acceptance rests more on other aspects such as the possible technological complexity and the fear of possible increases in haemolysis. Many workers have felt that pulsatile systems are substantially more complex to set up and run in routine cardiac surgical practice, thus the controversy continues. Familiarity and satisfaction with non-pulsatile perfusion create an inevitable barrier towards the introduction of new technology. The argument for the adoption of routine pulsatile perfusion does however rest on solid physiological foundations, and if pulsatile perfusion systems can be shown to produce the expected haemodynamic and metabolic superiority without compromising safety or reliability, then they may be incorporated into routine clinical practice with confidence. In this chapter, the role of pulsatile perfusion in modern cardiac surgical practice will be reviewed. In particular, consideration will be given to the underlying theories of the physiology of the pulse in the circulation, the pathophysiology of non-pulsatile perfusion and the haemodynamic and metabolic effects of pulsatility. Finally, the practical aspects of the incorporation of pulsatile systems into routine clinical practice will be discussed.

7.2 THEORIES OF THE PHYSIOLOGY OF PULSATILE ARTERIAL FLOW

In Mavroudis' (1978) comprehensive review of the subject of pulsatile perfusion, it is clear that though the existence of the pulse has been known from the time of Hippocrates, its physiological significance is still far from clear. There are however three principal theories proposed by which pulsatile arterial blood flow is considered to exert significant physiological effects. These principal theories are:

(1) The concept of energy equivalent pressure.
(2) Capillary critical closing pressure and microcirculatory patency.
(3) Neuroendocrine reflex mechanisms triggered by baroreceptor discharge.

7.2.1 The concept of energy equivalent pressure

This theoretical advantage of pulsatile over non-pulsatile flow was proposed by Shepard *et al.* (1966). He suggested that the production of pulsatile flow depends not on a pressure gradient but on an energy gradient. He defined an energy equivalent pressure to represent the energy content of the pulsatile arterial wave. Energy equivalent pressure was defined according to the following formula:

$$\text{eep} = \frac{\int \text{pfdt}}{\int \text{fdt}}$$

where p = pressure (mmHg), f = flow (ml s^{-1}), and dt = change in time at a specific point in time. The ratio of the power curve and the flow curve was taken at the end of the pressure and flow cycles. Using this formula, Shepard demonstrated that the energy needed to deliver pulsatile flow was 2.3 times that required to produce non-pulsatile flow for the same levels of mean flow and pressure. The extra energy inherent in pulsatile wave forms was thought to be available to tissues and it was suggested that this energy produced maintenance of capillary patency, increase in tissue lymph flow and, by creating oscillatory movements at cell level, an overall improvement in cell metabolism. These aspects of the fate of the available energy excess have not been well substantiated nor investigated, but Shepard's theory gains some support from the finding that a pulsatile arterial wave dissipates significantly more utilizable energy to tissues, than does a non-pulsatile wave of the same mean pressure (Wilcox *et al.*, 1967). Shepard's theory also predicts higher mean flow rates for pulsatile flow compared to non-pulsatile flow at equal perfusion pressures, and while this is true in clinical practice the significant reduction in peripheral vascular resistance associated with pulsatile perfusion could be an alternative explanation.

7.2.2 Capillary critical closing pressure and microcirculatory patency

The early studies of Parsons and McMaster (1938) demonstrated conclusively that non-pulsatile perfusion is associated with a reduction in the flow of lymph and interstitial fluid. Subsequent studies have indicated a reduction in capillary blood flow in general, and a significant reduction in cerebral capillary diameter with non-pulsatile as opposed to pulsatile flow. It has been suggested by Burton (1954) that as arterial pressure begins to fall at the end of systole, blood flow in the microcirculation will only continue until a critical closing pressure of the pre-capillary arterioles is reached when capillary perfusion ceases. Burton suggests that the peaks of pulsatile systolic pressure will ensure an effectively greater period of microcirculatory patency for equivalent levels of arterial pressure. This theory gained support from the observations by Takeda (1960), who demonstrated the presence of microcirculatory shunting and widespread capillary collapse during non-pulsatile perfusion. Microcirculatory shunting and reduced capillary perfusion do correlate well with the reported metabolic sequelae of non-pulsatile perfusion, i.e. reduced oxygen consumption, tissue acidosis and reduced metabolic uptake rates for oxygen and glucose.

7.2.3 Neuroendocrine reflex mechanisms triggered by baroreceptor discharge

It is well known that baroreceptors do respond to both static and pulsatile aspects of the arterial pressure wave. The change from pulsatile to non-pulsatile perfusion has been shown to result in a marked increase in the discharge frequency of carotid sinus baroreceptors (Angell-James and de Burgh, 1971). This central baroreceptor stimulus may possibly initiate reflex neuroendocrine responses which remain operative throughout the period of non-pulsatile perfusion. Previous authors have suggested that this baroreceptor mechanism may induce reflex vasoconstriction in the peripheral circulation, either by direct neural reflexes or by stimulating the release of humoral vasoconstrictors (e.g. angiotensin, vasopressin or catecholamines).

It does seem, however, that whatever mechanism or combination of mechanisms are operative, there is a final common pathway by which arterial pulsatility exerts its metabolic and haemodynamic effects, that is the maintenance of energy supply/demand equality at a cellular level by preserving capillary perfusion and maintaining basic cellular metabolic functions, for example, oxygen consumption and sodium–potassium pumping. When pulsatility is removed, despite maintenance of total arterial flow and mean arterial pressure, capillary perfusion is reduced, microcirculatory shunting develops and cell metabolism becomes disordered with reduced oxygen consumption, progressive acidosis and lactate accumulation. There is clearly a need for further research into the theoretical basis for pulsatile arterial flow and pressure. Such research is likely to promote the refinement of pulsatile systems in order that optimum characteristics of flow and pressure may be achieved.

7.3 HAEMODYNAMIC EFFECTS OF PULSATILE PERFUSION

There has been over the years a clear consensus among investigators that non-pulsatile perfusion is associated with a progressive elevation in peripheral vascular resistance levels. The period of vasoconstriction has also been followed into the post-perfusion period. The reports of Estafanous *et al.* (1973) in Cleveland have drawn attention to the associated hypertension/vasoconstriction phenomenon seen particularly in patients following coronary artery bypass graft procedures. The period of increase in peripheral vascular resistance persists for some hours after the end of the perfusion period. Awareness of the potentially hazardous consequences of unnecessarily high levels of peripheral resistance has been parelleled by the increased advocacy of vasodilator therapy in this particular period after non-pulsatile perfusion with vasodilator therapy such as epidural anaesthesia, sodium nitroprusside, or nitrate therapy (Stinson *et al.*, 1977). Though the occurrence of this syndrome is well described there is considerably less certainty in relation to its aetiology. Though increased catecholamine activity has been suggested by some authors, investigators have been unable to demonstrate a significant correlation between changes in catecholamine levels, and the haemodynamic changes seen during and after non-pulsatile perfusion. Additional evidence from Philbin's group has indicated that plasma ADH (vasopressin) levels are markedly elevated during non-pulsatile flow. Pulsatile perfusion is associated with significantly lower levels (Philbin *et al.*, 1979). There is, however, more evidence to suggest that renin–angiotensin activation may play a major aetiological role in the generation of this increase in peripheral vascular resistance. Furthermore, it has been suggested that the well-documented haemodynamic effect of pulsatile perfusion in maintaining lower levels of peripheral resistance is mediated through significantly lower degrees of renin–angiotensin activation compared with non-pulsatile perfusion.

7.3.1 Renin–angiotensin activation during cardiopulmonary bypass

Non-pulsatile perfusion is associated with marked elevation of plasma angiotensin II (AII) levels with persistence of elevated AII levels in the early postoperative period (Taylor *et al.*, 1977). Angiotensin II is an extremely powerful vasoconstrictor agent, and has been shown experimentally to produce increased arteriolar vasoconstriction and subendocardial ischaemia. A highly significant correlation between the rise in AII levels and the rise in peripheral vascular resistance during non-pulsatile perfusion has also been demonstrated. Following these initial studies renin–angiotensin activation during non-pulsatile perfusion has now been demonstrated by several other groups. In line with this theory of renin–angiotensin activation, the specific inhibitor substances of angiotensin II have been used after periods of non-pulsatile perfusion. The use of specific AII inhibitor has been shown by the author's group (Taylor *et al.*, 1979a), and by others, to be associated with a rapid and highly significant reduction in elevated levels of peripheral vascular resistance with a consequent increase in cardiac index (Fig. 7.1). These particular studies greatly strengthen the thesis that angiotensin II is a major factor in the development of increased vascular resistance during and after non-pulsatile perfusion (Taylor *et al.*, 1980a).

7.3.2 Peripheral vascular resistance during cardiopulmonary bypass

Whatever the precise aetiological factors involved, it has been clear for many years that pulsatile perfusion is associated with significantly lower levels of peripheral vascular resistance during and after the period of perfusion (Mandelbaum and Burns 1965; Dunn *et al.*, 1974).

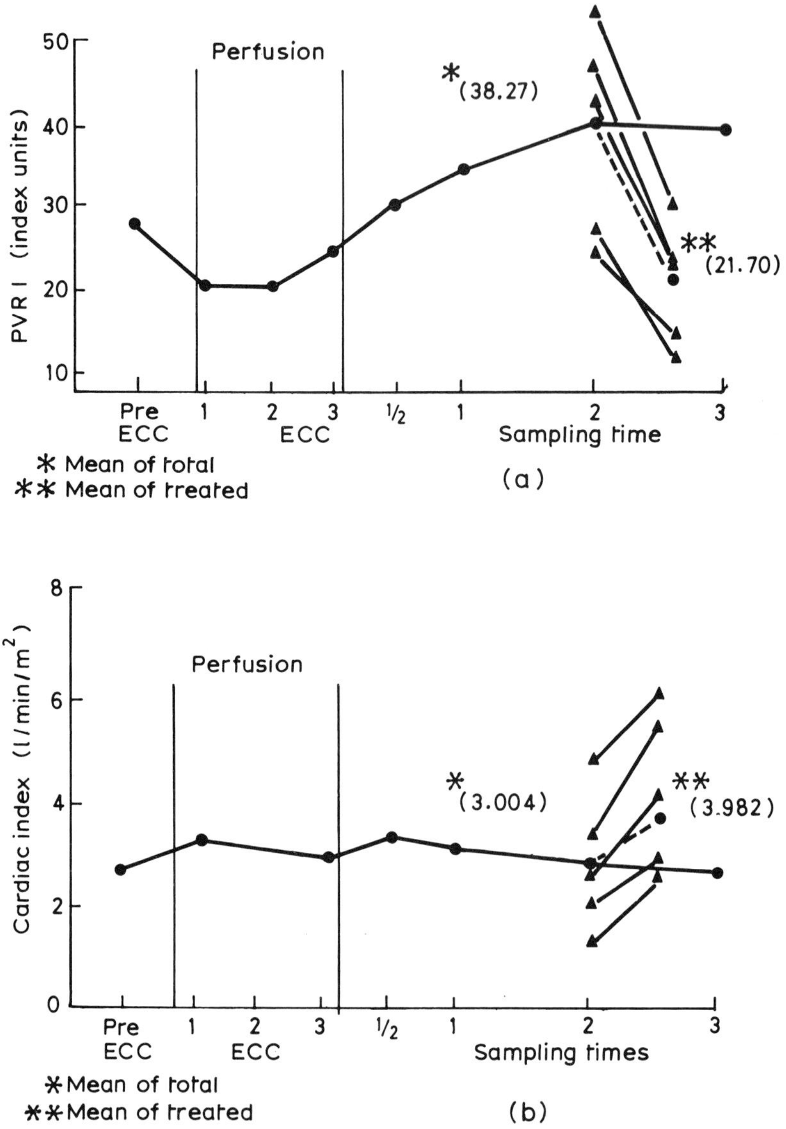

Fig. 7.1 Haemodynamic effects of angiotensin converting enzyme inhibitor (SQ14225) infused for 20 minutes intravenously 2 hours following conventional cardiopulmonary bypass. The mean levels of peripheral vascular resistance (a) and cardiac index (b) are shown for the control untreated group throughout the experimental period. The change in peripheral vascular resistance and cardiac index are shown for each individual subject at the start and end of the 20 minute infusion period. (Reproduced by permission from Taylor, *et al.*, *Cardiovasc. Res.*, **14**, 199–205, 1980.)

The haemodynamic benefits of pulsatile perfusion involve (1) the primary efect of reducing elevated levels of peripheral vascular resistance thus promoting improved tissue perfusion and (2) a secondary effect by which subsequent left ventricular performance is improved by exposing the left ventricle at the end of the perfusion period to a significantly lower level of peripheral vascular resistance, compared to that produced by non-pulsatile perfusion. This secondary effect relates to the concept of afterload as an important, even primary determinant of left ventricular performance (Sonnenblick and Downing, 1963).

This haemodynamic effect is distinct from any additional direct effect of pulsatile perfusion on the coronary circulation. The precise effects of pulsatile perfusion on the coronary circulation are currently under much investigation though no clear picture has as yet emerged. While some authors have demonstrated improved coronary artery and coronary graft flow and improvement in overall left ventricular performance (Bregman *et al.*, 1977), others have suggested that pulsatile perfusion is beneficial only in the fibrillating heart (Steed *et al.*, 1978). The introduction of clinically available pulsatile systems has been associated with some confusion in relation to these separate haemodynamic effects. We have previously indicated that the haemodynamic argument for the use of pulsatile perfusion rests principally on its peripheral effect, that is in preventing excessive rises in peripheral vascular resistance. While pulsatile systems may improve diastolic coronary filling by accurately synchronized counterpulsation modes, this is a separate and additional haemodynamic benefit which requires investigation in its own right.

If one accepts the thesis that non-pulsatile perfusion produces progressive elevation in peripheral vascular resistance levels, and that this is potentially hazardous in terms of increasing left ventricular work, the management of this haemodynamic situation is clearly of crucial importance. It has been stated that vasoconstriction may possibly be preventable if higher flow rates and perfusion pressures are employed. There is no convincing evidence that this is in fact so. Indeed, studies have shown that despite raising mean perfusion pressure to 70 mmHg (9.3 kPa) and flow to $3.5\,\mathrm{l\,m^{-2}\,min^{-1}}$ the pattern of rise in peripheral vascular resistance remains unaffected so long as non-pulsatile flow is employed. By contrast, the substitution of pulsatile flow even at a mean perfusion pressure of 50 mmHg (6.7 kPa) at conventional flow rates of $2.4\,\mathrm{l\,m^{-2}\,min^{-1}}$ is associated with preservation of normal levels of peripheral vascular resistance (Fig. 7.2). In parallel with these studies of vascular resistance during and after the period of perfusion, simultaneous measurement of cardiac index has indicated that cardiac index is not significantly improved with elevated flow rates and perfusion pressures during the period of non-pulsatile perfusion, but that the use of pulsatile perfusion is associated with significantly higher levels of cardiac index in the immediate post-perfusion period (Fig. 7.3).

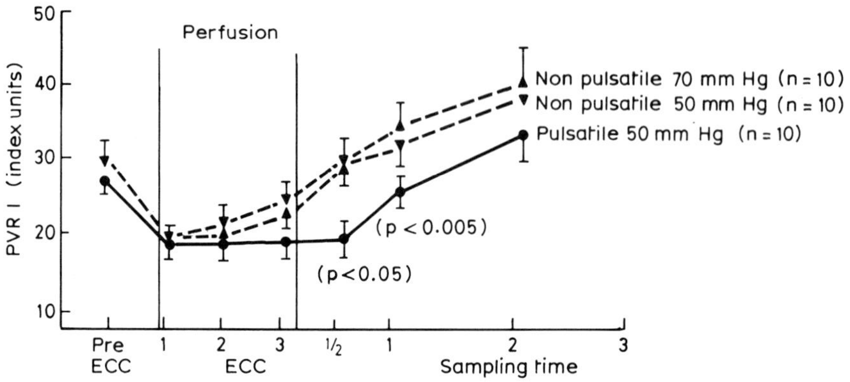

Fig. 7.2 Effect of pulsatile and non-pulsatile perfusion on peripheral vascular resistance index (PVRI). Note that both non-pulsatile groups exhibit persistent vasoconstriction during the perfusion period, continuing in the post-perfusion phase. Pulsatile perfusion is associated with maintenance of normal levels of PVRI during perfusion and significantly lower levels within the first hour post-perfusion.

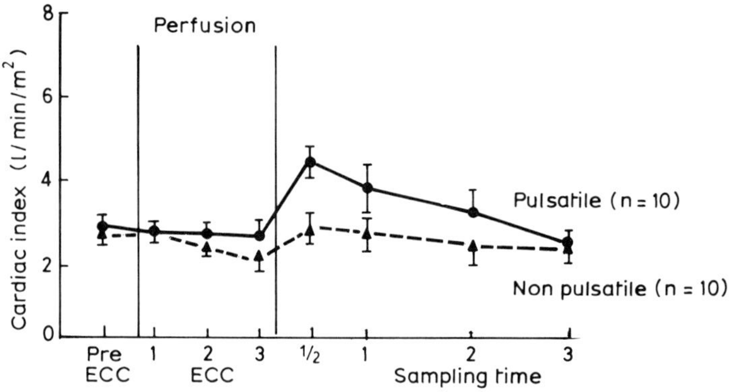

Fig. 7.3 Effect of pulsatile and non-pulsatile perfusion on cardiac index. These results are taken from the same experimental subjects as in Fig. 7.2. Note that cardiac index is significantly higher ($p<0.01$) within the first hour post-perfusion compared to the non-pulsatile group. Cardiac output determinations were obtained using indocyanine green dye-dilution technique.

The results of these experimental studies have been reflected in the findings of various groups using pulsatile perfusion in clinical practice. Improved haemodynamic status in the immediate postoperative phase after pulsatile perfusion has been associated with a reduced requirement for circulatory support, either with intra-aortic balloon counter pulsation (IABP) or with inotropic drugs. Bregman *et al.* (1977) have reported a reduction in the need for post-perfusion balloon pumping and a reduced incidence of peri-operative myocardial infarction in patients perfused with pulsatile flow. Pappas' group (Maddoux *et al.*, 1976), have reported similar findings and the author's group have found parallel reduction in the requirement for IABP support and in the use of inotropic drug infusions in the early postoperative period (Taylor *et al.*, 1979b). In continuing clinical studies the use of pulsatile perfusion has been associated with a significantly lower level of haemodynamic-related mortality with a lower incidence of intra-operative and low cardiac output associated deaths (Table 7.1). There is little doubt

Table 7.1 Mortality statistics in consecutive series of 1217 patients: Glasgow Royal Infirmary (1978–80)

	Pulsatile	*Non-Pulsatile*	*p*
Number of cases	763	454	
Total mortality (%)	3.5	8.1	<0.05
Elective mortality (%)	2.2	6.6	<0.05
On-table deaths*	18.3	32.2	<0.05
Deaths <24 h post-op.*	33.3	57.5	<0.05

Key * expressed as % of all deaths in that group.

that the haemodynamic superiority of pulsatile perfusion will be most evident in those patients who have impaired left ventricular function. In such patients excessive elevation in peripheral vascular resistance levels may exceed the already diminished reserve of left ventricular function, and so set up the essentials for a low cardiac output state in the post-perfusion period.

7.4 METABOLIC EFFECTS OF PULSATILE PERFUSION

The large numbers of previous studies in the literature concerning the metabolic effects of pulsatile as opposed to non-pulsatile perfusion are conveniently grouped into studies concerned with cell metabolism in general and specific organ function studies, principally those of the kidney, the brain and the pancreas.

The basic processes of cell metabolism, in particular oxygen consumption and the development of metabolic acidosis, have been considered to reflect the overall state of capillary flow and adequacy of tissue perfusion. Oxygen consumption was shown by many early workers to be significantly higher during pulsatile perfusion. Studies by Shepard and Kirklin (1969), Jacobs *et al.* (1969), and many others demonstrated progressive metabolic acidosis during non-pulsatile perfusion with a fall-off in oxygen consumption. Reduced cellular uptake of glucose has also been demonstrated with non-pulsatile flow. These disturbances in general cellular metabolism may reflect the reduction in capillary perfusion associated with a capillary closure effect of non-pulsatile perfusion previously discussed. Attempts have been made by some authors to overcome the fall-off in oxygen consumption with non-pulsatile perfusion by raising the mean flow rate. Although some studies have been unable to demonstrate significant differences at flow rates above 100 ml kg^{-1} min^{-1}, most authors, even with high flow rates, indicate that the metabolic superiority of pulsatile perfusion is demonstrable whatever the flow rate chosen.

It has been suggested that the increase in tissue water content during non-pulsatile perfusion may reflect a degree of cell membrane instability and sodium pump malfunction associated with impaired capillary perfusion. This concept has yet to be proven as has the proposed preventive action of pulsatile perfusion. It is however the feature of many studies that the integrity of the vascular compartment does seem to be better maintained with pulsatile perfusion, such that transfusion volumes and fluid replacement volumes are significantly less than those required with non-pulsatile flow. The studies of cellular metabolic effects of pulsatile perfusion are reflected in the function studies carried out by various groups into specific organs.

7.4.1 Brain function

Brain cells are considered sensitive to impaired perfusion. Studies of cerebral function in relation to open-heart procedures are however complicated, since in addition to any perfusion related insult the microembolic damage has for many years been considered an important feature in the overall cerebral damage picture. Microembolic damage may certainly produce focal brain lesions evident in previous histological studies. (Hill *et al.*, 1969). However, a pattern of diffuse ischaemic brain cell damage has been reported which may be related to perfusion. The studies of Wright and Sanderson (1972) have demonstrated that this diffuse brain cell damage syndrome associated with non-pulsatile flow may be prevented when pulsatile perfusion is used. In addition, recent studies have demonstrated a significant reduction in cerebral arteriolar and capillary diameter during non-pulsatile perfusion (de Paepe *et al.*, 1979). The autoregulation of cerebral blood flow has been assumed for many years to protect brain cells down to a mean perfusion pressure of 60 mmHg (8 kPa). The mechanisms maintaining autoregulation are, however, capable of modification by many factors, such as temperature, pattern of blood flow, blood viscosity, oxygen and carbon dioxide tensions in arterial blood and the effect of various drugs. In addition, cerebral blood flow is not distributed uniformly and certain areas of brain tissue do depend on a high blood flow pattern, and are thus at risk if autoregulation of cerebral blood flow does become compromised (Simpson, 1981). It is the author's increasing belief, however, that the use of non-pulsatile perfusion produces a functional disturbance in the brain, and not the picture of irreversible cell structural damage previously reported, unless severe carotid stenotic lesions are present (Fig. 7.4).

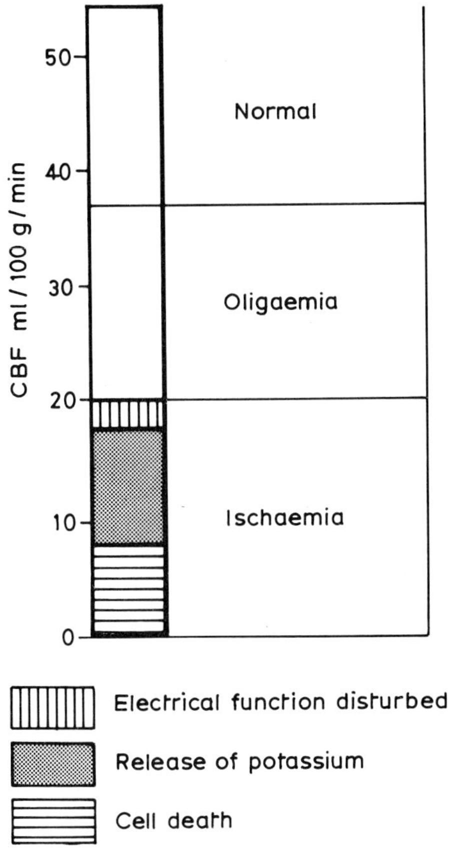

Fig. 7.4 Simplified thresholds of cerebral ischaemia. Note that cerebral blood flow (CBF) must fall to <20% of normal values before ischaemic cell death occurs.

The dynamic function of the hypothalamic–pituitary axis in relation to stress response patterns during open-heart surgery has proved to be a valuable and sensitive study model for cerebral function. The pattern of stress responses following general surgical procedures are well documented in the literature. During non-pulsatile perfusion however, significantly disordered response patterns are seen. The anterior pituitary fails to respond to a trophic stimulus of thyrotrophin-releasing hormone (TRH) in contrast to the normal response seen during major non-bypass surgery. Anterior pituitary secretion of ACTH falls to substress levels during non-pulsatile perfusion and the secretion of cortisol by the adrenal cortex is substantially reduced. Within sixty minutes of the end of non-pulsatile perfusion, however, pituitary TRH response returns to normal, ACTH secretion is restored and adrenal secretion of cortisol resumes. This syndrome of pituitary adrenal axis switch off during non-pulsatile perfusion is prevented when pulsatile flow is substituted (Figs 7.5 and 7.6). TRH response in the pituitary is normal and cortisol secretion

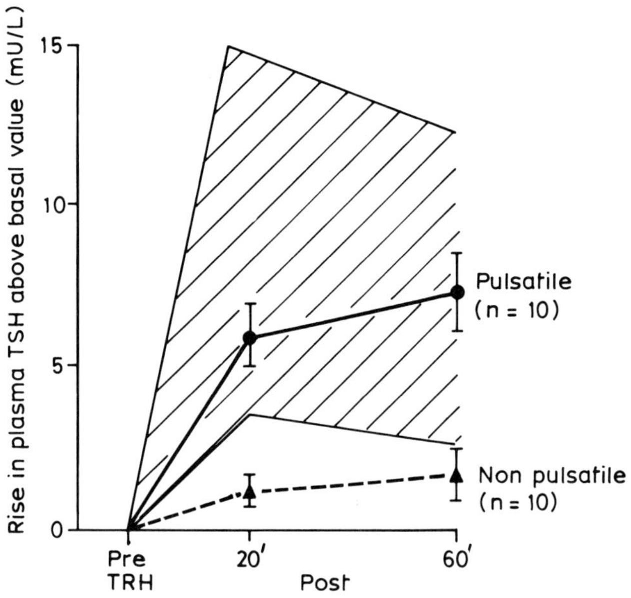

Fig. 7.5 Anterior pituitary response to thyrotropin releasing hormone (TRH) during pulsatile and non-pulsatile perfusion. Note that patients perfused with pulsatile flow in identical perfusion conditions exhibit restoration of a normal TRH test response (cross-hatched area). TRH response during non-pulsatile perfusion is subnormal. (Reproduced by permission from Taylor *et al.*, *J. Thorac. Cardiovasc. Surg.*, 75, 579–84, 1978.)

by the adrenal continues throughout the period of pulsatile bypass. These findings reflect a major physiological difference in response patterns by the hypothalamic pituitary axis during pulsatile and non-pulsatile perfusions for the same levels of mean flow and pressure (Taylor *et al.*, 1976, 1978a,b). Recent studies have also demonstrated a similar dysfunction pattern in relation to vasopressin secretion during non-pulsatile flow (Philbin *et al.*, 1979)

There is considerable interest at the present time in the area of cerebral damage during open-heart procedures. Psychometric testing and electrophysiological assessment have been used with some degree of success (Aberg, 1974). These methods are however difficult to quantitate and may not be

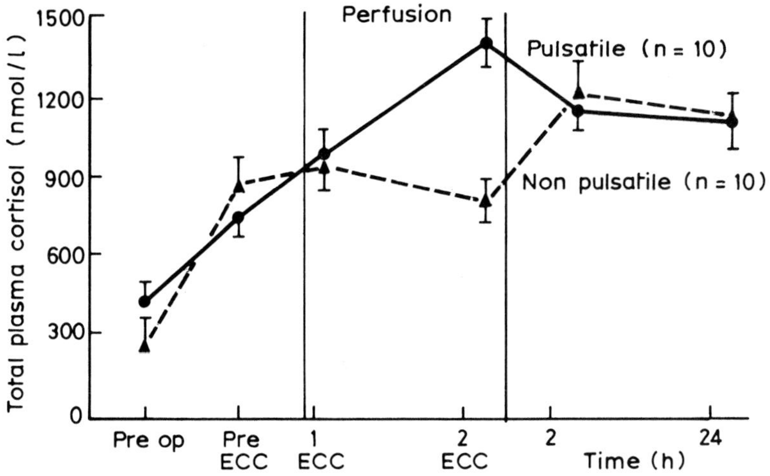

Fig. 7.6 Plasma cortisol levels corrected for haemodilution during pulsatile and non-pulsatile perfusion. Note that pulsatile perfusion preserves cortisol secretion during the perfusion period in contrast to the fall-off in cortisol secretion in the patients perfused with non-pulsatile flow. (Reproduced by permission from Taylor *et al.* *J. Thorac. Cardiovasc. Surg.*, 75, 574–8, 1978.)

sufficiently sensitive to allow accurate interpretation of results. The biochemical assessment of cerebrospinal fluid isoenzyme levels may prove to be a significant step forward in establishing an accurate and sensitive model for perfusion-related cerebral damage (Fig. 7.7). Early studies have demonstrated significant rises in creatine kinase isoenzymes in the cerebrospinal fluid during non-pulsatile perfusion (Taylor *et al.*, 1980b). Significantly lower levels were encountered when pulsatile flow was substituted. The continued refinement and search for accurate brain cell markers present in the cerebrospinal fluid, and hopefully in the peripheral blood may allow a more accurate assessment of the cerebral effects of different perfusion regimes.

7.4.2 Kidney function

Some of the earliest studies in the field of pulsatile and non-pulsatile perfusion were carried out in relation to renal function. Several authors have reported defects in renal excretory function during non-pulsatile perfusion. Tubular sodium excretion and a rise in the renal secretion of renin have been reported during non-pulsatile flow. A reduction in pulse pressure as opposed to a reduction in mean arterial perfusion pressure was suggested as the principal stimulus for renal renin release (Kohlstaedt and Page, 1940). In more recent studies the use of pulsatile perfusion has been reported to preserve renal

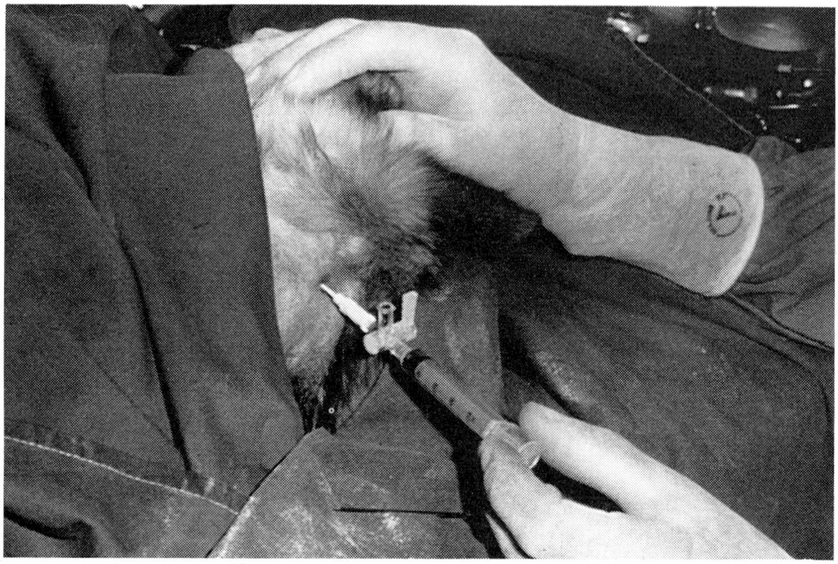

Fig. 7.7 Experimental technique of cisterna magna cannulation and aspiration of cerebrospinal fluid permitting assay of biochemical markers of brain injury.

cortical blood flow, renal venous return, and also renal tubular histology (Many *et al*., 1967). Pulsatile perfusion has also been shown to produce significantly lower plasma levels of renin and angiotensin II compared to the markedly elevated levels found during non-pulsatile perfusion. The significance of the pulse in renal physiology is also attested to by the widespread adoption of pulsatile perfusion in renal homograft preservation. It must be said however that in the author's opinion renal vascular autoregulation exerts a considerable protective mechanism by which the kidney is spared many of the deleterious effects of altered perfusion. In our experience relatively sophisticated tests of renal tubular function have to be used before significant differences may be demonstrated. It may be that the kidney is much more resistant to the perfusion differences between pulsatile and non-pulsatile flow than is, for example, the brain.

7.4.3 Pancreatic and liver function

There have been until recently few studies concerned with pancreatic, endocrine and exocrine function during and after open-heart surgery. Interest in the pancreas has however been stimulated by isolated findings indicating significant increases in plasma amylase levels after non-pulsatile perfusion. In addition, Feiner (1976) has reported a 16% incidence of ischaemic pancreatitis found in patients dying after open-heart surgery. Recent studies have now demonstrated that pulsatile perfusion is associated first with significantly lower levels of serum amylase and also with significantly lower incidence of elevated amylase creatinine clearance ratios, a more accurate index of pancreatic exocrine function (Murray *et al.*, 1982). As indicated, there have been relatively few studies in this area but the possibility does exist that the relatively frequent but generally ignored gastrointestinal upsets in the early postoperative period after open-heart surgery may reflect mild pancreatic damage and should be more widely investigated.

Current research into the effects of pulsatile and non-pulsatile perfusion on hepatic blood flow have shown the typical vasoconstrictive reponse to non-pulsatile perfusion and reduction in hepatic oxygen consumption (Fig. 7.8). Hepatic arterial flow and hepatic oxygen consumption fall to 50% of normal values with non-pulsatile flow, but are maintained at control levels with pulsatile perfusion (Mathie *et al.*, 1984).

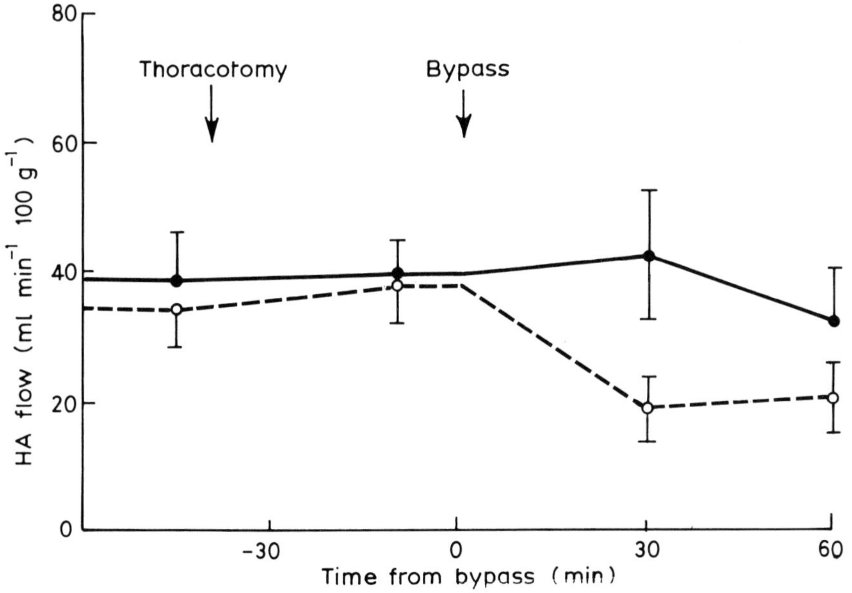

Fig. 7.8 Hepatic arterial blood flow during pulsatile (straight line) and non-pulsatile flow (dotted line). Pulsatile perfusion produces significant preservation of normal levels of hepatic arterial blood flow. At the same levels of mean pump flow and pressure, flow is reduced to about 50% of normal values during non-pulsatile perfusion.

It is possible therefore to obtain from the previous literature a clear consensus indicating the overall physiological superiority of pulsatile perfusion as opposed to the more conventional non-pulsatile flow. Significant improvements in haemodynamic status are evident. There is much evidence to suggest that capillary perfusion is preserved with pulsatile flow, and that this is reflected in preservation of cell metabolism in general and of specific organ metabolism in particular.

7.5 CLINICAL USE OF PULSATILE PERFUSION SYSTEMS

Although the theoretical basis for the adoption of pulsatile perfusion during open-heart surgery has been well established for some considerable time, there has not been the same consensus of opinion as to the optimum design of pulsatile pump systems. Indeed the technological problems associated with the development of pulsatile pump systems have been such that until very recently there were no acceptably reliable systems in commercial production. Although attempts were made in the early days of perfusion technology to produce clinically acceptable pulsatile pumps, development was hampered by technological complexity, and also the mistaken belief that the already high haemolysis index produced in early bypass circuits would be increased substantially with pulsatile pumps. These facts are of relevance when considering the clinical applicability of pulsatile perfusion. Although few workers would argue that pulsatile perfusion is not inherently more physiological than conventional non-pulsatile flow, many remain satisfied with non-pulsatile bypass, feeling that pulsatile perfusion may possibly introduce greater complexity for only a marginal benefit. Within the past few years those systems which have been developed represent the first commercially available truly pulsatile systems. Their availability has allowed certain groups including the author's to gain considerable experience in the clinical applicability of pulsatile perfusion in routine open-heart surgical practice. In this section pulsatile perfusion systems presently available and under development will be discussed. The results of studies concerning the haematological effects of pulsatile perfusion will be reviewed, together with the reported clinical experience of various cardiac surgical groups.

7.5.1 Pulsatile perfusion systems presently available

In the early development of pulsatile pump systems during the period of physiological studies, systems were often based on pneumatic or hydraulic pumps or on cam-driven piston pumps. Although such pumps have been shown to produce most acceptable pulsatile flow, few if any have proved sufficiently reliable and simple to commend them for routine clinical use. The systems which have been used most widely in clinical practice have been either modified roller pump systems or intermittent occlusive systems based on the intra-aortic balloon principle.

7.5.2 Modified roller pump systems

Modified roller pump systems have been used by several experimental groups and have been the subject of more recent clinical reports. Recent technological developments have resulted in the introduction of new modified roller pump systems which incorporate a pump head able to accelerate in the systolic phase, thus truly generating pulsatile flow and pressure (Figs 7.9 and 7.10). Studies of these pump systems considering the development of *in vitro* flow and pressure against variable circuit compliance and resistance have indicated that pump output is truly pulsatile throughout and beyond the

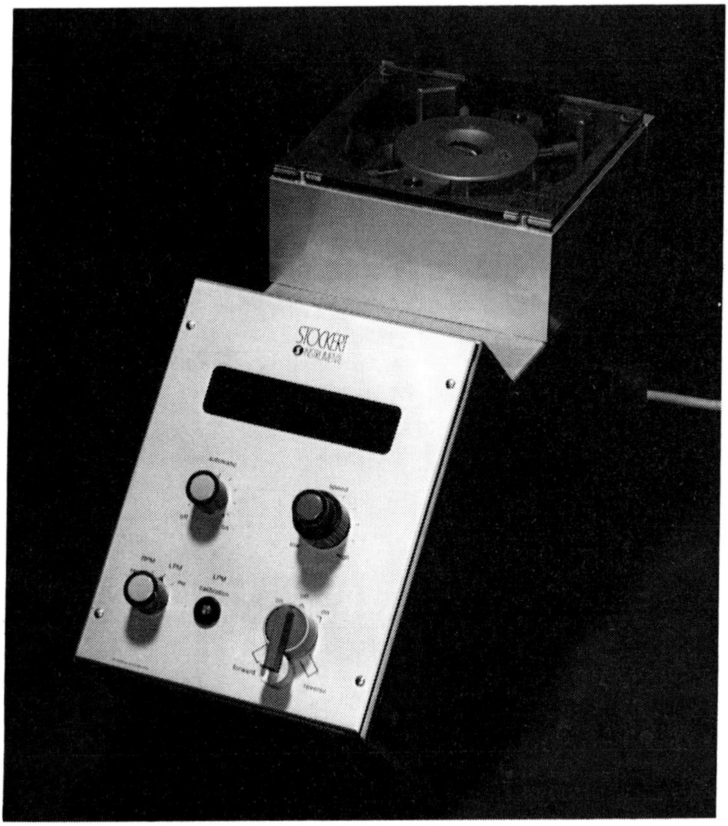

Fig. 7.9 The Stockert modified roller pump suitable for clinical pulsatile perfusion (a). The separate trigger module is shown (b) incorporating controls for internal triggering or ECG synchronized counterpulsation (*overleaf*).

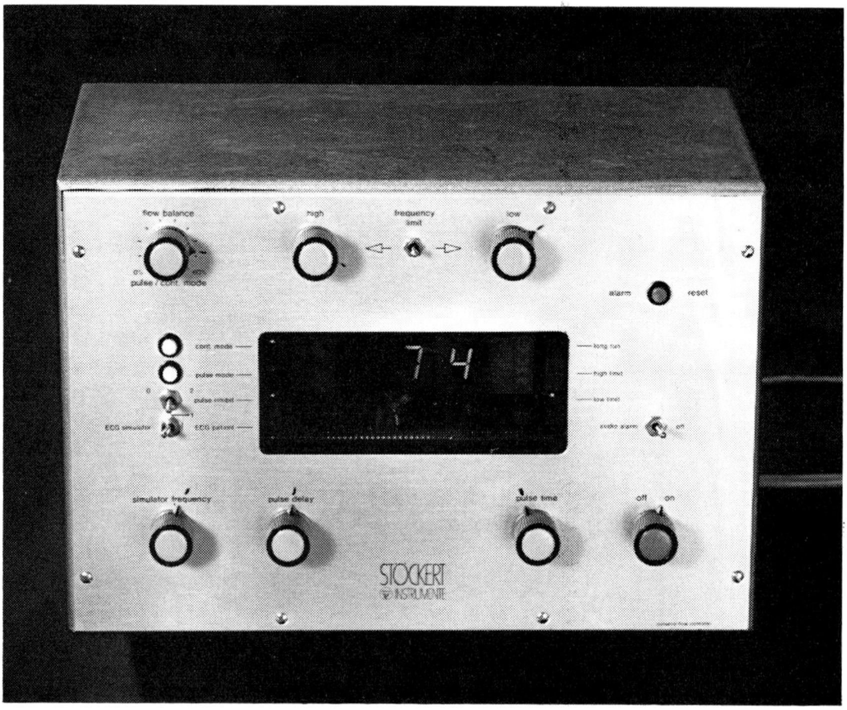

Fig. 7.9 *continued*

physiological range of these variables (Fig. 7.11). Modified roller pump systems are particularly attractive since the pump module effectively substitutes a pulsatile roller pump head for the conventional non-pulsatile head. Familiarity and belief in the safety and reliability of roller pumps make incorporation of these pulsatile systems easier than with systems involving greater degrees of complexity and possible unfamiliarity. Modified roller pump systems have the additional advantage in that they readily lend themselves to simple manual operation in case of electrical or mechanical break-down. This latter point is particularly relevant in relation to non-roller pulsatile pump systems which, depending on design characteristics, may be difficult if not impossible to operate manually in the event of break-down. Our experience in employing modified roller pump systems to produce pulsatile flow in excess of 3500 clinical cases has demonstrated our satisfaction with the safety, reliability and indeed simplicity of these particular systems. Furthermore, using a modified roller pump system to achieve pulsatile flow in general allows the individual surgeon and perfusion team to incorporate the pulsatile system into their existing circuitry and cannulae. Fears are sometimes expressed that very large bore aortic return cannulae will be required in order to achieve adequate pulsatile flow. This has not been the

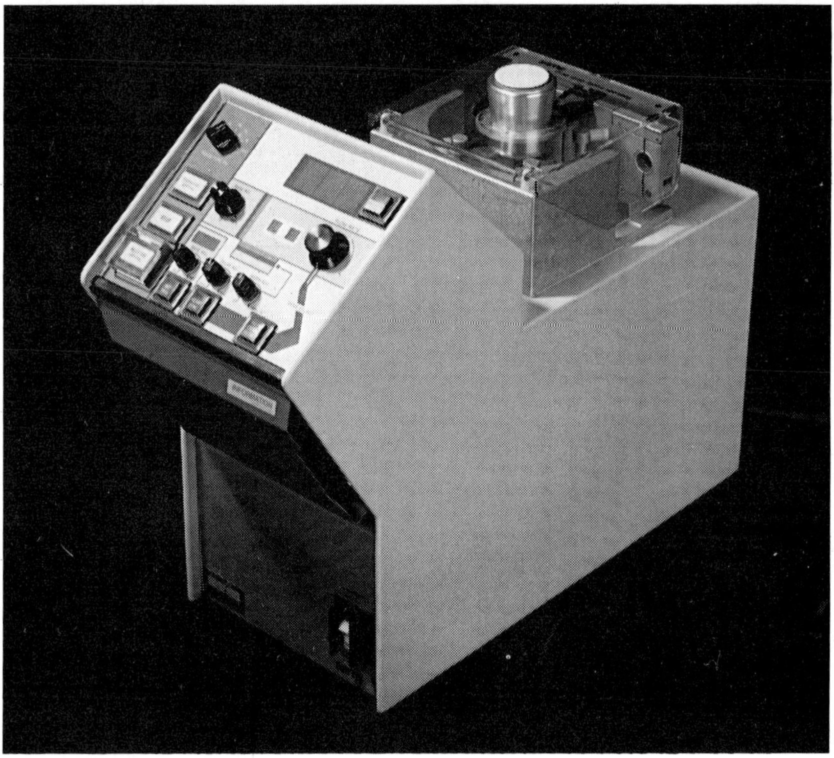

Fig. 7.10 The Sarns modified roller pump suitable for clinical pulsatile perfusion. All necessary controls are present on the pump face.

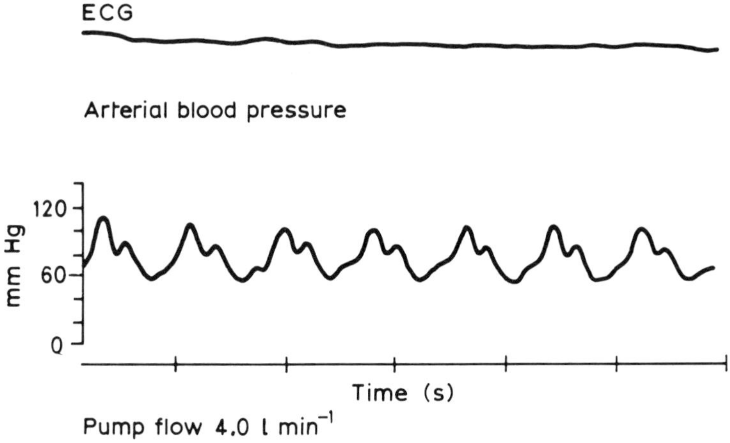

Fig. 7.11 Radial artery pressure trace from a patient during cardioplegic arrest with pulsatile perfusion produced by a Stockert modified roller pump system.

experience of our group or of other groups using these systems. The use of non-high-flow beak type aortic cannulae (8.0 mm diameter), or 20 to 22 gauge flexible aortic cannulae (Fig. 7.12) and indeed the use of femoral artery return for certain types of aneurysm surgery have all been associated with the achievement of good pulsatile flow wave patterns. With 8.0 mm arterial

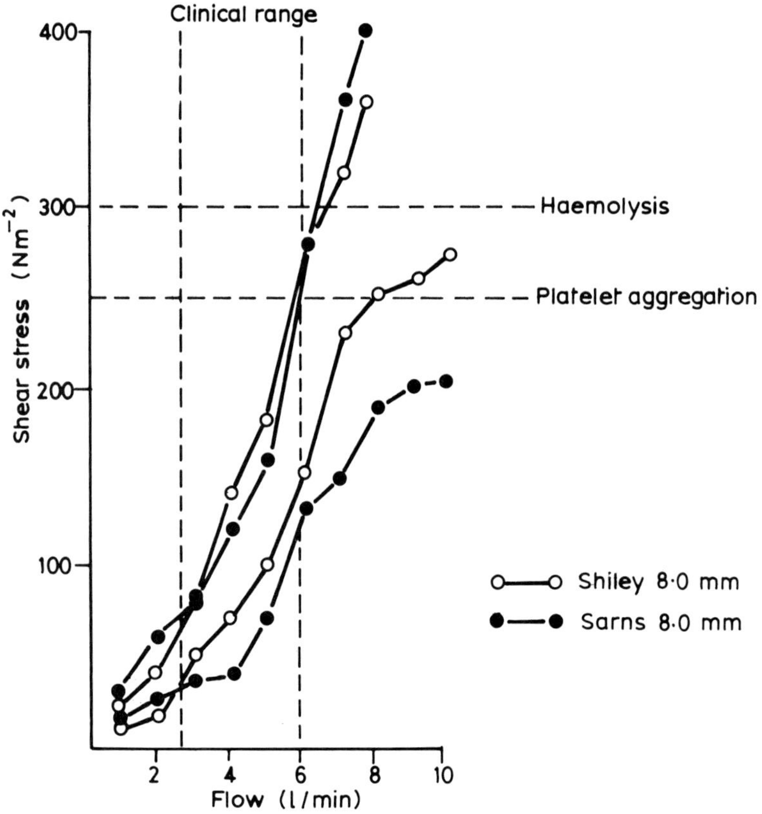

Fig. 7.12 Shear stress levels at incremental mean flow rates for two 8 mm arterial cannulae. Studies were carried out using pulsatile perfusion. Note that with pulsatile flow at a mean flow of four to five litres per minute, shear stress levels with both cannulae are acceptably low.

cannulae, the use of pulsatile flow is not associated with significant increase in haemolysis or excessive shear stress when compared with non-pulsatile flow (Gourlay and Taylor, 1984) Most modified roller pump systems presently available for clinical use comprise the modified roller pump itself and some form of electronic control module by which the amplitude, duration and frequency of pulse waves can be adjusted (Taylor *et al.*, 1978c). Most systems also incorporate in addition to the internal trigger for total cardiopulmonary bypass, a synchronization with the patient's ECG to allow a counter-pulsation facility (Fig. 7.13).

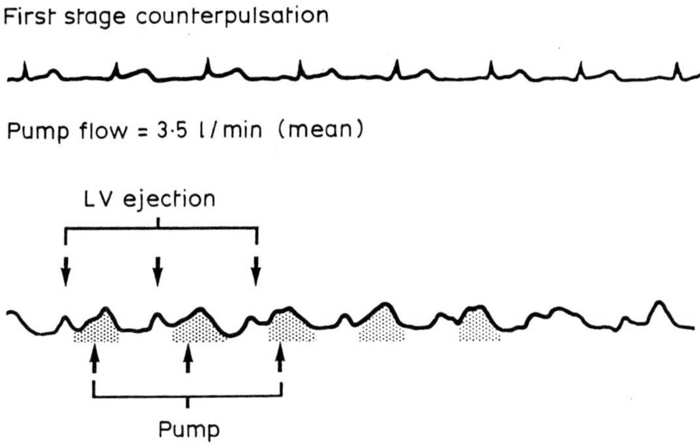

Fig. 7.13 Radial artery wave form in a patient during ECG synchronized counter-pulsation in the cardiac recovery period. Note the diastolic augmentation produced by synchronized timing of pump activity.

7.5.3 Intermittent occlusive systems–based on IABP principle

Intermittent occlusive systems based on the intra-aortic balloon pump principle have also been used extensively in clinical cardiac surgical practice (Bregman *et al.*, 1977; Maddoux *et al.*, 1976; Philbin *et al.*, 1979). The drive unit is connected, not to an intra-aortic balloon, but to an inflation/deflation chamber which is inserted into the arterial return line proximal to the aortic return cannula. The control module allows adjustable amplitude, duration and frequency of the pulsatile flow. It is obvious that these systems are inherently more invasive than modified roller pump systems in that the inflation/deflation chamber becomes an integral part of the arterial return line. Concern has been voiced in relation to these devices with regard to possible balloon leakage or rupture but those centres with considerable experience believe this to be a theoretical rather than a practical danger. The intermittent occlusive systems do however tend to be more complicated than modified roller pumps. Despite these features, experience with intermittent occlusive systems has undoubtedly proved their acceptability in producing pulsatile flow and pressure during routine cardiac surgical procedures. Clinical studies by Bregman's group have indicated that the use of balloon inflation-generated pulsatile flow has increased coronary flow and has improved renal function during cardiopulmonary bypass. Results have also indicated a reduction in the incidence of peri-operative myocardial infarction and in the need for postoperative intra-aortic balloon counterpulsation support. These results have been confirmed by Pappas' group in Denver also using a balloon pulsatile system (Maddoux *et al.*, 1976). It is of interest to note the essential similarity in the reported results of overall improvement in haemodynamics and reduction in haemodynamic related morbidity in those clinical studies of pulsatile perfusion using both modified roller pump systems and the modified intra-aortic balloon systems.

There are however possible negative factors related to the balloon inflation/deflation systems. In addition to the greater complexity previously mentioned, its use in synchronized counterpulsation in the cardiac recovery period after release of the aortic cross-clamp has been questioned. A recent study has indicated that although pulsatile flow generated by an inflation/deflation device increased mean coronary blood flow in the fibrillating heart, it was associated with overall decrease in mean coronary flow in the empty beating heart (Steed *et al.*, 1978). This effect was attributable to the occurrence of retrograde coronary flow during ventricular systole which was considered a possible effect of balloon deflation during ventricular systole exerting a suction effect on coronary blood flow. While it is clear that this report requires confirmation in order to substantiate coronary flow reversal in systole with balloon deflation systems, there may be no such problem present in modified roller pump systems which can be set to maintain a small but significant constant forward flow during ventricular systole and diastole. If systolic coronary flow reversal in the beating heart is confirmed in relation to the deflation phase of balloon systems, clearly this potential disadvantage does not apply to periods of total cardiopulmonary bypass. However, the ability of modified roller pump systems to maintain the small constant flow through the system throughout the pulsatile cycle may be considered a significant preferable feature to intermittent occlusive systems in this particular regard.

7.5.4 Recent developments in pulsatile perfusion pumps

The most recent literature on pulsatile perfusion is increasingly orientated towards reports from many groups using either modified roller pump systems or intermittent occlusive systems, both producing apparently acceptable physiological arterial flow and pressure. However, continued development of pulsatile pump systems is inevitable and indeed there are several systems currently under evaluation which may become available for clinical application in the near future. Some systems have reverted to pneumatic or hydraulic pumps which employ compression of distensible reservoirs (similar to a ventricle pumping principle) often employing an intervening diaphragm arrangement. This particular mode of producing pulsatile flow and pressure generates acceptable flow and pressure curves. These systems have however in the past proved to be unacceptably complex. It may be that future development will allow greater degrees of simplicity and reliability in these systems. Mechanical drive, moving-plate pulsatile systems have also been developed. These do not commend themselves at the present state of development because of inherent problems related to the change from pulsatile to non-pulsatile modes and to potential difficulties in manual maintenance of output in the case of mechanical break-down.

Continuing bioengineering studies centre on the important aspect of the nature of the pulsatile waveform produced by available and developing pulsatile systems. The author is of the opinion that an exact replica of the body's aortic flow and pressure waveforms does not require to be duplicated precisely by a pulsatile pump system. However, it is clear that certain features of pulsatile flow and pressure must be present in order for the flow generated by that system to be pulsatile in the physiological sense. The body would appear to be fairly tolerant in its definition of physiologically acceptable pulsatile flow, although it seems likely that the rate of rise in the flow and/or pressure curve in the aorta and possibly the total amplitude of pulsation, may be of importance in the determination of what constitutes physiologically acceptable pulsatile flow.

At the present time however there are commercially available pulsatile pump systems capable of producing physiologically acceptable pulsatile flow and pressure without significantly compromising reliability or safety in the cardiopulmonary bypass circuit. In this regard, anaesthetic techniques must not produce excessive vasodilatation with significantly subnormal peripheral vascular resistance levels. Maintenance of normal PVRI levels (around 20 to 25 index units) will allow excellent flow and pressure wave forms to be achieved routinely with modern pulsatile pump systems. The often varied complaint that teams have been unable to produce acceptable pulsatile perfusion with the new systems is almost always due to anaesthetic techniques which produce excessively vasodilated patients. Modern pulsatile pumps will *always* produce clinical pulsatile perfusion if peripheral vascular resistance is kept around normal levels.

7.6 HAEMATOLOGICAL EFFECTS OF PULSATILE PERFUSION

There is no doubt that certain of the pulsatile systems used in early experimental studies were associated with a high index of haemolysis. The actual contribution of the generation of pulsatile flow towards the total haemolysis index is, however, impossible to ascertain. It is increasingly acknowledged that the principal source of haemolysis in modern extracorporeal circulation originates in the high flow suction lines with air–blood interface trauma (see Chapter 15). Haematological studies recently reported in association with the use of modified roller pump systems have shown consistently that the use of pulsatile perfusion has not been associated with any significant increase in haemolysis or in blood cell depletion (Taylor, 1981a). In general, no group has reported plasma free haemoglobin levels at the end of clinical pulsatile perfusions in excess of 70 mg 100 ml^{-1}. Studies of depletion of white blood cells and platelets have also shown no significant difference between pulsatile and non-pulsatile perfusions. In a large clinical study of around 1000 clinical pulsatile perfusions we have failed to demonstrate any increase in requirement for homologous blood transfusion nor in the incidence of reopening for excessive haemorrhage in the postoperative period (Taylor, 1981b). Similar results in terms of haemolysis figures with pulsatile systems have been shown with some of the pneumatic and hydraulic ventricle pump systems, and although a report has demonstrated an increase in haemolysis with an intermittent occlusive system (Zumbro *et al.*, 1978), this finding has not been substantiated by other workers.

7.6.1 Arterial filters and pulsatile perfusion

The use of small-pore blood filters in association with pulsatile cardiopulmonary bypass has been studied by the author's group. Our previously expressed preference for arterial line 40 μm screen filtration allowed us to evaluate the effects of pulsatile as opposed to non-pulsatile flow on filter gradient and the incidence of filter blockage (Fig. 7.14). The design characteristics of the 40 μm screen filter with a large filter surface area and a small inherent gradient across the filter medium and housing were confirmed in studies which demonstrated that even at the peak of pulsatile flow, the gradient across the filter did not rise above 30 mmHg (4 kPa). Furthermore, the filter did not modify the pulsatile quality of flow and pressure transmitted to the patient. Filter blockage has not occurred with the 40 μm screen filter in our clinical experience. A comparative study of 20 μm screen filtration in the arterial return line did, however, produce higher levels of haemolysis with plasma free haemoglobin levels in some cases in excess of 100 mg 100 ml^{-1}. We have not studied the use of pure depth filters in the arterial return line in association with pulsatile flow in clinical practice, though *in vitro* studies confirm our belief that 40 μm screen filtration is optimal for pulsatile perfusion. (Gourlay *et al.*, 1984) (Fig. 7.15).

7.6.2 Clinical results with pulsatile perfusion

The ultimate argument for the use of pulsatile perfusion in clinical practice relates to a demonstrable improvement in morbidity and even in mortality. There are at present few comprehensive clinical studies. Indeed, the present

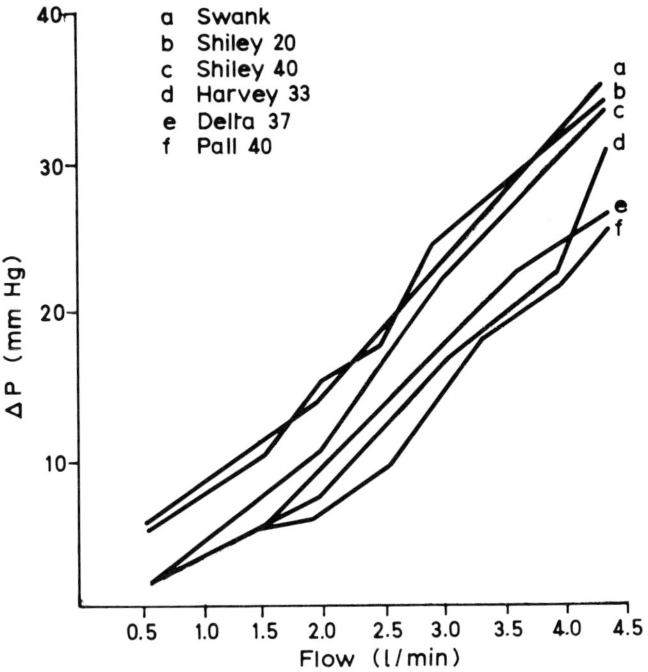

Fig. 7.14 Pressure drop across a range of arterial line filters with incremental pulsatile flow. Note that the highest levels of pressure drop are associated with the depth filter (Swank) and the 20 μm screen filter (Shiley 20).

low mortality with conventional techniques, particularly if the majority of the surgery is for elective coronary artery graft procedures, makes such studies difficult if not impossible to construct in such a way as to demonstrate significant improvement in mortality statistics. There is, however, a clear consensus in the literature in terms of improvement in haemodynamic morbidity. Previous studies have reported an improvement in left ventricular performance, a reduced incidence of peri-operative myocardial infarction, and a reduced requirement for postoperative intra-aortic balloon and inotropic drug support following the use of pulsatile bypass.

In our experience with routine pulsatile perfusion in over 3500 cases, of whom around 50% were valve replacement procedures, significant improvement in mortality with pulsatile perfusion has been demonstrated in two separate studies carried out in 1977–78, and 1978–80 respectively. Detailed consideration of those patients dying in pulsatile and non-pulsatile groups indicated a significantly higher occurrence of on-table deaths and low-output related deaths within the first 24 hours of surgery, in patients perfused with conventional non-pulsatile perfusion (Table 7.1). In addition, a consistent

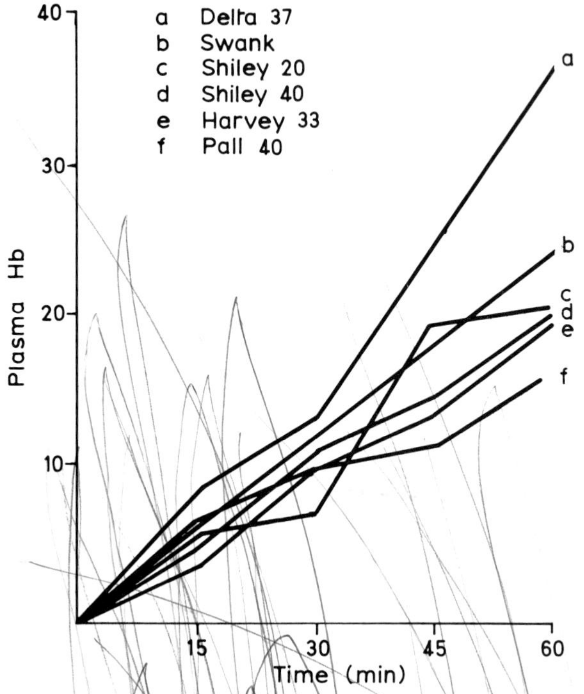

Fig. 7.15 Haemolysis associated with a range of arterial line filters during *in vitro* pulsatile perfusion. Note that haemolysis is low with the most commonly used arterial line filters although the range is considerable between the best (Pall 40 μm screen) and the worst (Delta 37 μm screen).

finding in our clinical studies has been the reduced requirement for intra-aortic balloon counterpulsation support in the post-bypass period. Overall mortality figures and a break-down of mortality figures between elective, urgent and emergency cases, indicates that for all categories, pulsatile perfusion is associated with a consistently lower mortality rate (Taylor *et al.*, 1979b). These results are in keeping with the experimental studies related to the effect of pulsatile perfusion in maintaining lower levels of peripheral vascular resistance, thus avoiding excessive increases in left ventricular work in the immediate post-perfusion period.

Considerable interest in the use of routine pulsatile perfusion has also been seen in relation to improvement in core cooling and rewarming in both adult and paediatric cardiac surgical practice (Williams *et al.*, 1979). Early reports are encouraging but further information is clearly required.

The present interest in cerebral function and cerebral damage during open-heart surgery has also focused attention on the possible benefits of pulsatile perfusion in this particular regard. In addition to the experimental studies of brain function previously described, clinical reports of improved cerebral function and increased requirement for anaesthetic agents during pulsatile bypass appear consistent with the view that pulsatile perfusion exerts a cerebral protective effect during cardiopulmonary bypass. Recent reports also advocate routine use of pulsatile perfusion in patients suffering from renal insufficiency. It is to be hoped that with the increasing adoption of pulsatile perfusion as the routine mode of perfusion during open-heart procedures, many of these questions and uncertainties regarding clinical experience and benefits will be resolved.

It is of interest that in this phase of development in cardiac surgical practice (one of refinement of existing techniques in an attempt to reduce morbidity) one of the principal areas of study has been the reawakening of interest in the use of pulsatile perfusion during open-heart surgical procedures (Taylor, 1984).

The argument for the adoption of pulsatile perfusion as routine rests on a sound physiological basis and is well supported by the results of numerous haemodynamic and metabolic studies carried out over many decades. A previous technological obstacle to developing pulsatile pump systems of acceptable reliability and simplicity has now, with technological advance, largely been overcome and there are presently available to the cardiac surgical and perfusion teams systems which will produce acceptable pulsatile flow and pressure without compromising the safety or reliability of the cardiopulmonary bypass circuit. The results of early clinical studies are encouraging and indicate, at the very least, that such systems may be employed as the routine mode of perfusion during open-heart procedures without compromising safety or reliability and without any significant increases in haemolysis or blood cell and platelet depletion. Indeed, those centres which have gained considerable experience in using pulsatile perfusion routinely have reported significant improvements in haemodynamic morbidity and mortality entirely in keeping with the results of experimental studies into the haemodynamic effects of pulsatile perfusion.

The author believes that the shift towards adopting routine pulsatile perfusion in open-heart surgical practice will continue and that it will prove a major contributory factor to the overall safety of cardiac surgical procedures.

REFERENCES

Aberg, T. (1974) Effect of open-heart surgery on intellectual function. *Scand. J. Thorac. Cardiovasc. Surg.*, Suppl. 15.

Angell-James, J. E. and de Burgh Daly, M. (1971) Effects of graded pulsatile pressure on the reflex vasomotor responses elicited by changes of mean pressure in the perfused carotid sinus-aortic arch regions of the dog. *J. Physiol.*, **214**, 51.

Bregman, D., Bowman, F. O., Parodi, E. N., Haubert, S. M., Edie, R. N., Spotnitz,

H. M., Reetsma, K. and Malm, J. R. (1977) An improved method of myocardial protection with pulsation during cardiopulmonary bypass. *Circulation* (*Suppl.* 11), **56**, 157.

Burton, A. C. (1954) Relation of structure to function of the tissues of the wall of blood vessels. *Physiol. Rev.*, **34**, 618.

De Paepe, J., Pomerantzeff, P. M. A., Nakiri, K., Armelin, E., Verginelli, G. and Zerbini, E. J. (1979) Observation of the microcirculation of the cerebral cortex of dogs subjected to pulsatile and non-pulsatile flow during extracorporeal circulation. In *A Propos du Debit Pulse*, Cobe Laboratories Inc, Belgium.

Dunn, J., Kirsh, M. M., Harness, J., Carroll, M., Straker, J. and Sloan, H. (1974) Haemodynamic, metabolic and haematologic effects of pulsatile cardiopulmonary bypass. *J. Thorac. Cardiovasc. Surg.*, **68**, 138.

Estafanous, F. G., Tarazi, R. C., Viljoen, J. F. and El Tawil, M. Y. (1973) Systemic hypertension following myocardial revascularisation. *Am. Heart. J.*, **85**, 732.

Feiner, H. (1976) Pancreatitis after cardiac surgery. *Am. J. Surg.*, **131**, 684.

Gourlay, T. and Taylor, K. M. (1984) In vitro evaluation of flow, haemolysis and shear stress in aortic cannulae. Unpublished data.

Gourlay, T., Becket, J. and Taylor, K. M. (1984) Arterial line filters. *Proc. C.E.C.E.C.* Paris.

Hill, J. D., Aguilar, K. J., Baranco, A., de Lanerolle, P. and Gerbode, F. (1969) Neuropathological manifestations of cardiac surgery. *Ann. Thorac. Surg.*, **7**, 409.

Jacobs, L. A., Klopp, E. H., Seamone, W., Topaz, S. R. and Gott, V. L. (1969) Improved organ function during cardiac bypass with a roller pump modified to deliver pulsatile flow. *J. Thorac. Cardiovasc. Surg.*, **58**, 703.

Kohlstaedt, K. G. and Page, I. H. (1940) The liberation of renin by perfusion of kidneys following reduction of pulse pressure. *J. Exp. Med.*, **72**, 201.

Maddoux, G., Pappas, G., Jenkins, M., Battock, D., Trow, R., Smith, S. C. and Steele, P. (1976) Effect of pulsatile and non-pulsatile flow during cardiopulmonary bypass on left ventricular ejection fraction early after aortocoronary bypass surgery. *Am. J. Cardiol.*, **37**, 1000.

Mandelbaum, I. and Burns, W. H. (1965) Pulsatile and non-pulsatile blood flow. *J. Am. Med. Assoc.*, **191**, 657.

Many, M., Soroff, H. S., Birtwell, W. C., Giron, F., Wise, H. and Deterling, R. A. (1967) The physiologic role of pulsatile and non-pulsatile blood flow: II Effects on renal function. *Arch. Surg.*, **95**, 762.

Mathie, R., Desai, J. and Taylor, K. M. (1984) Hepatic blood flow and metabolism during pulsatile and non-pulsatile cardiopulmonary bypass *Life Support Systems*. **2**, 303–5.

Mavroudis, C. (1978) To pulse or not to pulse. *Ann. Thorac. Surg.*, **25**, 259–71.

Murray, W. R., Mittra, S., Mittra, D., Roberts, L. B. and Taylor, K. M. (1982) The amylase creatinine clearance ratio following cardiopulmonary bypass. *J. Thorac. Cardiovasc. Surg.*, **82**, 248–53.

Parsons, R. J. and McMaster, P. D. (1938) The effect of the pulse upon the formation and flow of lymph. *J. Exp. Med.*, **68**, 353.

Philbin, D. M., Levine, F. H., Emerson, C. W., Coggins, C. H., Buckley, M. J. and Austin, W. G. (1979) Plasma vasopressin levels and urinary flow during cardiopulmonary bypass. *J. Thorac. Cardiovasc. Surg.*, **78**, 779.

Shepard, R. B. and Kirklin, J. W. (1969) Relation of pulsatile flow to oxygen consumption and other variables during cardiopulmonary bypass. *J. Thorac. Cardiovasc. Surg.*, **58**, 694.

Shepard, R. B., Simpson, D. C. and Sharp, J. (1966) Energy equivalent pressure. *Arch. Surg.*, **93**, 730.

Simpson, J. C. (1981) Cerebral perfusion during cardiac surgery using cardiac bypass. In *Towards Safer Cardiac Surgery* (ed. D. Longmore), MTP, Lancaster.

Sonnenblick, E. H. and Downing, S. E. (1963) Afterload as a primary determinant of ventricular performance. *Am. J. Physiol.*, **204**, 604.

Steed, D. L., Follette, D. M., Foglia, R., Maloney, J. V. and Buckberg, G. D. (1978) Effects of pulsatile assistance and non-pulsatile flow on subendocardial perfusion during cardiopulmonary bypass. *Ann. Thorac. Surg.*, **26**, 133.

Stinson, E. B., Holloway, E. L., Derby, G. C., Copeland, J. G., Oyer, P. E., Beuhler, D. L. and Griepp, R. B. (1977) Control of myocardial performance early after open-heart operations by vasodilator treatment. *J. Thorac. Cardiovasc. Surg.*, **73**, 523.

Takeda, J. (1960) Experimental study of peripheral circulation during extracorporeal circulation with a special reference to a comparison of pulsatile flow with non-pulsatile flow. *Arch. Jpn. Chir.*, **29**, 1407.

Taylor, K. M. (1981a) Pulsatile cardiopulmonary bypass. A review. *J. Cardiovasc. Surg.*, **22**, 561–8.

Taylor, K. M. (1981b) Why pulsatile flow during cardiopulmonary bypass? In *Towards Safer Cardiac Surgery* (ed. D. B. Longmore), MTP, Lancaster, pp. 481–500.

Taylor, K. M. (1984) The present status of pulsatile perfusion. *Current Med. Lit.-Cardiovasc. Med.*, **3**, 66.

Taylor, K. M., Bain, W. H., Davidson, K. G., Turner, M. A., Mittra, S. and Russell, M. (1979b) A comparative study of pulsatile and non-pulsatile cardiopulmonary bypass in 325 patients. *Proc. Eur. Soc. Artif. Org.*, **VI**, 238.

Taylor, K. M., Bain, W. H., Maxted, K. J., Hutton, M. H., McNab, W. Y. and Caves, P. K. (1978c) Comparative studies of pulsatile and non-pulsatile flow during cardiopulmonary bypass. I. Pulsatile system employed and its haematological effects. *J. Thorac. Cardiovasc. Surg.*, **75**, 569.

Taylor, K. M., Bain, W. H. and Morton, J. J. (1980a) The role of angiotensin II in the development of peripheral vasoconstriction during open-heart surgery. *Am. Heart J.*, **100**, 935–7.

Taylor, K. M., Casals, J., Morton, J. J., Mittra, S., Brannan, J. J. and Bain, W. H. (1979a) The haemodynamic effects of angiotensin blockade after cardiopulmonary bypass. *Br. Heart J.*, **41**, 380.

Taylor, K. M., Devlin, B. J., Mittra, S. M., Gillan, J. G., Brannan, J. J. and McKenna, J. M. (1980b) Assessment of cerebral damage during open-heart surgery. A new experimental model. *Scand. J. Thorac. Cardiovasc. Surg.*, **14**, 197–203.

Taylor, K. M., Jones, J. V., Walker, M. S., Rao, L. G. S. and Bain, W. H. (1976) The cortisol response during open-heart surgery. *Circulation*, **54**, 20.

Taylor, K. M., Morton, J. J., Brown, J. J., Bain, W. H. and Caves, P. K. (1977) Hypertension and the renin–angiotensin system following open-heart surgery. *J. Thorac. Cardiovasc. Surg.*, **74**, 840.

Taylor, K. M., Wright, G. S., Bain, W. H., Caves, P. K. and Beastall, G. H. (1978b) Comparative studies of pulsatile and non-pulsatile flow during cardiopulmonary bypass. III Anterior pituitary response to thyrotrophin-releasing hormone. *J. Thorac. Cardiovasc. Surg.*, **75**, 579.

Taylor, K. M., Wright, G. S., Reid, J. S., Bain, W. H., Caves, P. K., Walker, M. S. and Grant, J. K. (1978a) Comparative studies of pulsatile and non-pulsatile flow during cardiopulmonary bypass. II The effects on adrenal secretion of cortisol. *J. Thorac. Cardiovasc. Surg.*, **75**, 574.

Wilcox, B. R., Coulter, N. A., Peters, R. M. and Stacey, R. W. (1967) Power dissipation in the systemic and pulmonary vasculature of dogs. *Surgery*, **62**, 25.

Williams, G. Doyne, Seifen, A. B., Lawson, N. W., Norton, J. B., Readinger, R. I., Dungan, T. W. and Callaway, J. K. (1979) Pulsatile perfusion versus conventional high-flow nonpulsatile perfusion for rapid core cooling and rewarming of infants for circulatory arrest in cardiac operation. *J. Thorac. Cardiovasc. Surg.*, **78**, 667–77.

Wright, G. and Sanderson, J. M. (1972) Brain damage and mortality in dogs following pulsatile and non-pulsatile blood flows in extracorporeal circulation. *Thorax*, **27**, 738.

Zumbro, G. L., Shearer, G., Fishback, M. E. and Galloway, R. F. (1978) A prospective evaluation of the pulsatile assist device. *Ann. Thorac. Surg.*, **28**, 269.

8
Perfusion techniques for paediatric cardiac surgery

M. DE LEVAL

Perfusion techniques in paediatric cardiac surgery differ in several respects from standard techniques used for adults. Not all of the differences are related to the size of the patients to be operated on. Some relate to the complex nature of the anatomical abnormalities in the heart and some to the pathophysiology in young children with congenital heart disease. In this chapter, present techniques of cardiopulmonary bypass for cardiac surgery in infants and small children will be described.

Many units like ours employ extracorporeal circuits with either a bubble oxygenator or a membrane oxygenator, depending on the particular case. The use of membrane oxygenation with the potential reduction of blood trauma and the reduced priming volume make membrane oxygenators attractive in paediatric cardiac surgical practice. Some of the advantages of membrane oxygenation however may be lost in cases where excessive cardiotomy suction is required, due to the underlying anatomical nature of the defect.

For both bubble oxygenator and membrane oxygenator circuits, a shunt line is incorporated to allow recirculation during circulatory arrest and mixing of drugs administered. The pumps are set to respond to a line pressure in excess of 200 mmHg (26.7 kPa) at which point the occlusion will fail. Both circuits have a microfilter incorporated into the large capacity cardiotomy reservoir. Arterial line filters are not used routinely. Examples of the bubble oxygenator and membrane oxygenator circuits are shown in Figs 8.1 and 8.2.

8.1 PERFUSATE COMPOSITION

Moderate haemodilution to a haematocrit of around 30% is used routinely for all paediatric patients. It is important to base the calculation of perfusate composition on the patient's pre-operative haematocrit, calculated blood volume and the priming volume of the extracorporeal circuit. The haematocrit is measured routinely every 30 minutes during the period of

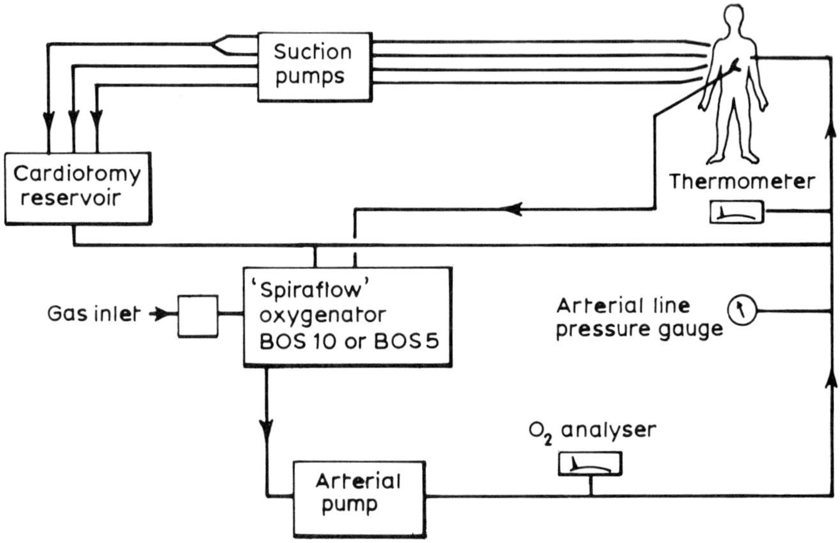

Fig. 8.1 Bubble oxygenator circuit.

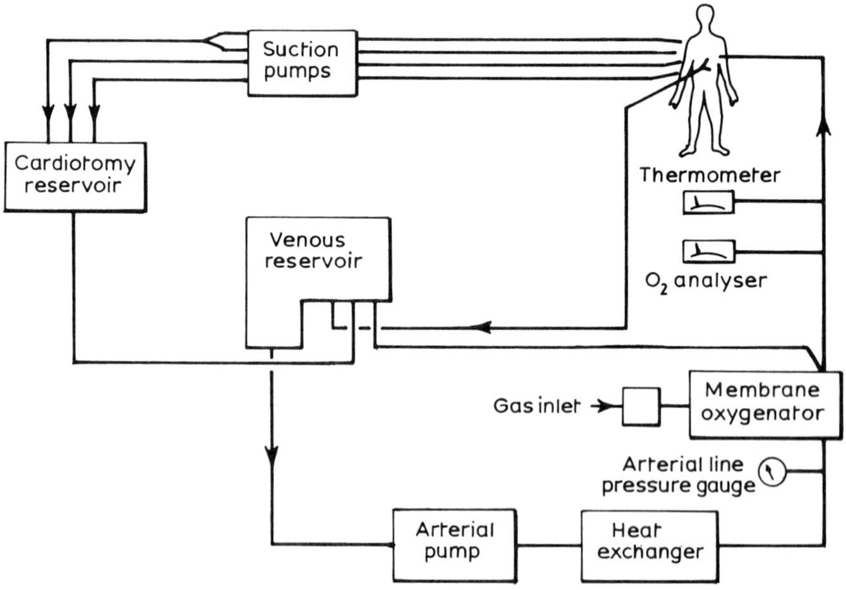

Fig. 8.2 Membrane oxygenator circuit.

cardiopulmonary bypass. The blood component of the perfusate is citrate phospate dextrose (CPD) drawn less than 48–72 hours before operation for neonatal cases, and no more than 5 days for older children. The CPD blood is heparinized by adding 25 mg of heparin to each unit of blood. This mixture is recalcified with 3 ml of 20% calcium chloride solution. The blood is diluted with Hartmann's solution, heparinized at 15 mg heparin per 500 ml of Hartmann's. The pH of the perfusate is adjusted by adding 8 mmol sodium bicarbonate for each unit of blood or Hartmann's solution.

Moderate haemodilution is particularly valuable in improving blood flow during hypothermia. However the greater increase in interstitial fluid (Pacifico *et al.*, 1970; Cohn *et al.*, 1971) is potentially an even greater problem in neonates (Mavroudis and Ebert, 1978). The addition of colloid to the perfusate is presently being studied, adding 100 ml salt-poor human albumin and 2.5 ml of 20% mannitol to the perfusate in infants.

8.2 CANNULATION TECHNIQUES FOR PAEDIATRIC CARDIAC SURGERY

Details of tubing diameters and cannulae size for paediatric cases are outlined in Tables 8.1 and 8.2.

Table 8.1 Choice of tubing diameters for various calculated pump flows (calculated as $2.4\,l\,m^{-2}\,min^{-1}$)

	Diameter (in)	*Calculated flow (ml min^{-1})*
Arterial line	0.25	0–1000
	0.375	>1000
Venous line	0.25	0–600
	0.375	600–3000
	0.5	>3000
Pump race line	0.25	0–600
	0.375	600–1500
	0.5	>1500

Table 8.2 Examples of arterial and venous cannulae size for various body surface areas (m^2) and calculated flow rates (calculated as $2.4\,l\,m^{-2}\,min^{-1}$)

BSA (m^2)	*Flow (ml min^{-1})*	*Arterial cannula (mm)*	*Venous cannula (mm)*
0.1	240	2.0	4.0
0.3	720	2.0	4.0
0.5	1200	2.0	4.0
0.7	1680	3.0	5.0
0.9	2160	3.5	6.0
1.0	2400	4.0	6.0
1.5	3600	4.5	6.0
1.6	3840	5.0	7.0

8.2.1 Arterial cannulation

Thin-walled, high-flow cannulae are used for arterial cannulation. The size of the cannula is selected so that the pressure gradient is less than 100 mmHg (13.3 kPa) at the highest anticipated flow rate. At present we use right-angled stainless-steel cannulae inserted into the ascending aorta within two concentric purse string sutures.

Femoral or iliac artery cannulation is required when the underlying condition leaves inadequate room for aortic cannulation. Such situations include aneurysm of the ascending aorta, or closure of a Pott's anastomosis when retrograde perfusion facilitates air evacuation from the aortic arch. Retrograde perfusion from the femoral or iliac arteries is also indicated when cooling is desirable before the sternal incision is made, for example in aneurysm or pseudoaneurysm of the right ventricle. Our preference is to use the external iliac artery, exposed extraperitoneally through a short transverse incision medial to the anterior superior iliac crest.

8.2.2 Venous cannulation

Most paediatric cardiac surgical procedures involving cardiopulmonary bypass require bicaval cannulation. Where intra-atrial rearrangement of the venous return is to be undertaken, for example a Mustard or Senning repair, and for the Fontan procedure, the superior and inferior cavae are cannulated directly.

When circulatory arrest and deep hypothermia are used, core cooling and rewarming is carried out using a single atrial cannula placed in the right atrium through the atrial appendage. In cases with anomalous systemic venous return, direct cannulation of the anomalous veins can be carried out with the patient on partial cardiopulmonary bypass. In small infants, or where the anomalies of systemic venous return are complex, deep hypothermia and circulatory arrest with a single cannula into the right atrium is often preferred.

When performing the Senning operation, the right atrial cannula is transferred to the left atrium once the superior and inferior caval pathways are constructed. The operation can then be carried out on conventional cardiopulmonary bypass.

8.2.3 Intracardiac suction

Our practice is to use four suction lines as routine. These are:

(1) Inserted into the left atrium or left ventricle after the onset of cardiopulmonary bypass to provide cardiac decompression. This vent is not

necessary in relatively short procedures when the left heart is not emptied of blood.

(2) Suction line connected to the aortic needle utilized to infuse the cardioplegic solution. We use 1 mm bore needles for infants, and 2 mm bore for older children.
(3) Suction line connected to a sump sucker.
(4) Suction line connected to a hand-held sucker, for aspirating blood from the operating field.

Control of suction on all four suction lines is important and a well-controlled occlusive pump is employed fitted with a pressure release valve limiting the negative pressure. Only blood from the cardiac chambers is returned to the extracorporeal circuit. Blood spilled into the pericardial sack is discarded.

8.3 ASPECTS OF PERFUSION PRACTICE IN PAEDIATRIC CARDIAC SURGERY

The first point of importance is that large systemic to pulmonary artery anastomoses must be dissected before cardiopulmonary bypass begins, and should be closed before cooling at the onset of bypass to avoid distension of the heart and over-perfusion of the lungs. Other important points specific to paediatric practice are that even a small patent ductus arteriosus must be closed if the operation involves a period of circulatory arrest. If the ductus is not closed there is a risk of cerebral air embolism when the heart is open. For aortopulmonary window repair and repair of persistent truncus arteriosus, the pulmonary arteries must be occluded during perfusion to avoid flooding of the lungs and distension of the heart.

Most intracardiac repairs in paediatric cardiac surgical practice are performed with moderate to profound hypothermia, that is less than 25°C perfusate temperature. The exceptions to this rule are short procedures for which only mild to moderate hypothermia is used (25°C–>32°C).

Cooling is achieved by commencing perfusion with the perfusate temperature at 25°C. For some small infants, where surgery is performed under deep hypothermia and circulatory arrest, the nasopharyngeal temperature is lowered to 26–28°C by surface cooling before commencing the sternotomy. Surface cooling is achieved using ice bags placed on the lower chest and abdomen, axillae and groins, avoiding the precordial area and the extremities. For other patients, who are less sick and more haemodynamically stable, cooling is achieved by core cooling alone. All patients are laid on a water blanket which provides additional means of cooling and rewarming.

The use of moderate or profound hypothermia and total circulatory arrest allow improved operating conditions, particularly in cases of excessive blood return to the heart. In addition, low arterial flow rates reduce collateral coronary circulation and contribute to myocardial protection. During hypothermia, we accept periods of reduced flow rates or total circulatory arrest periods (Kirklin *et al.*, 1973). The suggested minimal safe arterial flows in hypothermia and the estimated safe duration times of total circulatory arrest are outlined in Tables 8.3 and 8.4.

Table 8.3 Suggested minimal safe arterial flow in hypothermia

Temperature (nasopharyngeal)	*Flow* ($l\ min^{-1}\ m^{-2}$)	*Safe duration (min)*
28°C	1.6	120
28°C	0.5	20
26°C	0.5	30
22°C	0.5	45

Table 8.4 Estimated safe duration of total circulatory arrest

Temperature (nasopharyngeal)	*Duration (min)*
28°C	20
26°C	30
22°C	45
19°C	60

During the rewarming phase, after the intracardiac repair has been completed, we maintain a gradient of no more than 12°C between the water bath and the arterial blood leaving the oxygenator. The perfusate temperature should not be raised above 39°C and the water temperature not above 42°C (Kirklin *et al.*, 1976). During cooling and rewarming periods, the caval tapes are left unsnared and central venous pressures maintained at around 4–5 mmHg (0.5–0.67 kPa) by adjusting the venous drainage and suction in the left vent. During these periods therefore the heart is allowed to eject and produce a pulsatile flow with improved peripheral organ perfusion (Mavroudis, 1978; Taylor, 1982). The provision of pulsatile flow during these periods has also been shown to provide more rapid and more uniform cooling and rewarming (Williams *et al.*, 1979). Subendocardial perfusion in the heart itself is also better maintained under conditions of pulsatile flow (Steed *et al.*, 1978).

During the period of cardiopulmonary bypass, ventilation is discontinued although a constant positive pressure of 5 cm H_2O is applied to the lungs to keep some degree of inflation and reduce pulmonary atelectasis.

8.4 MYOCARDIAL PROTECTION IN PAEDIATRIC CARDIAC SURGERY

We have used crystalloid cardioplegic myocardial protection since 1977 (Braimbridge *et al.*, 1974). The solution (see Table 8.5) is administered into the aortic root by a simple pressure bag infusion set. A myocardial thermistor probe is used for continuous recording of the myocardial temperature. Initial cardioplegic dose is approximately 30 ml kg^{-1} body weight, aiming to lower the myocardial temperature to below 10–12°C. Cardioplegic solution is reinfused if myocardial temperature reaches 20°C, or if electrical activity reappears after 30–40 minutes (Bull *et al.*, 1980). As has already been indicated, myocardial protection is undoubtedly improved by the combined use of profound core hypothermia and reduced pump flow during the period of cardiopulmonary bypass.

Table 8.5 St Thomas' cardioplegic solution No. 1

Chemical	*Ringer's solution (mmol)*	*Cardioplegic solution (mmol)*	*Final concentration* (*mmol* l^{-1})*
Calcium chloride	2.25	0	2.20
Potassium chloride	4.02	15.96	19.59
Sodium chloride	147.13	0	144.25
Magnesium chloride	0	15.99	15.968
Procaine hydrochloride	0	1	0.98
Distilled water	1000 ml	20 ml	1020 ml

* Concentration corrected for fluid volume of 1020 ml
Osmolarity = approximately 300 mmol/kg H_2O

8.5 REMOVAL OF SURGICAL AIR

In addition to conventional techniques to remove surgical air which are employed in both paediatric and adult cardiac surgical practice, specific care must be taken in particular cases because of the anatomical configuration of the heart and great arteries. After intra-atrial repair for transposition with a Mustard or Senning procedure, specific precautions are required because the anterior ventricle (right) is the systemic ventricle. When the aorta is unclamped, a 15 or 18 gauge needle is inserted into the most anterior part of the right ventricle, and the aortic needle is connected to a suction line. If the pulmonary venous atrium is not closed when the aortic cross-clamp is released, a vent is introduced through the right atrial appendage, across the tricuspid valve into the right ventricle to make the systemic atrio-ventricular valve incompetent.

For intracardiac repairs performed in very small hearts using circulatory arrest, intracardiac vents may not be used. Removal of surgical air is then accomplished by placing the aortic needle vent on gentle suction when the aorta is unclamped, and when the ventricle begins to contract the heart is elevated and a needle introduced into the left ventricular apex, with the usual measures of obstructing the venous return line to fill the heart and manually inflating the lungs with positive pressure. In particularly small infants, the needle vent must not be too large since excessive suction on a large bore vent may be sufficient dangerously to reduce the perfusion pressure.

8.6 PRESSURE MONITORING DURING PAEDIATRIC CARDIAC SURGERY

A systemic arterial cannula and a central venous cannula are routinely inserted after induction of anaesthesia. A left atrial pressure monitoring line is routinely inserted at completion of the intracardiac repair, with the exception of simple cases, such as secundum atrial septal defect (ASD), pulmonary stenosis, or uncomplicated ventricular septal defect. The left atrial catheter is inserted through a purse string suture at the junction of the right upper pulmonary vein and the left atrium. In small infants, a similar catheter can be placed through the right atrial appendage purse string, the catheter being brought out to the right epigastrium.

8.7 HEPARIN DOSAGE AND REVERSAL IN PAEDIATRIC CARDIAC SURGERY

As with other units, we have found that more precise control of heparinization is possible using regular monitoring of the activated clotting times (ACT) (de Leval *et al.*, 1972). We are in agreement with Bull *et al.* (1975a,b) and aim for an activated clotting time of 480 s. Over the years we have found that heparin requirements during hypothermic cardiopulmonary bypass are less than those for normothermic perfusion. At present we determine the baseline ACT before bypass and administer an initial heparinizing dose of 3 mg per kg body weight. ACT determinations are repeated every 45 minutes during bypass, and incremental heparin given if required, to raise ACT to 480 s. Most patients require only the single initial dose of heparin. Protamine reversal is based on the ratio of 1.3–1.5 mg protamine to 1 mg circulating heparin. In practice, this appears often to be an underestimate of the protamine requirement, and increments of protamine are given to return the ACT to the pre-cardiopulmonary bypass level.

REFERENCES

Braimbridge, M., Chayen, J., Bitensky, L., Hearse, D., Jynge, P. and Cankovic-Darracott, S. (1974) Cold cardioplegia or continuous coronary perfusion? *J. Thorac. Cardiovasc. Surg.*, **74**, 900.

Bull, B., Korpman, R., Huse, W. and Briggs, B. (1975a) Heparin therapy during extracorporeal circulation. I. Problems inherent in existing heparin controls. *J. Thorac, Cardiovasc. Surg.*, **69**, 685.

Bull, B., Hase, W., Brauer, F. and Korpman, R. (1975b) Heparin therapy during extracorporeal circulation. II. The use of a dose response curve to individualize heparin and protamine dosage. *J. Thorac. Cardiovasc. Surg.*, **69**, 685.

Bull, C., Cooper, J. and Stark, J. (1980) Myocardial and biophysical assessment of myocardial protection in children. Proc. International Symposium *Cardioplegia – The First 100 Years*. Futura Publications, London, p. 200.

Cohn, L., Angell, W. and Shumway, N. (1971) Body fluid shifts after cardiopulmonary bypass. I. Effect of congestive heart failure and haemodilution. *J. Thorac. Cardiovasc. Surg.*, **62**, 423.

de Leval, M., Hill, D., Dontigny, L. and Gerbode, F. (1972) Contrôle de l'héparinisation continue par le temps de coagulation activé (ACT). *Ann. Chir. Thorac. Cardiovasc.*, **11**, 287.

Kirkwood, J. W., Pacifico, A., Hannah, H. III, and Allarde, R. (1973) Primary definitive intracardiac operations in infants. Intraoperative support techniques. In *Advances in Cardiovascular Surgery* (ed. J.W. Kirklin) Grune & Stratton, New York, London, p. 85.

Kirklin, J. W., Lell, W., Bexley, J. and Appelbaum, A. (1976) Cardiopulmonary bypass for cardiac surgery. In *Surgery of the Chest*, 3rd edn, W. B. Saunders, Philadelphia, Ch. 29.

Mavroudis, C. (1978) To pulse or not to pulse? *Ann. Thorac. Cardiovasc. Surg.*, **25**, 259.

Mavroudis, C. and Ebert, P. (1978) Hemodilution causes decreased compliance in puppies. *Circulation* (Suppl. 1), **58**, 155.

Pacifico, A., Digerness, S. and Kirklin, J. (1970) Acute alterations of body composition after open intracardiac operations. *Circulation*, **41**, 331.

Steed, D., Follette, D., Foglia, R., Maloney, J. and Buckberg, G. (1978) Effects of pulsatile assistance and non-pulsatile flow on subendocardial purfusion during cardiopulmonary bypass. *Ann. Thorac. Surg.*, **26**, 133.

Taylor, K.M. (1982) Why pulsatile flow? In *Towards Safer Cardiac Surgery* (ed. D. B. Longmore) MTP, Lancaster.

9
Counterpulsation techniques

DAVID BREGMAN and PETER KASKEL

Mechanical circulatory assist techniques, which either impart energy to the circulatory system or reduce the work load of the heart, have been developed by a multitude of investigators in the twentieth century. The principle which has most successfully underlined the vast majority of these techniques is counterpulsation, a term coined by Harken in 1958.

The origins of counterpulsation began with 'phase shift diastolic augmentation' originated by Kantrowitz and Kantrowitz in 1953. In 1958 Kantrowitz created an early analogue of balloon pumping by wrapping diaphragmatic muscle around the thoracic aorta, timed to contract in diastole, thereby retarding the arterial pulse (Kantrowitz and McKinnon, 1958).

It is the purpose of this chapter to describe the multitude of counter- and co-pulsation techniques, which have been derived and developed from this basic concept.

9.1 ARTERIO-ARTERIAL COUNTERPULSATION

The earliest form of counterpulsation was called arterio-arterial counterpulsation, described by Harken (1958). The procedure involved a mechanical system (Figs 9.1 and 9.2), which removed blood from the femoral artery during ventricular systole, and rapidly reinfused the same blood during diastole, to increase coronary perfusion pressure. By this method, in the normotensive preparation, one could decrease left ventricular work and increase coronary blood flow, thereby improving the balance between myocardial oxygen supply and oxygen demand. This concept was initially received with great enthusiasm and several investigators reported some success with its initial clinical application (Jacobey *et al.*, 1968; Rosensweig *et al.*, 1970; Jacobey, 1971). However, the method had three major drawbacks:

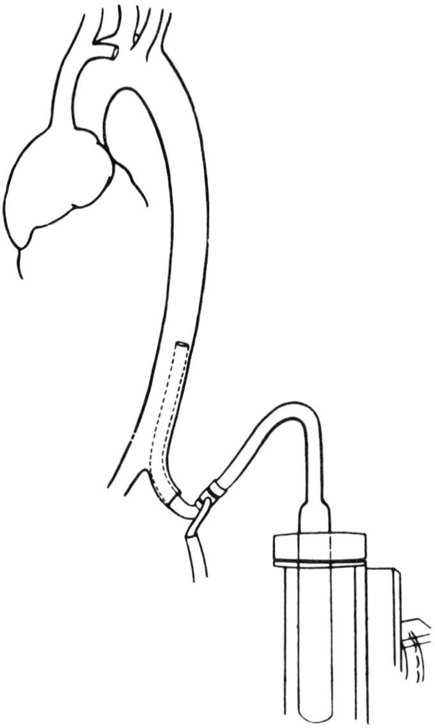

Fig. 9.1 Schematic representation of arterio-arterial counterpulsation to the circulation. (From Clauss *et al.* (1961) *J. Thorac. Cardiovasc. Surg.*, 4, 447. Used by permission.)

(1) Excessive turbulence was caused by the rapid withdrawal and reinfusion of blood through narrow cannulae caused appreciable haemolysis, and therefore limited the duration of clinical application of the procedure.
(2) The procedure required either bilateral femoral or iliac arteriotomies, so that enough blood could be withdrawn and reinfused during each cardiac cycle.
(3) It was shown by Dormandy *et al.* (1971) that in the hypotensive state counterpulsation by the femoral route produced no increase in coronary blood flow. It was only when the animal or the patient was made more normotensive with volume and/or pressor agents that, in fact, there was an increase in coronary blood flow, with peripheral arterio-arterial counterpulsation.

The procedure was also employed by Jacobey (1968, 1971) through the subclavian approach.

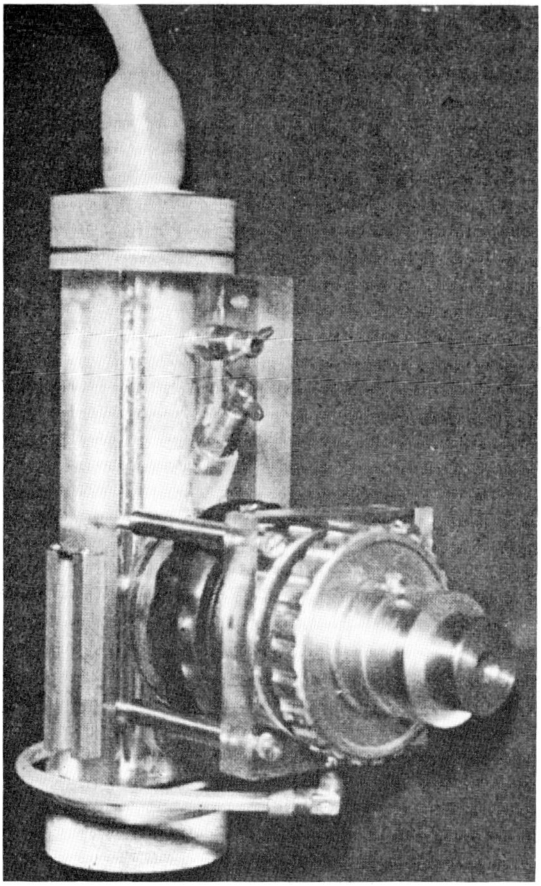

Fig. 9.2 The arterial counterpulsator device used by Harken and associates. (From Clauss *et al.* (1961) *J. Thorac. Cardiovasc. Surg.*, 4, 447. Used by permission.)

9.2 INTRA-AORTIC BALLOON PUMPING

In 1962 Moulopoulos *et al.* suggested the use of a single chambered intra-aortic balloon, positioned in the descending thoracic aorta, to accomplish the same haemodynamics as did arterial counterpulsation, but without its drawbacks. The balloon was inflated in diastole, beginning with closure of the aortic valve, and was held in inflation until the onset of ventricular systole, when the balloon was rapidly deflated. The inflation of the balloon displaced intra-aortic blood towards the coronary tree, thereby augmenting coronary perfusion and myocardial oxygen supply. The collapse of the balloon created a 'sink' which decreased the impedance to left ventricular ejection (i.e. decreased left ventricular afterload), and consequently reduced myocardial oxygen demand. The first clinical trial in man of intra-aortic balloon pumping was reported by Kantrowitz *et al.* (1968).

The main advantages of intra-aortic balloon pumping (IABP) over conventional arterio-arterial counterpulsation are:

(1) Assistance is possible for extended periods of time with IABP since there is minimal haemolysis.
(2) Only a single femoral arteriotomy is required.
(3) Coronary blood flow is augmented even in the hypotensive state.

There are two additional significant advantages of either arterio-arterial counterpulsation or intra-aortic balloon pumping:

(1) As demonstrated by Jacobey *et al.* (1963) after a short period of counterpulsation, dormant intercoronary collateral beds are opened, and these channels remain open after the procedure is terminated.
(2) Nachlas and Sieband (1967), Cox *et al.* (1968), Maroko *et al.* (1972) and Sugg *et al.* (1969) have shown that the early institution of intra-aortic balloon pumping minimizes the size of the resultant myocardial infarction after coronary occlusion.

Initially three types of surgically inserted intra-aortic balloons became available (Figs 9.3):
(1) a single chambered balloon; (2) a dual chambered balloon; and (3) a tri-segment single-chambered balloon. All of these balloon designs have now been replaced by a single-chambered percutaneous intra-aortic balloon.

9.2.1 The percutaneous intra-aortic balloon

In 1980 a method was described to modify the standard surgically inserted balloon and enable it to be inserted by the Seldinger technique into the arterial tree (Bregman *et al.*, 1980). The catheter section within the balloon membrane was replaced with a straight wire, enabling the balloon membrane to be wrapped around the wire and therefore passed through a sheath into the aorta (Figs 9.4 and 9.5). Several models of this balloon have now been developed. In its initial form the standard balloon (Percor) was wrapped manually. Subsequently the Percor DL balloon could be wrapped automatically. The Percor DL II balloon has the advantage that it may be passed over a guide wire or inserted directly through an arterial sheath. Arterial pressure may also be monitored through the balloon. Both balloons have an automatic wrapping mechanism. We have also learned that a longer 12 french dilator sheath is advantageous for insertion, and a standard 11 inch sheath is now

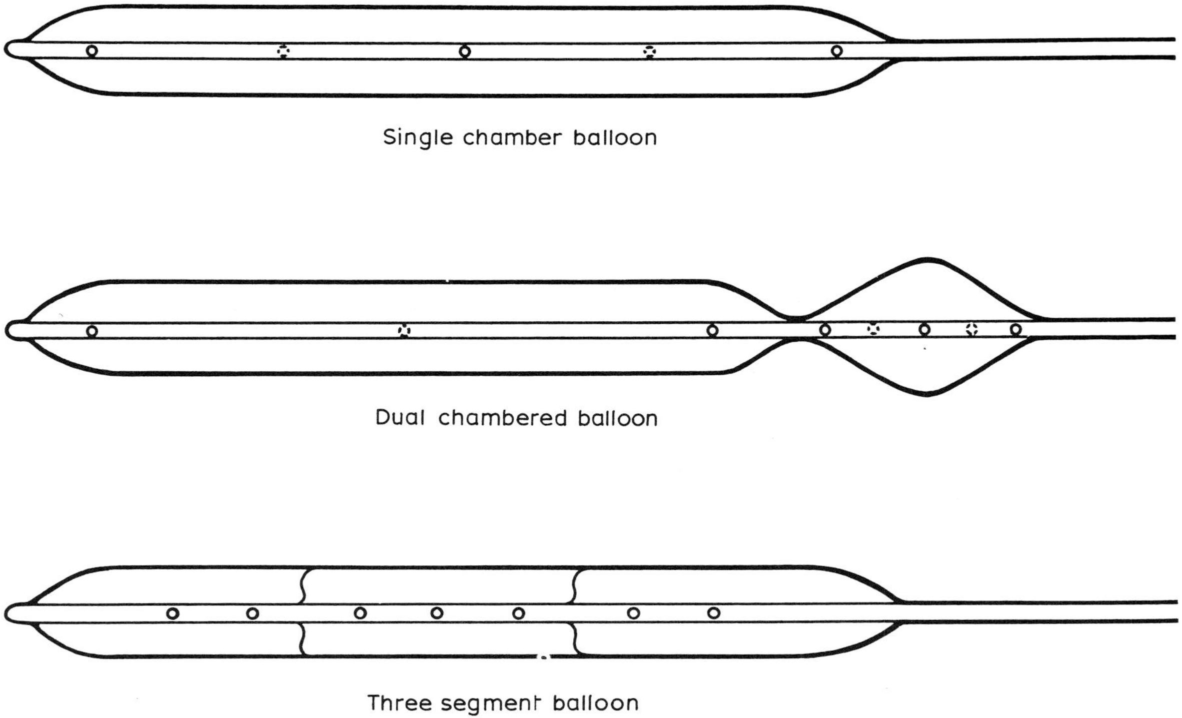

Fig. 9.3 Single, dual, and three segment intra-aortic balloons.

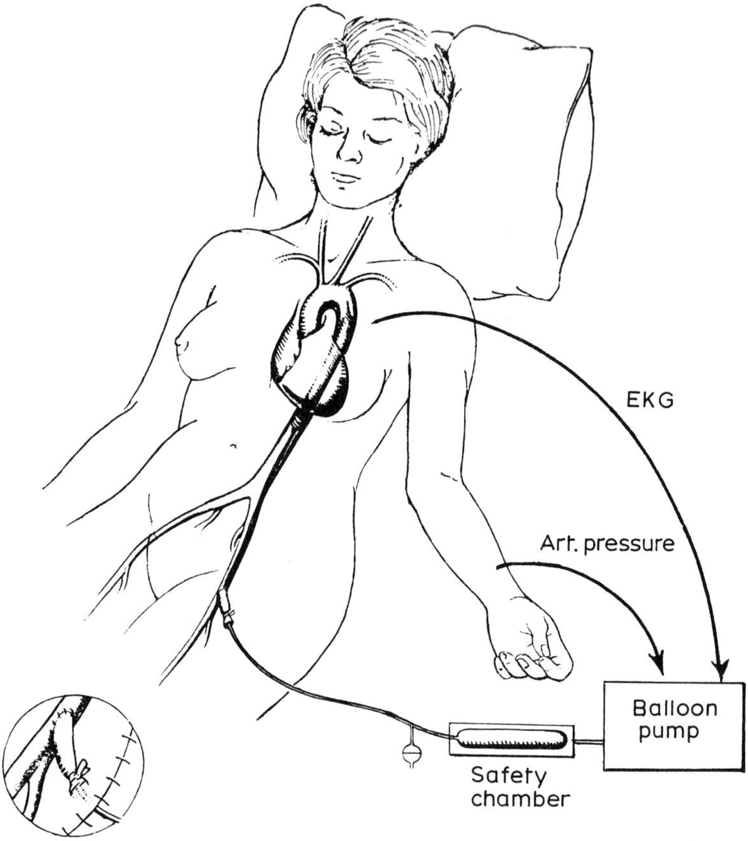

Fig. 9.4 The intra-aortic balloon inserted surgically through a sidearm graft into the common femoral artery.

packaged with each balloon. Finally a 40 ml percutaneous balloon mounted on an 8 french catheter is now available for use in patients with smaller arterial trees.

9.3 EXTERNAL COUNTERPULSATION

External counterpulsation (ECP) theoretically provides assistance to the heart by diastolic pressure augmentation and reciprocal systolic pressure unloading (Fig. 9.6). As first conceived by Dennis *et al.* (1963) and Osborn *et al.* (1963) this method has the advantage of achieving counterpulsation in a relatively non-invasive fashion. Pressure variations are applied to the legs synchronous with the heart beat, thereby utilizing the femoral arterial tree as a pumping chamber in diastole. The initial clinical trials of external counter-

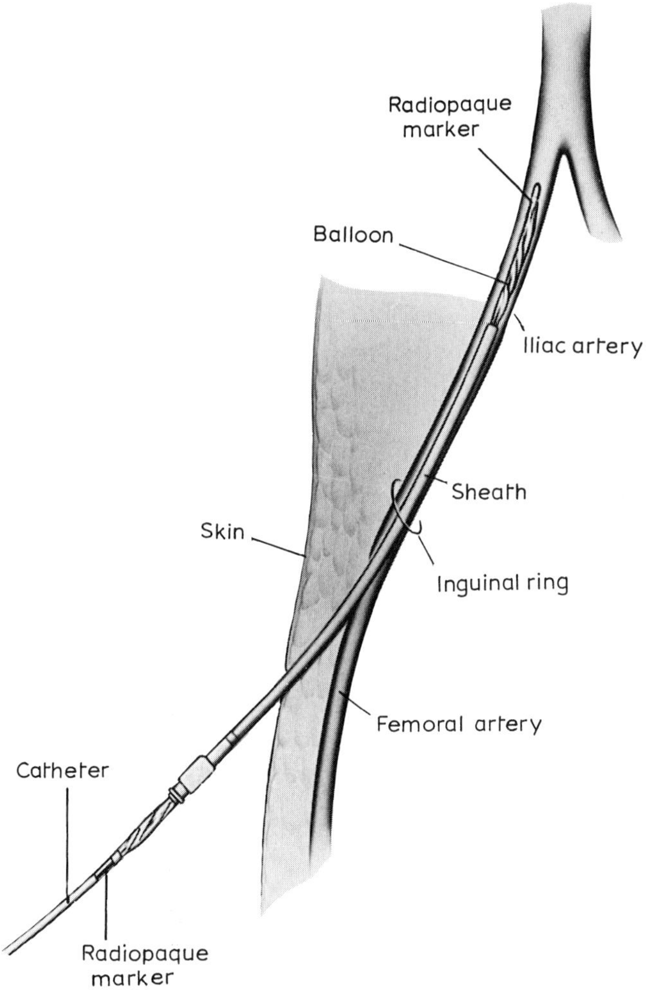

Fig. 9.5 Schematic diagram showing insertion of furled percutaneous intra-aortic balloon through a 12F sheath in the common femoral artery.

pulsation have shown that it does produce an effective arterial diastolic augmentation (though somewhat less than the balloon), but the observations concerning systolic unloading are not consistent, and some investigators have actually reported an increase in left ventricular afterload (Beckman *et al.*, 1973). The volume status of the patient during these clinical trials appears to be extremely important, since external counterpulsation is haemodynamically much more effective in a volume loaded situation. A cooperative study on the clinical assessment of external counterpulsation appeared to

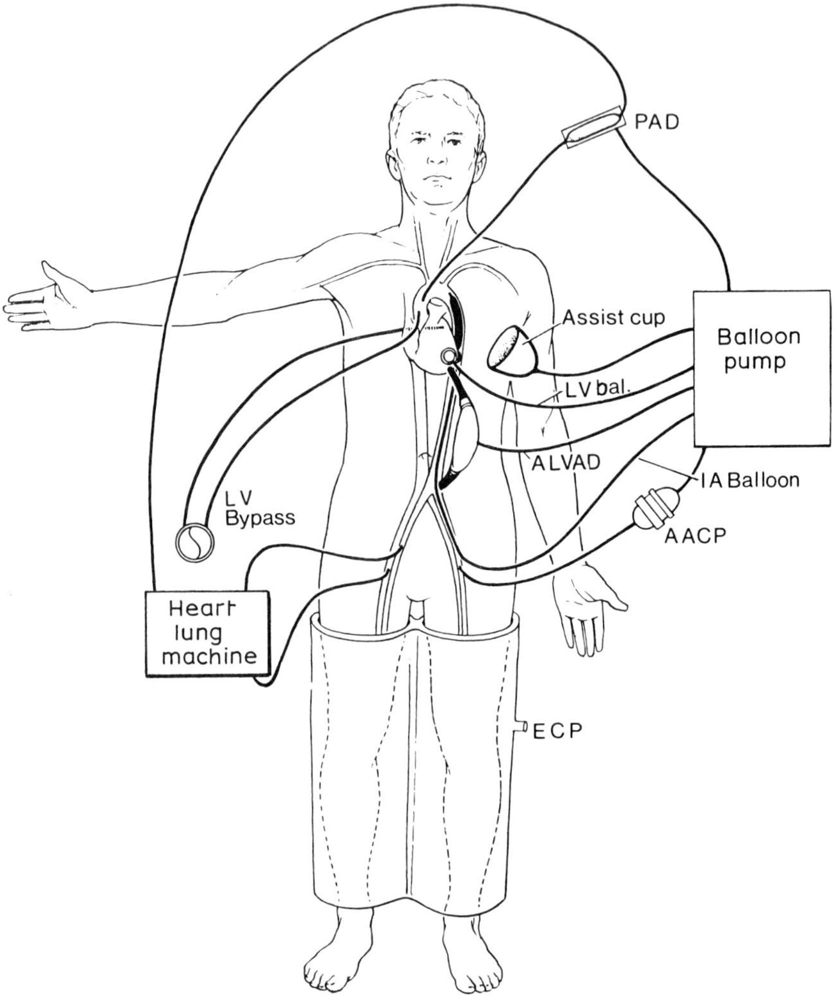

Fig. 9.6 Schematic drawing of current clinical temporary mechanical cardiac assist techniques.

demonstrate that it reduced mortality and morbidity in patients with acute myocardial infarction (Amsterdam *et al.*, 1976).

9.4 DYNAMIC AORTIC PATCH

Kantrowitz *et al.* (1972) felt that a permanently implanted in-series cardiac assist device may represent a promising approach to the treatment of chronic left ventricular failure. A dynamic aortic patch was fabricated which represents a 'permanent' configuration of an intra-aortic balloon pump (Fig. 9.7). Short-term studies have shown that the haemodynamic effects of the patch correspond closely with those of the intra-aortic balloon pump. The device is implanted in the descending thoracic aorta and its blood interface consists of Electrolour (dacron velour backed by bio-electric polyurethane). The initial results in three patients are somewhat encouraging. Further clinical trials are needed to determine if this technique is a reasonable alternative to more conventional medical therapy.

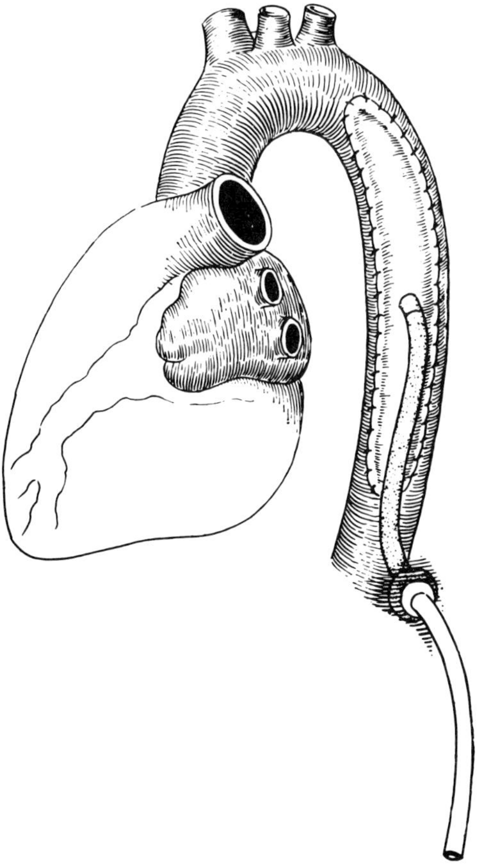

Fig. 9.7 Permanent in-series cardiac assistance with the dynamic aortic patch. (From Schraut *et al.* (1976) *Surgery*, **79**, 193. Used by permission.)

9.5 INFERIOR VENA CAVA BALLOON PUMPING

To model the clinical setting of external counterpulsation, a unidirectional intra-aortic balloon was placed in the inferior vena cava, at the junction of the right atrium, in combination with an intra-aortic balloon pump, in a canine cardiogenic shock preparation (Bregman *et al.*, 1974) (Figs 9.8 and 9.9). Both balloons were timed to the electrocardiogram to inflate during diastole. Inferior vena cava balloon pumping alone improves circulatory haemodynamics (aortic flow, aortic pressure and coronary sinus flow) only in a volume-loaded cardiogenic shock preparation. If the animal were hypovolaemic, the balloon was found to be detrimental. Vena cava balloon pumping in combination with intra-aortic balloon pumping simulated external counterpulsation and together, in a hypervolaemic setting, were found to provide no additional haemodynamic benefit compared to the vena cava balloon. This technique has not therefore been adopted in clinical practice.

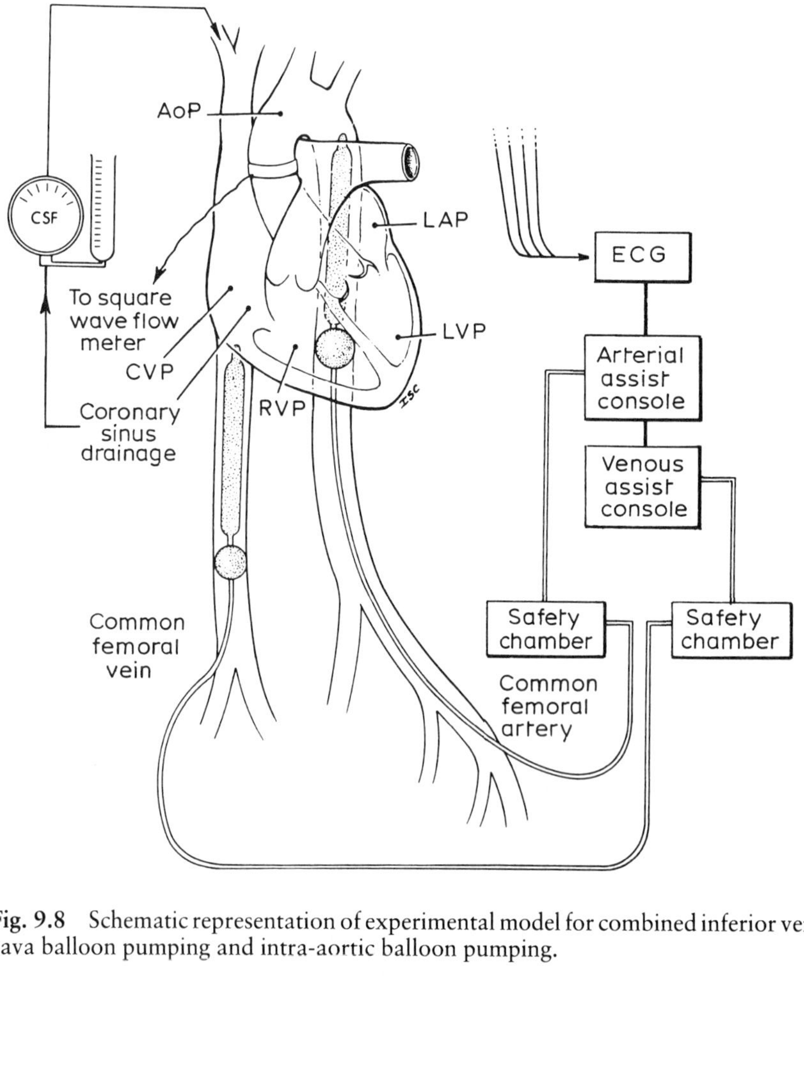

Fig. 9.8 Schematic representation of experimental model for combined inferior vena cava balloon pumping and intra-aortic balloon pumping.

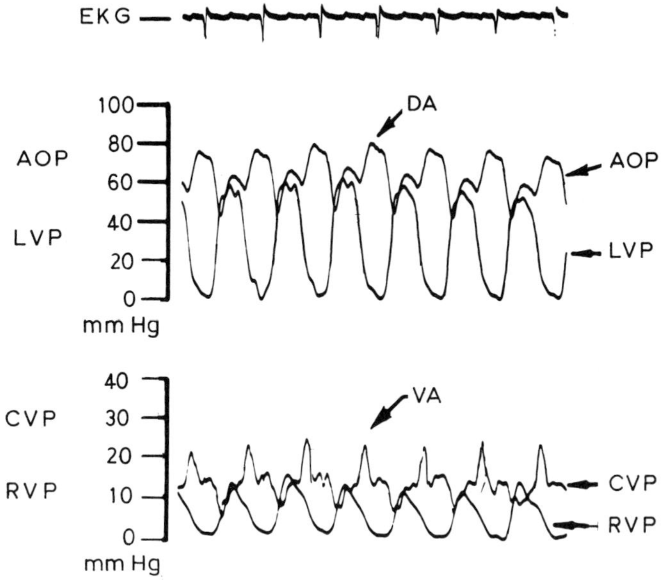

Fig. 9.9 Wave forms characterized by simultaneous balloon pumping in the inferior vena cava and the aorta. Note venous augmentation (VA) in the central venous pressure (CVP) tracing. EKG, electrocardiogram; AOP, aortic pressure; LVP, left ventricular pressure; RVP, right ventricular pressure; DA, arterial diastolic augmentation.

9.6 RIGHT VENTRICULAR BALLOON PUMPING

Right ventricular balloon pumping was used in an experimental model of right ventricular failure induced by elevating pulmonary vascular resistance in a pulmonary embolus model. A spherical balloon was introduced into the right ventricular cavity via the right ventricular apex (Spotnitz *et al.*, 1967). It was synchronized to the cardiac cycle to inflate during systole and deflate during diastole (right ventricular co-pulsation). Right ventricular balloon pumping was shown to increase cardiac output by increasing right ventricular peak systolic pressure, while at the same time lowering right ventricular end diastolic pressure. Perhaps one detrimental effect of this balloon might be the generation of subendocardial ischaemia in the right ventricle, and in the clinical setting it might be advisable to use an intra-aortic balloon pump in combination with the right ventricular balloon to offset this possibility.

9.7 LEFT VENTRICULAR BALLOON PUMPING

Petrovsky and Shumakov (1967) first described the experimental use of a left ventricular balloon device. Schupbach *et al.* (1969) described an experimental prosthetic myocardium which was a dynamic left ventricular balloon patch. Donald and McGoon (1971) reported the experimental use of a left ventricular balloon. The left ventricular balloon is a pear or spherical-shaped balloon mounted on a catheter (Fig. 9.10). The balloon is inserted experimentally into the left ventricular cavity via a stab wound at the apex of the left ventricle and

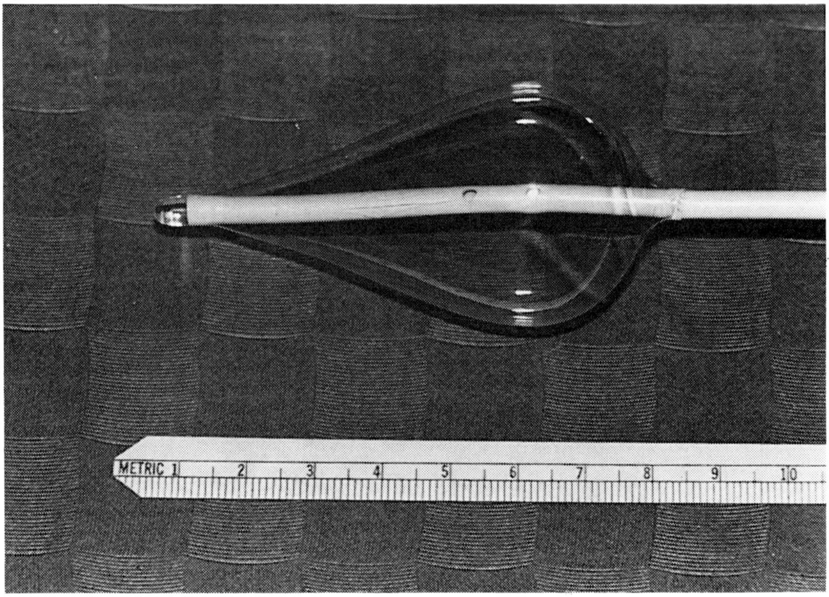

Fig. 9.10 Left ventricular balloon.

is positioned so as not to obstruct the left ventricular outflow tract or distort the mitral valvular apparatus. The left ventricular balloon is inflated synchronously with left ventricular systole (co-pulsation), and is deflated during ventricular diastole. Haemodynamically, left ventricular balloon pumping caused haemodynamic changes similar to a balloon in the right ventricle. Increases in left ventricular systolic pressure, forward cardiac output, and coronary blood flow were produced in conjunction with a rapid fall in left ventricular end diastolic pressure and left atrial pressure, in the experimental low output state (Figs 9.11 and 9.12). There is an increase in myocardial wall tension associated with the inflation of the left ventricular balloon, and myocardial oxygen consumption is increased. For this reason, left ventricular balloon pumping was combined with intra-aortic balloon pumping to offset this imbalance in myocardial oxygen supply and demand (Bregman *et al.*, 1974). One problem with balloon pumping in either ventricular cavity is that it is volume limited. In addition, it does cause multi-focal ventricular premature contractions.

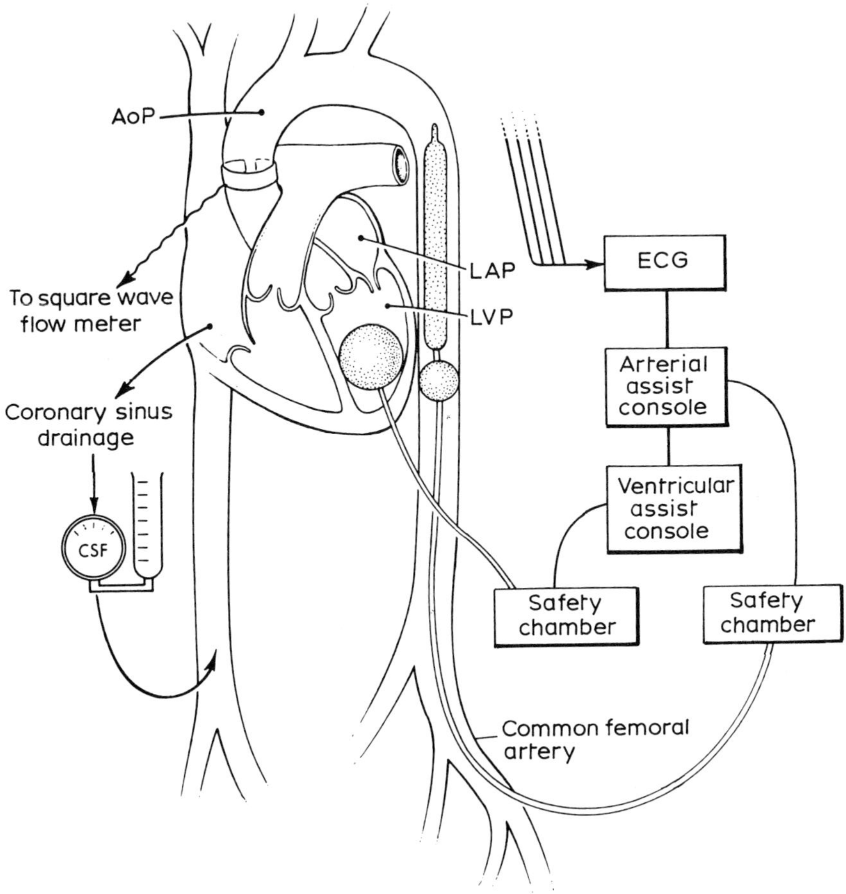

Fig. 9.11 Schematic representation of experimental model for left venticular balloon pumping and intra-aortic balloon pumping.

9.8 PULSATILE ASSIST DEVICE

A pulsatile assist device was developed in 1976 for use during cardiopulmonary bypass to create pulsatile flow during extracorporeal circulation and arterio-arterial counterpulsation either at the beginning or the end of an open-heart surgical procedure (Figs 9.13 and 9.14) (Bregman *et al.*, 1977). This device has been found to have a multitude of other uses. The use of such devices to produce pulsatile perfusion is discussed more fully in Chapter 7. With the distal aspect of the device clamped off, it may be used as a blood counterpulsator. One such application is arterial counterpulsation through the femoral artery when a balloon pump cannot be inserted because of tortuosity of the iliac or femoral system (Fig. 9.15).

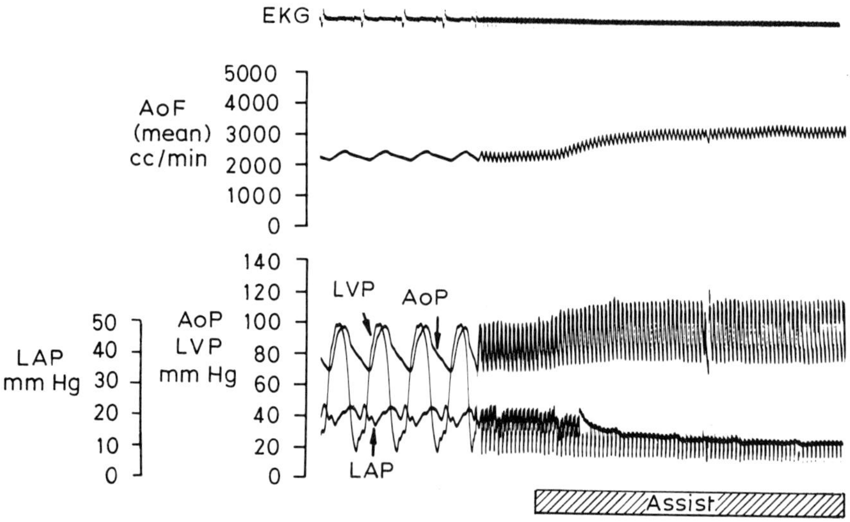

Fig. 9.12 The effect of left ventricular balloon pumping in canine cardiogenic shock. With onset of assist, note the prompt fall in left atrial pressure (LAP) and left ventricular end-diastolic pressure, with a concomitant rise in aortic flow (AoF), aortic pressure (AoP), and left ventricular pressure (LVP).

9.8.1 Left ventricular co-pulsation

In this procedure the pulsatile assist device is used as an auxiliary ventricle by connecting it to a cannula positioned either through the apex of the left ventricle or through the superior pulmonary vein across the mitral valve apparatus into the body of the left ventricular cavity (Marrin *et al.*, 1982). The advantage of using the pulsatile assist device instead of a left ventricular balloon to effect left ventricular co-pulsation, is that a larger blood volume is available (80 ml). In addition, no ventricular arrhythmias are generated with this procedure. Left ventricular co-pulsation in a cardiogenic shock preparation produced a 35.6% increase in mean aortic blood pressure, a 32.3% reduction of mean left atrial pressure, a 66.7% increase in cardiac output and a 76.2% increase in coronary blood flow. In all parameters it was markedly superior to intra-aortic balloon pumping, but it is of course more invasive. Similar experimental observations have been made in the right ventricle.

9.9 PULMONARY ARTERY COUNTERPULSATION AND BALLOON PUMPING

For several years investigators have been interested in supporting the right side of the heart via counterpulsation techniques in the pulmonary arterial

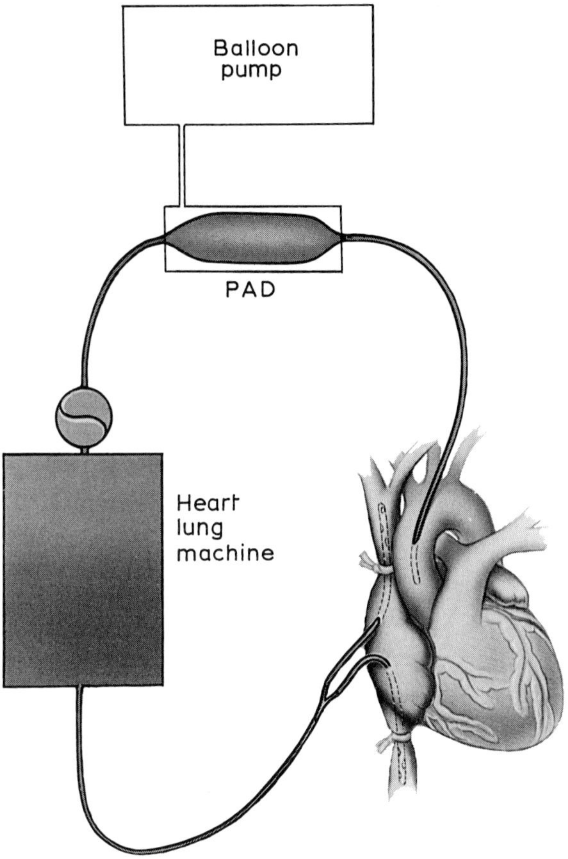

Fig. 9.13 The pulsatile assist device (PAD) in a cardiopulmonary bypass circuit. Oxygenated blood flows through the valveless balloon within the PAD and on into the aorta. The balloon pump pneumatically squeezes the PAD balloon to effect synchronous counterpulsation or pulsatile cardiopulmonary bypass.

circuit. Kralios *et al.* (1970) experimentally placed a balloon pump in the main pulmonary artery and one of its branches. They demonstrated excellent haemodynamics when the balloon was timed to inflate during diastole. A better appreciation of the effects of synchronized counterpulsation of the pulmonary artery on right ventricular haemodynamics was demonstrated by Spotnitz *et al.* (1971). Avery *et al.* (1977) demonstrated that pulmonary artery counterpulsation could easily be established by utilizing the pulsatile assist device. In these experiments a pulmonary embolus model was created in a canine preparation, and the PAD was clamped at its distal aspect to effect

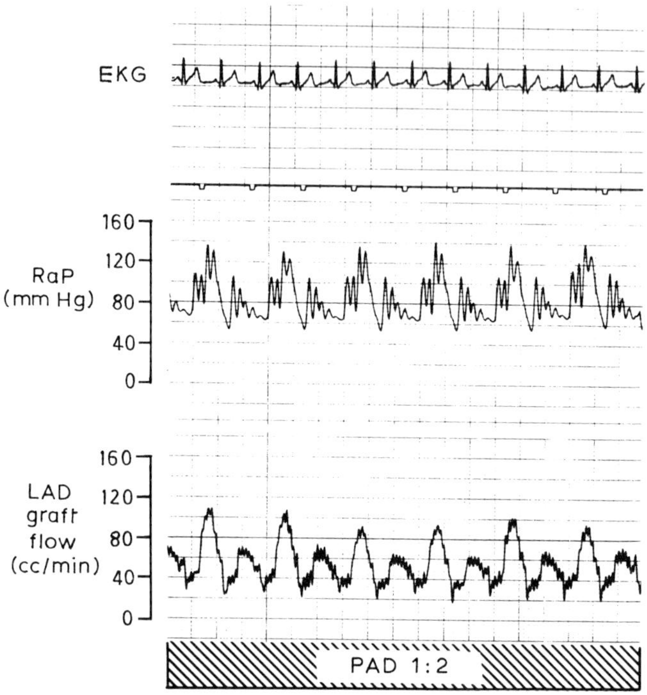

Fig. 9.14 Effect of the PAD in creating synchronous pulsatile cardiopulmonary bypass. Assist is on every other beat. Note pulse pressure at 40 mmHg (5.3 kPa) during total cardiopulmonary bypass and marked increase in LAD graft flow with the device. RaP = right artery pressure. LAD = blood flow in left anterior descending saphenous vein bypass graft.

counterpulsation in the pulmonary artery. In these experiments, pulmonary artery systolic pressure decreased 36%, pulmonary vascular resistance decreased 30%, while the cardiac output increased by 17% (Figs 9.16 and 9.17).

A further extension of these experiments was reported by Brutel *et al.* (1982) by creating a Fontan canine model, counterpulsating the conduit just distal to the valve and utilizing the same pulsatile assist technique. In these experiments improvement in forward cardiac output through the conduit was readily demonstrated. In the clinical setting a recent application of pulmonary artery counterpulsation for acute right ventricular failure was reported (Miller *et al.*, 1980). A dacron side-arm graft was attached to the main pulmonary artery and an intra-aortic balloon pump was placed within this graft with its distal end ligated so that the balloon could counterpulsate

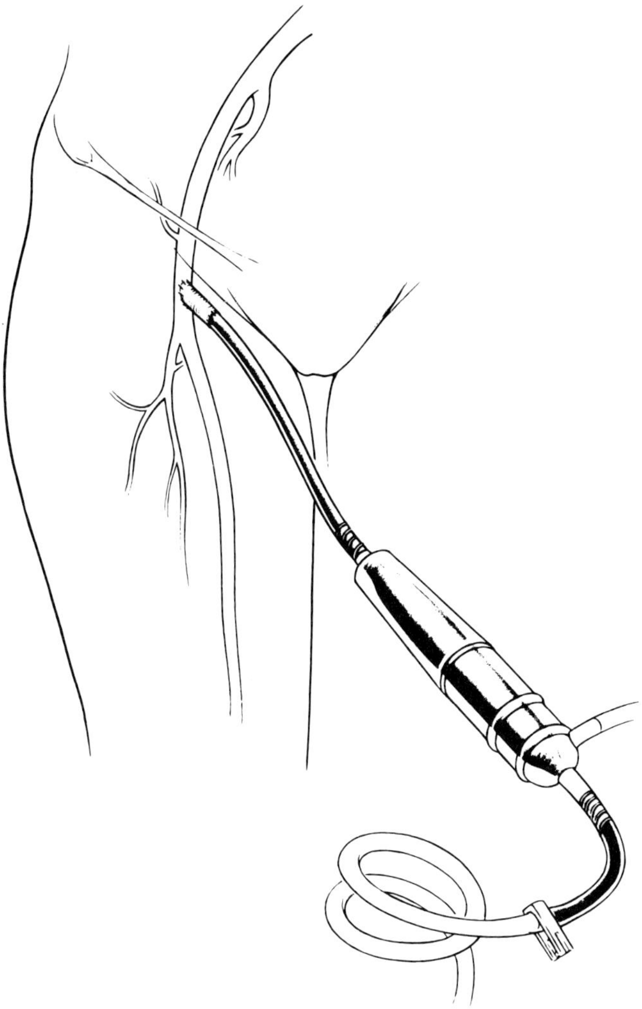

Fig. 9.15 Arterio-arterial counterpulsation through the femoral artery with a pulsatile assist device (PAD).

the pulmonary tree. With this system, a patient with profound right ventricular failure could be separated from cardiopulmonary bypass.

9.10 COUNTERPULSATION DURING RESUSCITATION

Norman reported in 1972 a unique way of employing the principles of counterpulsation during open chest cardiac massage (Molokhia *et al.*, 1972)

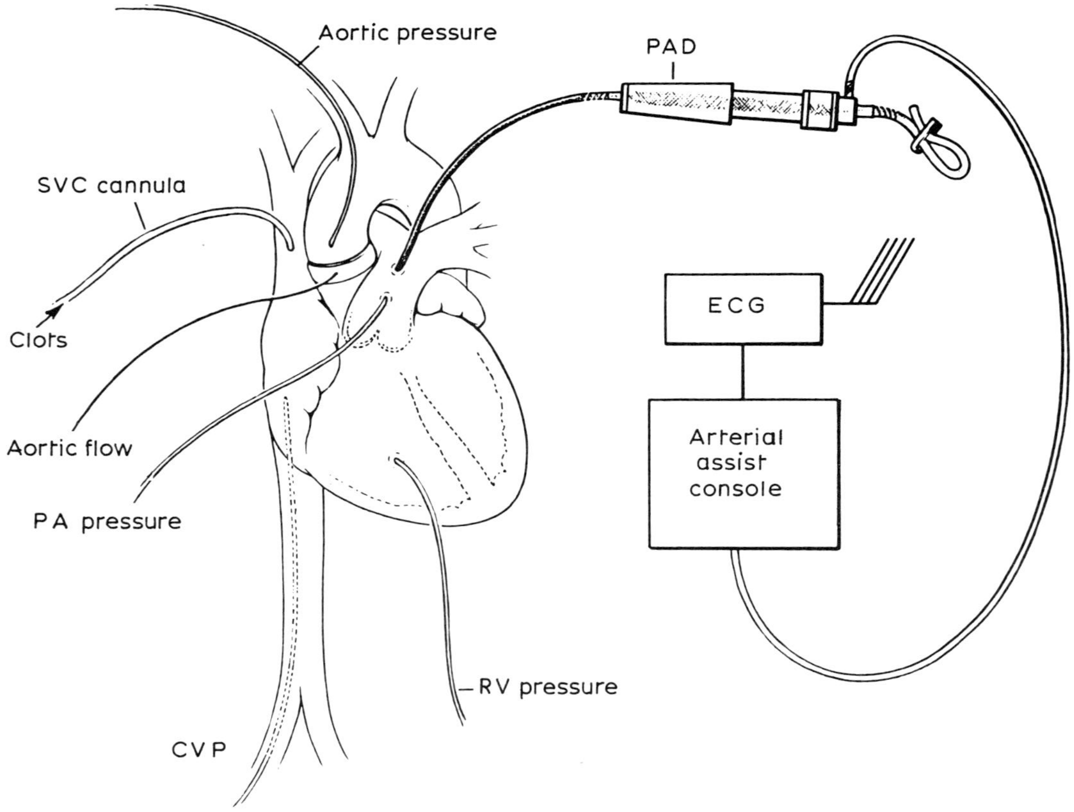

Fig. 9.16 Experimental preparation for use of pulsatile assist device (PAD) to effect pulmonary artery (PA) counterpulsation. SVC = superior vena cava; CVP = central venous pressure; RV = right ventricular.

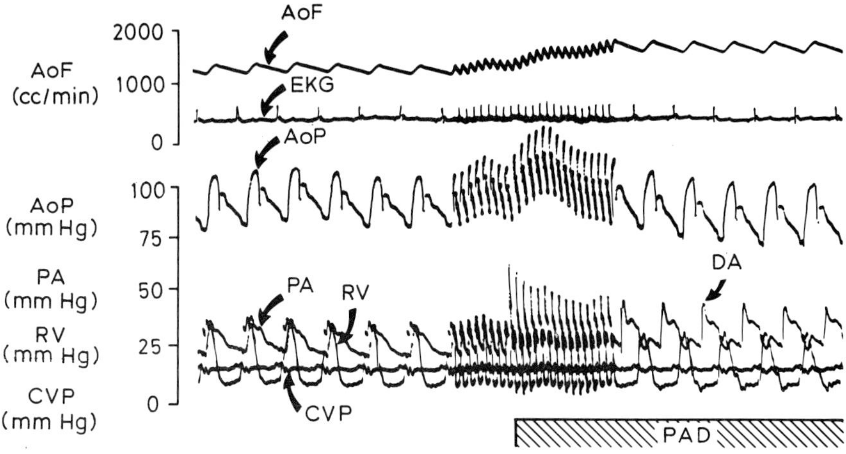

Fig. 9.17 Representative tracing of the effects at pulmonary artery (PA) counterpulsation with the pulsatile assist device (PAD). Note the increase in aortic flow (AoF) and aortic pressure (AoP) and fall in Pa and RV systolic pressure in the PA tracing with PA counterpulsation.

(Fig. 9.18). By massaging the heart with one hand and alternately pinching the aortic root with the opposite hand one would in effect counterpulsate the aortic root during cardiopulmonary resuscitation. In a series of ten mongrel dogs the findings consistently showed easier defibrillation and improvement in coronary sinus flows when this method of augmenting coronary perfusion was employed. Coletti *et al.* (1983) have recently extended this concept by measuring coronary blood flow during open chest cardiac compression with flow augmentation by intra-aortic balloon pumping.

9.10.1 Abdominal counterpulsation

Abdominal counterpulsation is a new and more central application of external counterpulsation. In a canine preparation manual abdominal counterpulsation was applied in a cardiogenic shock setting (Figs 9.19 and 9.20). The findings showed that the diastolic augmentation achieved with abdominal counterpulsation was not quite as significant as with intra-aortic balloon pumping. Nevertheless common carotid blood flow was much more significantly increased with abdominal counterpulsation than with intra-aortic balloon pumping (Coletti *et al.*, 1982). Also important is that with abdominal counterpulsation there is an improvement in central venous pressure whereas the effect of intra-aortic balloon pumping on this parameter is negligible. Currently this technique is gaining in popularity and has begun

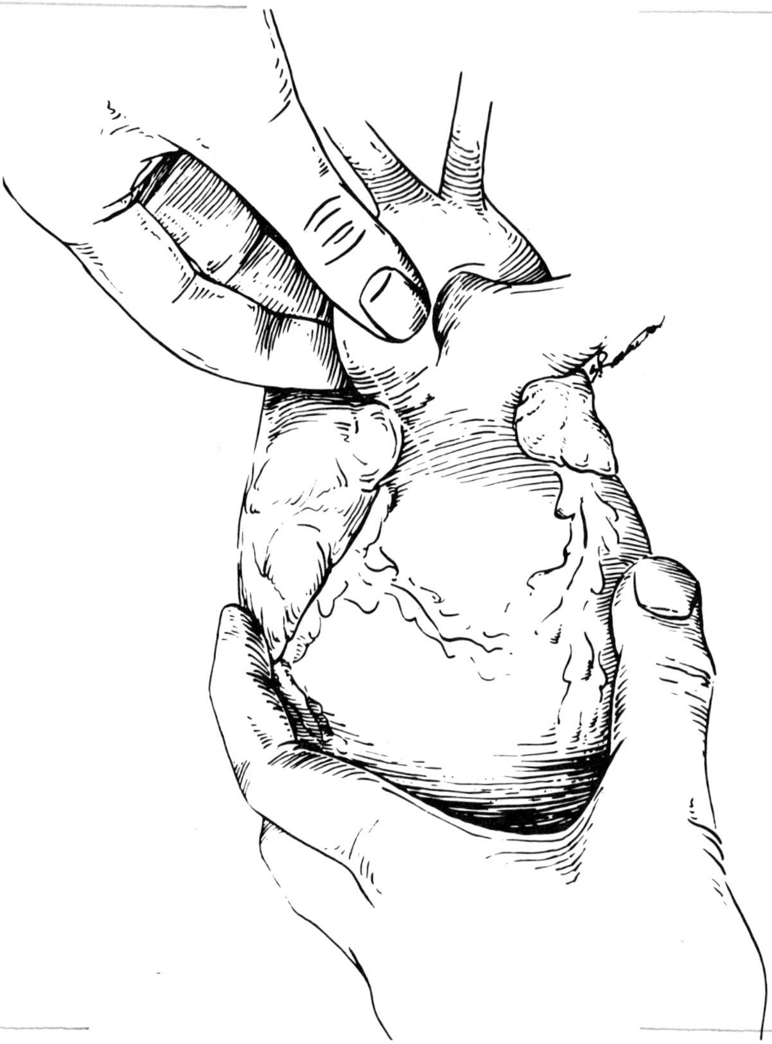

Fig. 9.18 Technique for manual cardiac massage and aortic countercompression. (From Norman *et al.* (1972) *Chest*, **62**, 610. Used by permission.)

to be used during cardiopulmonary resuscitation in conjunction with closed chest cardiac massage in an asynchronous fashion (Voorhees *et al.*, 1982).

9.10.2 Direct mechanical cardiac massage

Anstadt *et al.* (1966) described a cup which is placed over the apex of the right ventricle to encompass the entire heart. A vacuum holds the apex of the heart

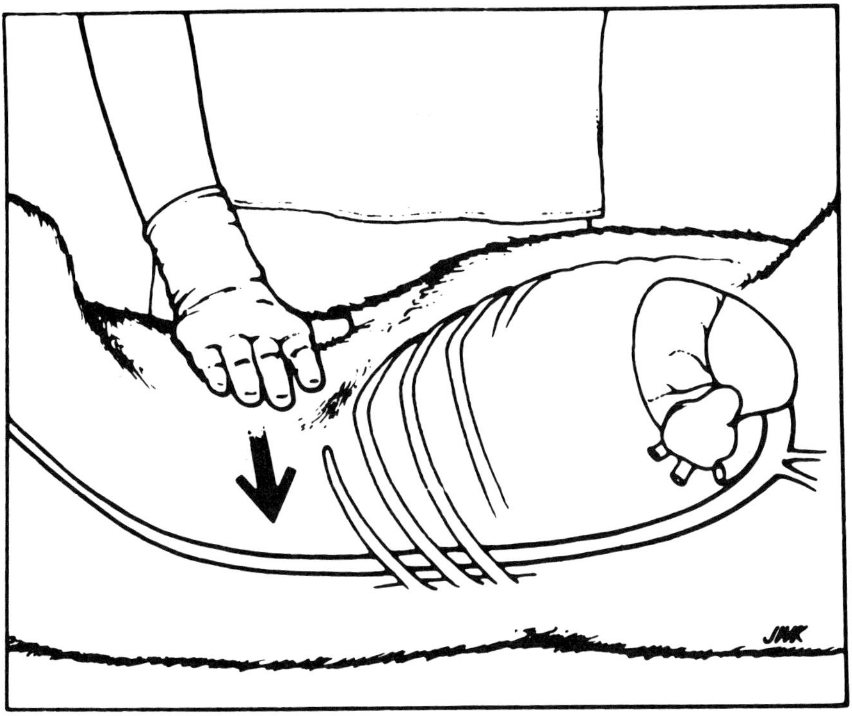

Fig. 9.19 Schematic presentation of the canine application of manual abdominal counterpulsation (AC).

within the cup and manual compression of the heart is then afforded by the membrane within the cup as well as relaxation. The device shows great promise in the laboratory for improving forward haemodynamics from both ventricles, but in the clinical setting the device has not produced very favourable results (Fig. 9.6).

9.11 CONCLUSIONS

Multiple mechanical devices and techniques are now available for use to assist the failing heart for a period of hours to days employing the basic principle of counterpulsation or co-pulsation. It is important to realize that many of these techniques can be *combined* with each other so that more than one can be used in the same individual at the same time. At the present time the most widely used of these devices are the percutaneous intra-aortic balloon pump and the pulsatile assist device. Perhaps a permanent compact application of one or more of these techniques might be a solution to cardiac failure in man.

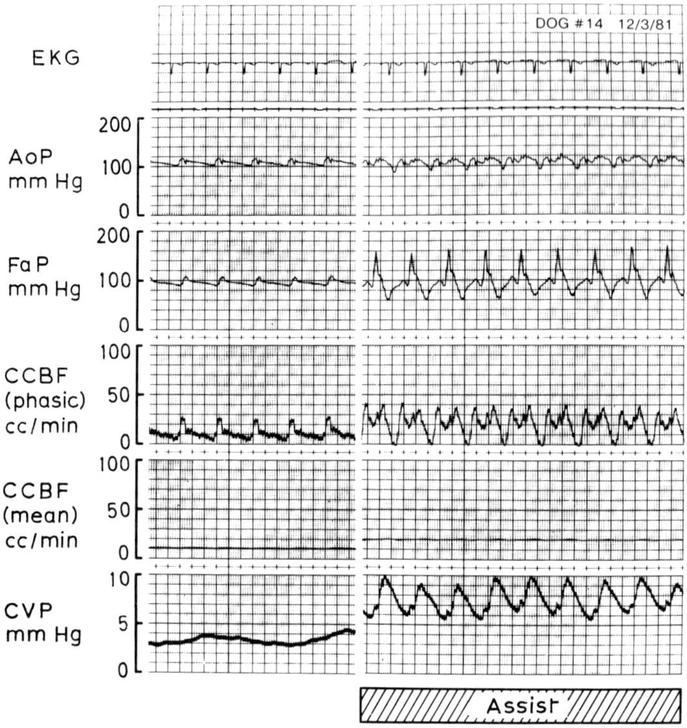

Fig. 9.20 Effects of abdominal counterpulsation in the canine preparation. AoP (aortic pressure), FaP (femoral artery pressure), CCBF (common carotid blood flow), CVP (central venous pressure).

REFERENCES

Amsterdam, E. A., Messer, J. V., Willerson, J. W., Loeb, H. S., Criley, M., Banas, J. S., and Mason, D. T. (1976) Clinical assessment of external pressure circulatory assistance in acute myocardial infarction. *Am. J. Cardiol.*, **37**, 116.

Anstadt, G. L., Blakemore, W. S., and Baue, A. E. (1966) Prolonged circulatory support by direct mechanical ventricular assistance. *Trans. Am. Soc. Artif. Int. Org.*, **12**, 72.

Avery, G. J., II, Spotnitz, H. M., Reemtsma, K., Malm, J. R. and Bregman, D. (1977) A new counterpulsation device for the treatment of acute pulmonary embolus – canine circulatory dynamics. *Trans. Am. Soc. Artif. Int. Org.*, **23**, 103.

Beckman, C. B., Romero, L. H., Shatney, C. H., Nicoloff, D. M ., Lillehei, R. C. and Dietzman, R. H. (1973) Clinical comparison of the intra-aortic balloon pump and external counterpulsation for cardiogenic shock. *Trans. Am. Soc. Artif. Int. Org.*, **19**, 414.

Bregman, D., Bailin, M., Bowman, F. O., Jr, Parodi, E. N., Haubert, S. M., Edie, R. N., Spotnitz, H. M., Reemtsma, K. and Malm, J. R. (1977) A pulsatile assist device (PAD) for use during cardiopulmonary bypass. *Ann. Thorac. Surg.*, **24**, 574.

Bregman, D., Nichols, A. B., Weiss, M. B., Powers, E. R., Martin, E. C. and Casarella,

W. J. (1980) Percutaneous intra-aortic balloon insertion. *Am. J Cardiol.*, **46**, 261.
Bregman, D., Parodi, E. N. and Malm, J. R. (1974) Left ventricular and unidirectional intra-aortic balloon pumping. *J. Thorac. Cardiovasc. Surg.*, **68**, 677.
Bregman, D., Parodi, E. N., Reemtsma, K. and Malm, J. R. (1974) Unidirectional balloon pumping in the inferior vena cava and aorta. *J. Thorac. Cardiovasc. Surg.*, **67**, 553.
Brutel De La Riviere, A., Haasler, G., Malm, J. R. and Bregman, D. (1982) Mechanical assistance of the pulmonary circulation after right ventricular exclusion. *Ned. T. Geneesk.*, **126**, 1613.
Coletti, R. H., Kaskel, P. S. and Bregman, D. (1983) Measurement of coronary blood flow during open chest cardiac compression with flow augmentation by intra-aortic balloon pumping. (Abstr) *Am. Soc. Artif. Int. Org.*, **12**, 1.
Coletti, R. H., Kaskel, P. S., Cohen, S. R. and Bregman, D. (1982) Abdominal counterpulsation a new concept in circulatory assistance. *Trans. Am. Soc. Artif. Int. Org.*, **28**, 563.
Cox, J. L., McLaughlin, V. W., Flowers, N. C. and Horan, L. G. (1968) The ischemic zone surrounding acute myocardial infarction: Its morphology as detected by dehydrogenase staining. *Am. Heart J.*, **76**, 650.
Dennis, C., Moreno, R. Jr, Hall, D. P., Grosz, C., Ross, S. M., Wesolowski, S. A. and Jenning, A. (1963) Studies on external counterpulsation as a potential measure for acute left heart failure. *Trans. Am. Soc. Artif. Int. Org.*, **9**, 186.
Donald, D. E. and McGoon, D. C. (1971) Circulatory support by a left ventricular balloon pump. *Circulation*, **43**, (Suppl. I), 96.
Dormandy, J. A., Goetz, R. H. and Kripke, D. C. (1971) Hemodynamics and coronary blood flow with counterpulsation. *Surgery*, **65**, 311.
Harken, D. E. (1958) Presentation at the International College of Cardiology Meeting, Brussels, Belgium.
Jacobey, J. A. (1971) Results of counterpulsation in patients with coronary artery disease. *Am. J. Cardiol.*, **27**, 137.
Jacobey, J. A., Craddock, L. D., Wolf, P. S. and Beckwitt, H. L. (1968) Clinical experience with counterpulsation in coronary artery disease. *J. Thorac. Cardiovasc. Surg.*, **56**, 846.
Jacobey, J. A., Taylor, W. J., Smith, G. T., Doorlin, R. and Harken, D. E. (1963) A new therapeutic approach to acute coronary occlusion: Opening dormant coronary collateral channels by counterpulsation. *Am. J. Cardiol.*, **11**, 218.
Kantrowitz, A. and Kantrowitz, A. (1953) Experimental augmentation of coronary flow by retardation of arterial pressure pulse. *Surgery*, **34**, 628.
Kantrowitz, A., Krakauer, J., Rubenfire, M., Jaron, D., Freed, P. S., Welkowitz, W., Cascade, P., Wayszczuk, W. J., Lipsius, M., Ciborski, M., Phillips, S. J. and Hayden, M. T. (1972) Initial clinical experience with a new permanent mechanical auxiliary ventricle: The dynamic aortic patch. *Trans. Am. Soc. Artif. Int. Org.*, **28**, 159.
Kantrowitz, A. and McKinnon, W. M. P. (1958) The experimental use of the diaphragm as an auxiliary myocardium. *Surg. Forum*, **9**, 266.
Kantrowitz, A. Tjonneland, S., Freed, P. S., Phillips, S. J., Butner, A. N. and Sherman, J. L. Jr (1968) Initial clinical experience with intra-aortic balloon pumping in cardiogenic shock. *J. Am. Med. Assoc.*, **203**, 135.
Kralios, A. C., Zwart, H. H. Jr, Moulopoulos, S. D., Collan, R., Kwan-Gett, C. S. and Kolff, W. J. (1970) Intrapulmonary artery balloon pumping. *J. Thorac. Cardiovasc. Surg.*, **60**, 215.

Maroko, P. R., Bernstein, E. F., Lippy, P., Delaria, G. A., Covell, J. W., Ross, J., Jr and Braunwald, E. (1972) Effecs of intra-aortic balloon counterpulsation on the severity of myocardial ischemic injury following acute coronary occlusion. *Circulation.*, **45**, 1150.

Marrin, C. A. S, Rose, E. A., Spotnitz, H. M. and Bregman, D. (1982) Mechanical circulatory support via the left ventricular vent – The concept of left ventricular copulsation. *J. Thorac. Cardiovasc. Surg.*, **84**, 426.

Miller, C. D., Moreno-Cabral, R. J., Stinson, E. B., Shinn, J. A. and Shumway, N. E. (1980) Pulmonary artery balloon counterpulsation for acute right ventricular failure. *J. Thorac. Cardiovasc. Surg.*, **80**, 760.

Molokhia, F. A., Ponn, R. A., Robinson, W. J., Asimacopoulos, P. J. and Norman, J. C. (1972) A method of augmenting coronary perfusion during internal cardiac massage. *Chest*, **62**, 610.

Moulopoulos, S. D., Topaz, S. and Kolff, W. J. (1962) Diastolic balloon pumping (with carbon dioxide) in the aorta – a mechanical assistance to the failing circulation. *Am. Heart J.*, **63**, 669.

Nachlas, M. M. and Sieband, M. P. (1967) The influence of diastolic augmentation on infarct size following coronary artery ligation. *J. Thorac. Cardiovasc. Surg.*, **53**, 698.

Osborn, J., Main, J., Beachley, F. and Gerbode, F. (1963) Circulatory support by leg and airway pulses in experimental mitral insufficiency. *Circulation*, **28**, 781.

Petrovsky, B. V. and Shumakov, V. I. (1967) Artificial heart implanted into the organism. *Kardiologia*, **8**, 14.

Rosensweig, J., Chatterjee, S. and Merino, F. (1970) Treatment of acute myocardial infarction by counterpulsation: Experimental rationale and clinical experience. *J. Thorac. Cardiovasc. Surg.*, **59**, 243.

Schupbach, P., Suyansky, E., Tomecek, J., Santa, A., Freed, P. S., and Kantrowitz, A. (1969) An experimental prosthetic myocardium. *Trans. Am. Soc. Artif. Int. Org.*, **15**, 434.

Spotnitz, H. M., Berman, M. A., Reis, R. L. and Epstein, S. E. (1971) The effects of synchronized counterpulsation of the pulmonary artery on right ventricular hemodynamics. *J. Thorac. Cardiovasc. Surg.*, **61**, 167.

Spotnitz, A., Bregman, D., Spotnitz, H. M., Parodi, E. N., Scott, G. and Malm, J. R. (1967) Right intraventricular balloon pumping: Hemodynamic effect in embolus induced ventricular failure (abstr). *Am. Soc. Artif. Int. Org.*, **4**, 59.

Sugg, W. L., Webb, W. R. and Ecker, R. R. (1969) Reduction of extent of myocardial infarction by counterpulsation. *Ann. Thorac. Surg.*, **7**, 311.

Voorhees, W. D., Niebauer, M. J. and Babbs, C. F. (1982) Improved oxygen delivery during CPB with manual abdominal counterpulsation. *Circulation*, **66** (Suppl. II), 168.

10

Oxygenation – general review

J. C. SIMPSON

The present success of cardiac surgery, especially surgery of complicated congenital heart disease and extensive myocardial revascularization relies heavily upon extracorporeal perfusion techniques, employing amongst other things an efficient gas-exchange mechanism. The piece of apparatus, known as the oxygenator, supplants the patient's pulmonary function for gas exchange (but not for pharmacological filtration or immune mechanisms) during the period of extracorporeal circulation. The requirements for the oxygenator include (1) efficient oxygenation of desaturated haemoglobin, and (2) simultaneous control of carbon dioxide tension and homeostasis. The oxygenator thus acts as an artificial 'alveolar – pulmonary capillary system' for gas exchange, in two principal clinical situations:

(1) Short-term circulatory and pulmonary support for patients undergoing open-heart surgery.
(2) Long-term support in the group of patients who have acute severe pulmonary insufficiency (Zapol *et al.*, 1972). (See Chapter 13.)

Two groups of oxygenator are presently in widespread clinical use:

(1) Direct gas interface oxygenators – such as rotating disc oxygenators, screen or bubble oxygenators. In this group there is direct contact between the circulating fluid of the system and the delivered gas mixture.
(2) Membrane oxygenators – in this group there is a 'gas porous' membrane between the circulating fluid and the gas mixture.

Though the specific characteristics of bubble and membrane oxygenators are considered in detail in Chapters 11 and 12, it is reasonable to consider briefly the functional differences between these two groups with respect to their efficiency as oxygenators. The direct gas interface oxygenators depend on matching of gas flow to blood flow on whatever surface the oxygenator system provides (Galletti *et al.*, 1972). They are efficient for relatively short time periods, measured in hours, but are associated with progressive damage to cellular elements and platelets in the perfusate, protein denaturation and deposition and the production of gaseous microemboli. Membrane oxygenators eliminate this direct trauma to the blood, and unless there is major protein deposition on the membrane surface, remain efficient for periods of up to several days.

10.1 THEORETICAL CONSIDERATIONS

Assuming that gas flow and blood flow through the oxygenator are matched, according to manufacturer's specifications to produce fully saturated blood in the arterial line, oxygen will be conveyed to the patient's tissues both as oxygen dissolved in the plasma and as saturated oxyhaemoglobin. Oxygen is distributed to perfused cells from the capillaries down the concentration gradient between the oxyhaemoglobin and plasma, through the capillary wall, across the interstitial space, through the cell membrane to the target enzyme system of the cell. The overall adequacy of cellular oxygenation is thus influenced, during extracorporeal circulation, by numerous factors affecting both oxygen supply to the cells, the oxygen demand of the cells and the ability of the cells to take up oxygen.

The adequacy of tissue perfusion will be affected by other variables, including vasoconstriction, pulsatility of blood flow etc. The metabolic demands of the tissues will be affected by temperature change, e.g. induced hypothermia. Oxygen uptake by tissues will be influenced by factors affecting the oxygen dissociation curve, e.g. temperature, PCO_2, and will also be affected by intracellular pH, sodium/potassium balance etc.

These factors may be further influenced by many interactive variables including changes in blood viscosity and in colloid osmotic pressure during perfusion. The generation of 'tissue damaging factors' during perfusion may also affect tissue oxygenation. Such substances include vasoactive agents, e.g. histamine, serotonin, derivatives of complement activation and liberation of free radical species.

10.2 TISSUE PERFUSION

Cardiopulmonary bypass pumps deliver a set flow into the patient's arterial circulation and thus eventually to the cells of the tissues (Fig. 10.1). Conventional techniques have employed non-pulsatile flow, but systems are increasingly available which deliver pulsatile flow (see Chapter 7). The advantages of pulsatile flow include better tissue perfusion for a given flow rate. This may be due to preservation of myogenic tone at an arteriolar level (Shepherd and Kirklin, 1969), and to preservation of perfusion autoregulation in organs until this is lost due to hypothermia.

The actual flow of oxygenated prime through an organ or tissue is

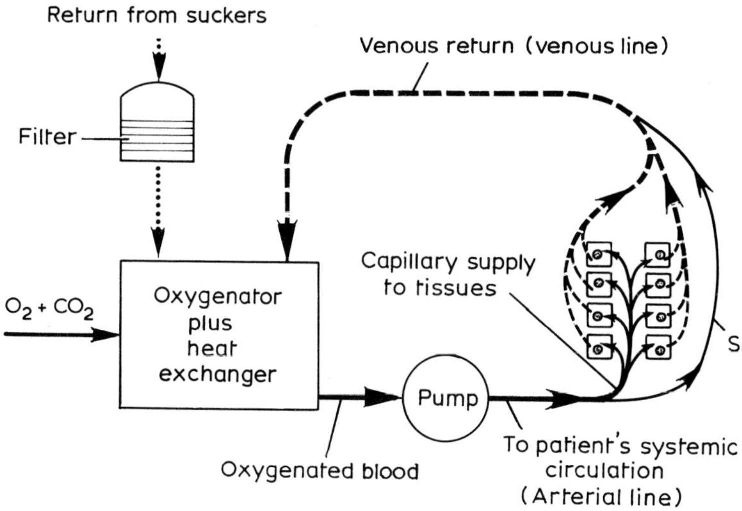

Fig. 10.1 Oxygen transport during conventional cardiopulmonary bypass. Vasoconstriction will be associated with increase in shunt flow, and proportional reduction in true oxygen delivery through the capillary supply to the tissues.

proportional to the degree of afferent arteriolar tone, which is itself a direct result of any change in myogenic tone in the arteriolar wall. Myogenic arteriolar tone is directly influenced by vasoactive drugs, changes in locally occurring natural hormone levels, tissue temperature, local tissue metabolic activity and any degree of local tissue acidosis. It is frequently impossible to be certain which is the most important of these factors. However, increased vasoconstriction will increase shunting through larger arterio-venous channels in the tissues with the net result that an apparently adequate tissue flow may still lead to poor cellular oxygenation. (See Fig. 10.1). The use, almost routinely, of hypothermic perfusion will cool all tissues thus reducing the oxygen demands *pro rata* with the local fall of temperature, but in the face of vasoconstriction and reduced tissue flow, the local temperature may not fall and tissue oxygenation be compromised by poor flow and normal cellular activity.

This concept has led to the use of vasodilator therapy during extracorporeal circulation. Avoidance of vasoconstriction allows oxygenated blood to reach tissue capillary networks, minimizing temperature gradients within these tissues and possibly reducing shunting, although this is difficult to quantitate *in vivo*. The use of moderate haemodilution, as in current practice, reduces the viscosity of the circulating fluid, and may also secondarily improve tissue perfusion. However this benefit to perfusion may be achieved at the expense of other negative effects of moderate haemodilution.

The first is dilution of oxygen-carrying capacity due to reduced haemoglobin (as red cell mass) per volume of fluid (Niinikoski *et al.*, 1981). The second is a fall in colloid pressure of the perfusate with the extrusion of fluid into the interstitial spaces of the tissues (Utley *et al.*, 1981). Haemodilution, is controllable, however, and when utilizing hypothermia, more oxygen dissolves in the fluid phase of the prime (a significant factor for oxygen transport to the cell). During lengthy perfusion this benefit may be lost due to massive leakage of fluid and, later, proteins, cells and degraded cells into the interstitial space. This phenomenon increases the distance for the diffusion of oxygen towards the cell interior (Rosenkranz *et al.*, 1980), compounding cellular hypoxia and local acidosis.

Certain deviations from the ideal scheme of oxygen delivery (shown in Fig. 10.2) have already been mentioned. It is now necessary to consider those

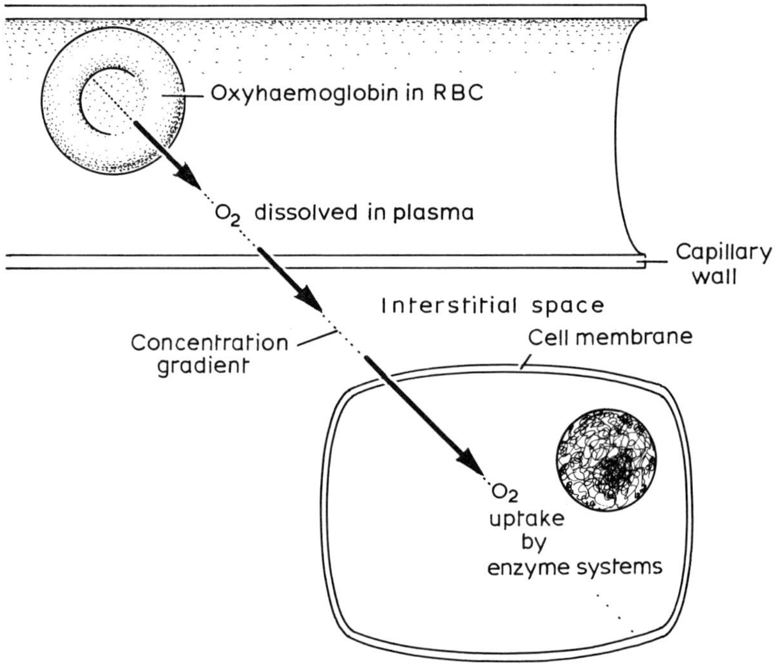

Fig. 10.2 Oxygen delivery to the tissues. Oxygen diffuses down the substantial concentration gradient between the red blood cell (RBC) and the tissue cell mitochondria.

factors, given a steady blood flow in undamaged tissue capillaries, which influence oxygen delivery to the enzyme systems within the cell membrane. The oxygen contained within the haemoglobin matrix will physically diffuse down the concentration gradient, from plasma, across the capillary wall into solution in interstitial fluid, and thence into the cell through the cell's semi-permeable membrane. The oxygen tension gradient, from red cell to mitochondria, is very high, the mitochondria having a PO_2 of 1–2 mmHg, (0.13–0.26 kPa), the red cell a PO_2 in excess of 100 mmHg (13.3 kPa). The speed of diffusion of oxygen down this gradient is time related and takes longer for any increase in physical distance.

The net availability of oxygen for this transfer process is controlled by alterations to the shape and position of the oxygen dissociation curve (Fig.

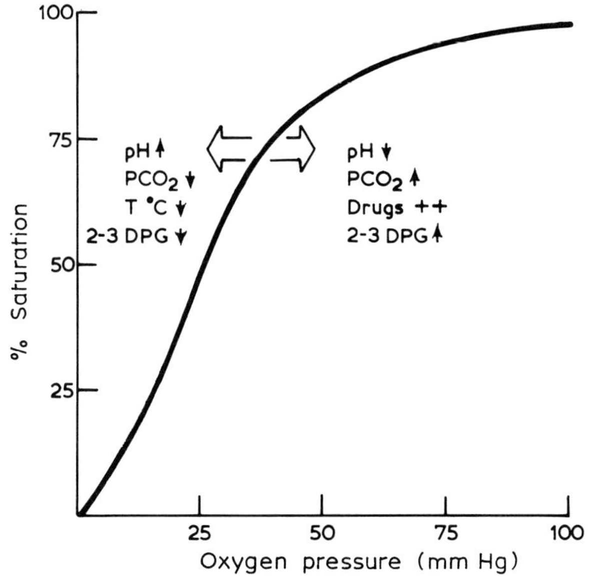

Fig. 10.3 Factors affecting the oxygen dissociation curve during cardiopulmonary bypass.

10.3), and is altered by local tissue environmental factors. Hypothermia, an increase in pH, a decrease in PCO_2 and in 2,3-diphosphoglycerate (DPG) will shift the curve to the left (Bordiuk *et al.*, 1973), shifting the P_{50} (the oxygen tension present when the haemoglobin is 50% saturated) to the left at the same time, with a net decrease in oxygen available to the tissues. However a local decrease in pH, an increase in local CO_2 tension, the effect of some anaesthetic agents and an increase in 2,3-diphosphoglycerate will shift the curve to the right, together with the P_{50}. This results in a reduction in haemoglobin's affinity for oxygen with a consequent increase in oxygen availability for transfer to the internal chemical matrix of the cell (Valeri *et al.*, 1980). The carbon dioxide, in solution from cellular metabolism, will diffuse down its concentration gradient into solution in plasma and be transported via the serum as bicarbonate ion (HCO_3^-) and as a carbamino moiety within the red cell.

10.3 MEASUREMENT

It is obvious therefore that during extracorporeal circulation there are many variables which will influence tissue oxygenation. It is, therefore, mandatory to attempt to monitor whether an adequate amount of oxygen is reaching the cells to preserve cellular function and integrity. The ideal measurement to make is that of intracellular PO_2, pH and possibly potassium (K^+) concentration, preferably in all cells and preferably continuously. This idealistic concept is hopelessly impractical, invasive and tissue destructive, as well as being technically impossible, at the present time except for *in vitro* research preparations. A compromise must be sought, which with minimal invasion and tissue destruction gives comprehensible results, using a reliable machine system which is easily calibrated, simple to operate and preferably capable of continuous data display so that trends may be detected and analysed.

The most important questions to be answered are (1) what parameter is the best one to monitor? (2) how best should this be done? (3) in what mode should the results be displayed? and (4) what are the operating limits of the system?

As far as oxygenation is concerned, there are two principal areas of interest.

(1) Is the oxygenator working adequately – as an oxygenator?
(2) Are the body tissues adequately oxygenated and perfused by the fluid environment provided by the extracorporeal circulation?

It is important to consider whether 'oxygenating potential' of the perfusate should be measured as partial pressure, saturation or oxygen content. Ideally oxygen content would be the most informative measurement (Valeri *et al.*, 1972), but with the present state of the methodology, this is a cumbersome and time-consuming measurement, if the results are to be reproducible and meaningful. Most units rely on the measurement of partial pressure of oxygen and a derived value for oxygen saturation. Modern blood-gas analysis machines are programmed to report partial pressures and also to apply a temperature correction so that the results on a sample of blood at the patient's temperature are presented after conversion to 'normal' body temperature (Kelman and Nunn, 1966). Samples thus analysed on the arterial side of the circulation, either from the arterial line from the pump, or from an indwelling arterial cannula, will indicate if the oxygenator is itself efficient and will indicate what environmental oxygen is perfusing the tissues. Similar samples taken from the venous side of the extracorporeal circulation will indicate the fall in oxygen tension occurring during tissue perfusion. From these results it is possible to determine if tissues are extracting oxygen adequately, and to gain some idea of oxygen consumption, with respect to temperature gradients, change in metabolic rate, perfusion pressure, and flow rate. Accurate determination of oxygen consumption is only realistically obtained if arterial and venous blood oxygen content are accurately measured, and when the respiratory quotient is known or assumed at a given body temperature. Repeated measurements of oxygen consumption, presented as a trend recording will give valuable information as to the efficiency of tissue oxygenation.

If, during perfusion, tissue hypoxia occurs, then there will be a fall in pH, and a secondary fall in plasma bicarbonate (HCO_3^-),due to increase in anaerobic metabolism. These two values (pH and HCO_3^-) are part of routine measurement during blood gas analysis and they give further evidence of tissue hypoxia (Kessler *et al.*, 1976). Unless severe damage has been done to the cellular elements of the blood by passage through the oxygenator, both measurements are minimally affected during artificial oxygenation unless there has also been a considerable change in carbon dioxide tension during gas exchange in the oxygenator. A fall in bicarbonate (HCO_3^-) in the arterial blood samples analysed may indicate poor tissue oxygenation despite an adequate venous oxygen tension. This result may indicate shunting in the tissues, or some other cause of under-perfusion, and should be dealt with appropriately.

It appears that the simplest method for assessing adequacy of oxygenation is the repeated, reliable measurement of arterial O_2 tension and pH in arterial blood samples taken from the patient. Currently this is the practice most widely used in cardiac units, but it should not be forgotten that it is relatively incomplete and does not give continuous real time information.

10.4 ON-LINE TECHNIQUES FOR OXYGENATION ASSESSMENT

Recent developments in miniaturization, and perfection of blood interfacing membranes have made possible the use of polarographic electrodes, sampling catheters attached to gas chromatograph systems, mass spectrometers and oximeters for continuous and on-line real-time estimation of PO_2, pH, oxygen saturation and PCO_2. The sensors may be inserted into the artificial cardiopulmonary bypass circuit or directly into patient tissues. Whilst still being invasive and potentially tissue destructive, the usefulness of the resulting data may offset the disadvantages. These techniques have, however, many other technical problems and need a high level of capital investment to ensure their success and further refinement.

10.4.1 Polarographic systems

The development by Clark of the bipolar oxygen measuring electrode system into a single unit has given the facility of intravascular measurement of PO_2 with a reasonable degree of accuracy. This system has been miniaturized and used as a direct intravascular monitoring system. Polarographic cells may be inserted into the arterial side of the oxygenator and pump circuit and also into the venous side. Function of these electrodes depends on the type of membrane covering the system. This in turn determines response time, stability and sensitivity. The function of the system is also altered by changes in perfusate temperature and by deposition of blood-derived debris on the catheter tip. This latter problem of deposition can partially be overcome by using a silicone membrane or a heparin-impregnated membrane. It has been shown that some anaesthetic agents affect electrode function (Hahn *et al.*, 1975). These problems will be overcome, and this system remains a potentially viable standard system for measuring PO_2 continuously, or in two locations (arterial and venous) with the facility to derive oxygen consumption.

10.4.2 Oximetry

A modification of the type of catheter containing the oxygen sensitive electrode system offers the possibility of adding other sensors, such as an oximeter. Using fine-bore fibre-optic systems it is possible to illuminate blood with one fibre-optic cable and to monitor its reflection with another, displaying the resultant signal as O_2 saturation (Parker, 1981). Such a catheter can also have a sampling channel – for blood sampling and *in vitro* analysis, for estimation of pH, PCO_2 and (HCO_3^-). It is possible to add a pH measuring module to the catheter, the difficulty at present being the lack of a suitably stable sensor at the catheter tip.

10.4.3 Mass spectrometry

Providing funds are available to purchase, maintain and service the central machine, mass spectrometry can be adapted to measure oxygen tension in tissues and blood. The ideal reference gas is argon (Lundsgaard and Degn, 1981) which enables *in situ* calibration of the special probe. Although these systems are in their infancy they lend themselves to the monitoring of other parameters such as cardiac output, oxygen consumption etc. after the cardiac surgical procedure, e.g. in the intensive care unit.

10.4.4 Gas chromatography

In an attempt to bypass the hazards and difficulties of intravascular polarographic systems, and to obtain 'continuous' reading of PO_2 during extracorporeal oxygenation Moffit *et al.* (1979) used gas chromatography. The sensor was a semi-permeable membrane, using helium as a carrier gas, inserted into the brachial artery. The results demonstrated good correlation between gas chromatography as an applied monitor, and standard *in vitro* measurement of the same parameters (PCO_2 and PO_2) in blood samples.

The foregoing methods are essentially concerned with perfusate gas tensions. As indicated earlier in this chapter it is useful to know what are tissue oxygenation, oxygen consumption and oxygen supply, in local tissues, with respect to their theoretical environment (the perfusate). This may be done using miniaturized oxygen electrodes.

10.4.5 Invasive oxygen electrode systems

It is claimed that miniaturized electrodes are relatively non-destructive in tissue. A tissue PO_2 histogram may be constructed by plotting signals from the micro-electrode system against insertion depth of the micro-electrode within the tissue. One reason to pursue research into this type of monitoring system is that change in the shape of the tissue PO_2 histograms will occur, before any other system change, in the presence of tissue hypoxia from any cause (Pranger *et al.*, 1980). Thus such a monitoring device should act as an early warning system. However, the question yet to be answered is in which tissue should it be located?

10.4.6 Non-invasive tissue oxygen measurement systems

The need for a non-invasive system for monitoring tissue oxygenation is thus obvious. The future probably lies in the development of transcutaneous oxygen monitoring devices. Such a monitoring system has been used in the care of sick babies especially after surgery, as a continuous monitor of tissue oxygenation and has been shown to work well and reliably (Peabody *et al.*, 1978). To obtain reasonable results with such a system using a modified polarographic electrode (platinum), and a special membrane with maximal diffusing capacity, the capillaries in the skin beneath the sensor need to be vasodilated (e.g. with local heat). This system enables the polarographic system to 'see' capillary blood and give an index of tissue oxygenation. Apparently the system works comparatively well in normothermic adults, but not efficiently during cardiopulmonary bypass – presumably due to the inevitably low capillary blood flow through the skin during extracorporeal circulation, particularly when hypothermia and non-pulsatile flow are used. These problems may prove difficult to solve unless there is radical re-thinking of cardiopulmonary bypass perfusion technique.

Whatever system of monitoring is developed, it must be easy to handle and calibrate, produce reproducible results and comprehensible data about tissue and blood oxygenation, since extracorporeal circulatory techniques have many potential dangers. These need to be recognized before irreversible hypoxic tissue damage occurs.

10.5 SUMMARY

There is little doubt that extracorporeal circulatory techniques can augment or replace the patient's own pulmonary function for oxygenation. The effect of this procedure on tissue function needs to be monitored continuously, preferably giving guidance as to changes in oxygen consumption, with respect to tissue blood flow. Perhaps the best system, yet to be developed, will be based upon multi-purpose solid-state sensors (Stetter, 1978) measuring PO_2, PCO_2, pH, ion concentrations, in both arterial blood and venous blood, with tissue probes in selected locations, inserted with minimal trauma, measuring the same variables. All signals would be fed into a computer which recognizes trends and gives appropriate information in real time, as a readily understandable signal.

REFERENCES

Bordiuk, J. H., McKenna, P. J., Giannelli, S. R. and Ayers, S. M. (1973) Alterations in 2-3 DPG and O_2 haemoglobin affinity in patients undergoing open heart surgery. *Circulation*, **43** (Suppl. I), 141.

Galletti, P. M., Richardson, P. D., Snider, M. T. and Friedman, L. I. (1972) A standardised method for defining the overall gas transfer performance of artificial lungs. *Trans. Am. Soc. Artif. Int. Org.*, **18**, 389–92.

Hahn, C. E. W., Davis, A. and Albery, W. J. (1975) Electrochemical improvement of the performance of PO_2 electrodes. *Resp. Physiol.*, **25**, 109–33.

Kelman, G. and Nunn, J. F. (1966) Nomograms for correction of blood PO_2, PCO_2, pH and base excess for time and temperature. *J. Appl. Physiol.*, **21**, 1484.

Kessler, M., Hoper, J. and Krumme, B. A. (1976) Monitoring of tissue perfusion and cell function. *Anaesthesiology*, **45**, 184.

Lundsgaard, J. S. and Degn, D. (1981) Use of argon as an internal standard in mass spectrometry for monitoring oxygen in *Monitoring Vital Parameters during Extracorporeal Circulation* (ed. H. P. Kimmich), S. Karger, London.

Moffit, E. A., McLaren, R. G., Imrie, D. D., Allen, T. B., Kinley, C. E. and Barrat, J. (1979) In line blood gas analysis by gas chromatography in patients during and after coronary artery surgery. *Can. Anaesth. Soc. J.*, **26**, 157–61.

Niinikoski, J., Laaksonen, V., Meretoja, O., Jalonen, J. and Inberg, M. (1981)

Oxygen transport to tissues under normovolaemic, moderate and extreme haemodilution during coronary bypass operation. *Ann. Thorac. Surg.*, **31**, 134–9.

Parker, D. (1981) Continuous measurement of blood oxygen tension and saturation in *Monitoring of Vital Parameters during Extracorporeal Circulation* (ed. H. P. Kimmich), S. Karger, London.

Peabody, J. L., Gregory, G. A., Willis, M. M. and Tooley, W. H. (1978) Transcutaneous oxygen tension in sick infants. *Am. Rev. Resp. Dis.*, **118**, 83–6.

Pranger, R. L., Hook, P. H., Elstrodt, J., Kessler, M., Lubbers, D. and Wildevuur, C. (1980) Improved tissue perfusion (PO_2 histograms) in extracorporeal circulation using membrane instead of bubble oxygenators. *J. Thorac. Cardiovasc. Surg.*, **79**, 513–17.

Rosenkranz, E. R., Utley, J. R., Menninger, F. J., Dembitsky, W. P. and Hargens, A. (1980) Interstitial fluid pressure changes during cardio-pulmonary bypass. *Ann. Thorac. Surg.*, **30**, 536–42.

Shepherd, R. B., Kirklin, J. W. (1969) Relation of pulsatile flow to oxygen consumption and other variables during cardio-pulmonary bypass. *J. Thorac. Cardiovasc. Surg.*, **58**, 694.

Stetter, J. R. (1978) A surface chemical view of gas detection. *J. Colloid Interface Soc.*, **64**, 432–43.

Utley, J. R., Wachtel, C., Cain, R. B., Spaw, E. A., Collins, J. C. and Stephen, D. B. (1981) Effect of hypothermia, haemodilution and pump oxygenation on organ water content, blood flow, oxygen delivery and renal function. *Ann. Thorac. Surg.*, **31**, 121–8.

Valeri, C. R., Yarnoz, M., Vecchione, J. J., Dennis, R. C., Anastasi, J., Valeri, D. A., Pilack, L. E., Hechtman, H. B., Emerson, C. P. and Berger, R. L. (1980) Improved O_2 delivery to the myocardium during hypothermia, by perfusion with 2-3 DPG enriched red blood cells. *Ann. Thorac. Surg.*, **30**, 527.

Valeri, C. R., Zaroulis, C. G., Marchionni, L. and Patti, K. L. (1972) A simple method for measuring oxygen content in blood. *J. Lab. Clin. Med.*, **79**, 1035–40.

Zapol, W., Pontoppidan, H., McCullough, N., Schmidt, V., Bland, J. and Kitz, R. (1972) Clinical membrane lung support for acute respiratory insufficiency. *Trans. Am. Soc. Artif. Int. Org.*, **18**, 553–61.

11
Bubble oxygenation

D. W. BETHUNE

The principle of using artificial circulation to perfuse tissue and maintain its function has been recognized for many years. Ingenious machines for the oxygenation of blood were described in the mid nineteenth century. The clinical application of these principles were possible once Landsteiner (1901) had described the blood groups and McLean (1916) had isolated heparin and made the control of coagulation possible.

Gibbon's final machine used a stationary screen oxygenator (Gibbon, 1953). It was a sophisticated expensive device which required several litres of blood to prime the circuit and oxygenator. It provided a high flow of oxygenated blood and remarkably good clinical results were achieved in the early years of intracardiac surgery using Gibbon type oxygenators (Kirklin *et al.*, 1957). However, the capital expense coupled with the problems of resterilizing the oxygenator meant that this type of device could not have supported the explosive growth of cardiac surgery which has occurred in the last 30 years.

The scientific observations by Andreasen and Watson (1952, 1953) on the ability of animals to survive with a greatly reduced cardiac output formed the basis for an extraordinary and unparalleled programme of experimental and clinical work in Minneapolis which in three years resulted in the description of the successful clinical use of a bubble oxygenator. The initial clinical reports in 1954 (Warden *et al.*, 1954) from the Minneapolis team led by Lillehei described the use of cross circulation to support children during intracardiac surgery. The following year (Warden *et al.*, 1955) saw a description of another novel approach using reservoir perfusion. Finally in 1956 (DeWall *et al.*, 1956) a description of a bubble oxygenator appeared together with reports of its successful clinical use. The DeWall–Lillehei bubble oxygenator was a major breakthrough. The simplicity of the basic concept was linked to simple construction and disposability, the oxygenator was made up from plastic tubing which could be disposed of at the end of the case. The numerous bubble oxygenators which have been commercially made since that time have all depended on the same functional compartments (Fig.11.1).

11.1 COMPARTMENTS OF BUBBLE OXYGENATORS

11.1.1 Oxygenating column

The initial compartment consists of a mixing chamber where oxygen is dispersed into the venous blood. The oxygen is passed through small holes in

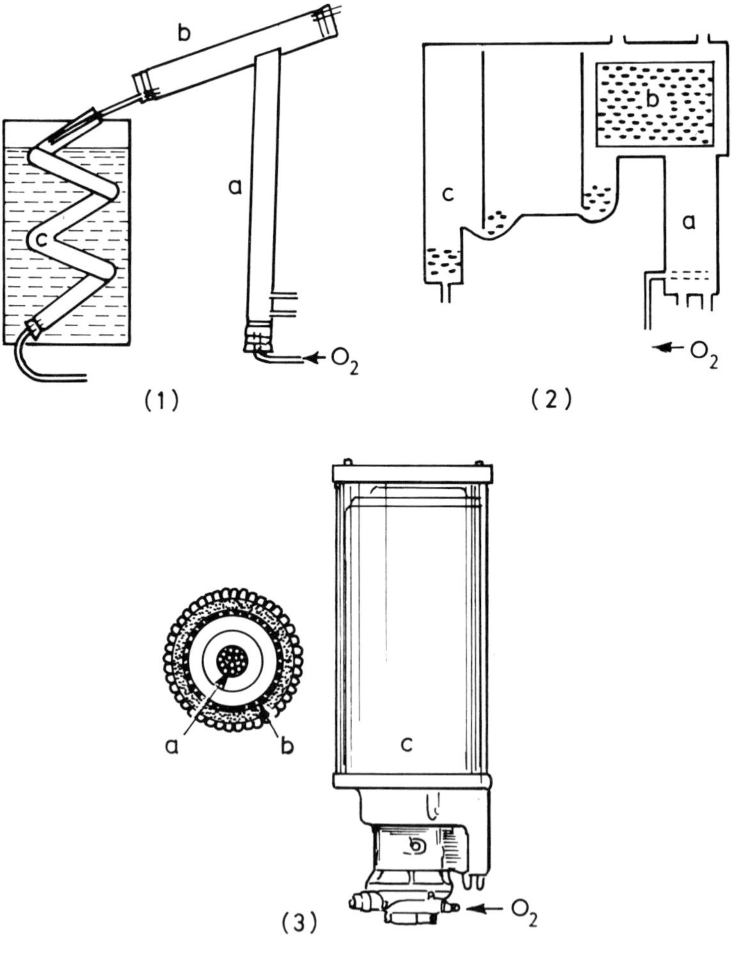

Fig. 11.1 Bubble oxygenators. (1) DeWall–Lillehei pattern (1956); (2) Rygg Kyvsgaard oxygenator (1956); (3) Harvey concentric column (1975). a: Oxygenating column; b: defoaming compartment; c: arterial reservoir.

a plate or tube. The size of the bubbles has a fundamental effect on the function of the device (small bubbles give a larger surface area per unit of oxygen which increases the oxygenating capacity). However, carbon dioxide removal is dependent on the volume of oxygen ventilating the device. A compromise is needed to balance the desire for low oxygen flows and therefore smaller bubbles against the need for efficient carbon dioxide removal. There has been a regrettable tendency for manufacturers to equate low oxygen to blood flow ratios with oxygenator 'efficiency'. This has led to the production of devices which can just maintain homeostasis at normothermia when used with 100% oxygen. Such a device may lead to problems in clinical practice as moderate hypothermia during perfusion is routinely used in most cardiac surgical units. During hypothermia at a constant PCO_2 the total carbon dioxide content of the body will rise as a result of the increase in solubility. In addition, many perfusionists maintain a relative hypercarbia during hypothermic perfusions to ensure some degree of cerebral vasodilatation. Recent experimental work in our unit has shown that during clinical perfusions when normocapnoea (corrected for temperature) has been maintained, the ratio between carbon dioxide elimination and oxygen uptake at 30°C is 'normal' at about 0.8. On rewarming the ratio alters as the blood warms and carbon dioxide elimination exceeds oxygen consumption. Ratios in the order of 1.4:1 have been observed during the active rewarming phase and with some modern bubble oxygenators it has proved impossible to maintain physiologically normal blood gas tensions. Maintaining the PO_2 in the range 12.5–15 kPa results in a high PCO_2 and increasing the ventilation to maintain a normal PCO_2 results in an unacceptably high PO_2. These experimental results would suggest that manufacturers should aim to produce devices which have the capacity to exchange more carbon dioxide than oxygen at a given oxygen flow rather than devices which have small bubbles and a limited capacity for carbon dioxide removal. The importance of the total dissolved gas tensions will be considered in the section on clinical use. Changing the size of the bubble column will alter the characteristics of the oxygenating compartment. In most commercial devices the column size is fixed and with hard shell devices the complexities introduced by having a variable column may outweigh any advantage, though research in this field is continuing (Tamiya *et al.*, 1982). In the bubble oxygenators constructed from sheet film it is comparatively easy to adjust the column size by using external slats.

11.1.2 Defoaming compartment

The mixture of blood and gas which emerges from the bubble column must be defoamed. The method established by DeWall and Lillehei has not been altered fundamentally. An open sponge or mesh coated with antifoam is placed in the path of the oxygenated blood. The defoaming stage must have sufficient capacity to cope with the rated blood flow of the device. The defoamer is a critical part of the oxygenator and defects in its preparation cannot be determined by visual inspection. For this reason the methodology used by manufacturers to ensure a uniform coating of the mesh is critical. In the early use of bubble oxygenators worries regarding the ability of the defoaming column to function for anything other than a short period were a major limiting factor in their use for patients expected to need more than 30 minutes of cardiopulmonary bypass. That this is no longer the case probably reflects both improvements in the manufacturing process and the undoubted increase in the expertise of perfusionists.

11.1.3 The arterial reservoir

The final compartment of any bubble oxygenator is a reservoir used to store the arterial blood. The design of the reservoir must allow larger microbubbles to float away from the outlet port, and there must be a smooth flow of blood through the reservoir since any turbulence or sudden change in level may cause splashing and the generation of further bubbles. The outlet from the reservoir must be designed to prevent vortex formation which would entrain air. The original helical reservoir on the DeWall–Lillehei oxygenator (DeWall *et al.*, 1956) functioned well at the low flows used in the original technique. Attempts to make the technique more physiological by increasing the flow (Diesh *et al.*, 1957) probably failed because at higher flows microbubbles would not be able to float up against the increased downward flow of blood. Such failure to allow upward movement of bubbles resulted in major gaseous microembolization. The Gott adaptation (Gott *et al.*, 1957) in sheet film of the three-dimensional spiral of the original DeWall–Lillehei, while successfully used for many years, had the failing that if the level in the reservoir fell there was a waterfall effect at each turn of the arterial reservoir.

Considering the basic simplicity of the bubble oxygenator the range of physical appearance is now extremely wide. Only one design from the early devices has stood the test of time virtually unchanged, the original Rygg device (Rygg and Kyvsgaard, 1956). This device is still commercially available as the Polystan Venotherm Oxygenator (Fig. 11.2) the only visible change being the incorporation of an integral heat exchanger. The fitting of heat exchangers as an integral part of bubble oxygenators has not only made for simpler circuits but when they are placed in the oxygenating column heat exchange becomes much more efficient. The Polystan bubble oxygenator was at one time available with an integral heat exchanger fitted in either the arterial reservoir or in the oxygenating column. The latter siting increased the efficiency of heat exchange by 60% (Bethune *et al.*, 1975).

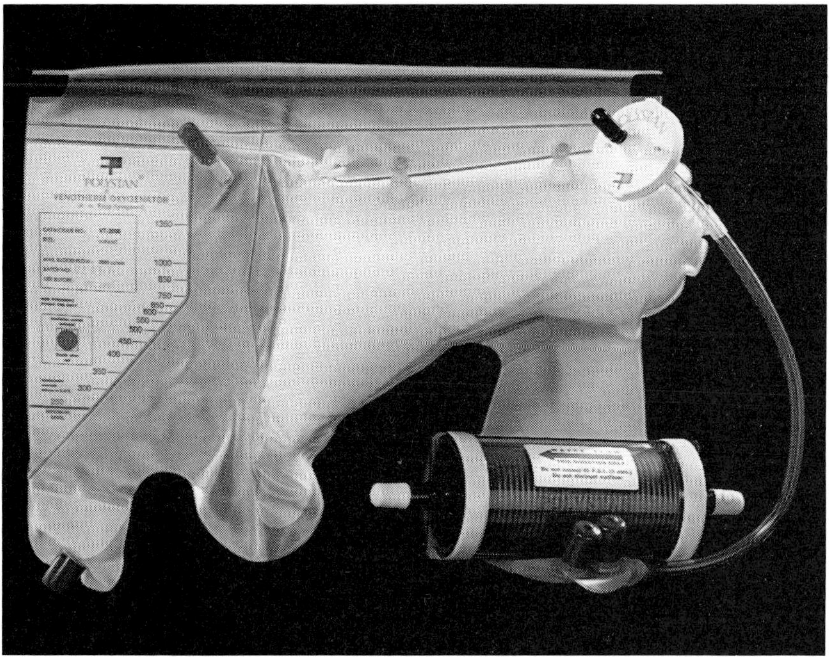

Fig. 11.2 Polystan Venotherm oxygenator.

11.2 CLINICAL USE OF BUBBLE OXYGENATORS

With all devices comprehensive 'Instructions for use' will be provided by the manufacturer. These should be studied carefully before any equipment is assembled. There are however general principles which apply to all bubble oxygenators. In practice the construction of a particular device may mean that a set method of use or assembly must be followed.

11.2.1 Priming

The technique used to prime an oxygenator will have a considerable effect on the volume, tension and composition of any dissolved gases. Following the studies of Branthwaite (1975) which identified the start of cardiopulmonary bypass as a time when marked changes occur in the electrical activity of the brain, and the demonstration of the large number of gaseous microemboli originating from the oxygenator at the start of bypass (Clark *et al.*, 1976), techniques have evolved for priming which result in the lowest possible gas content and tension (Bethune, 1976). Details of the technique may be applied to any oxygenator or circuit. The device is flushed with carbon dioxide to

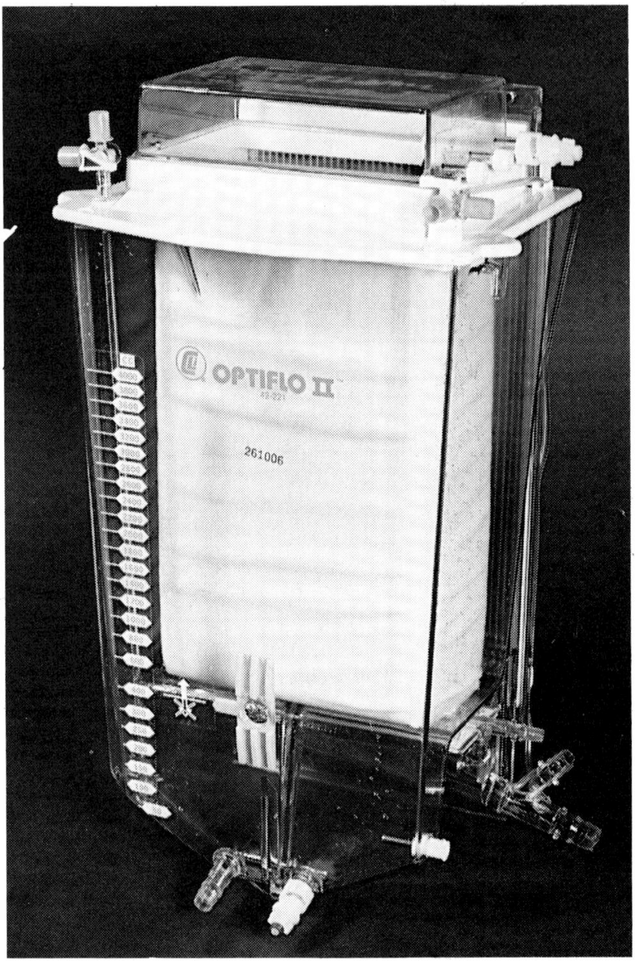

Fig. 11.3 The Cobe Optiflo II bubble oxygenator.

remove the relatively insoluble air and replace it with a more soluble gas. The fluids used to prime the circuit are stored at 50°C as the volume of gas in solution is less at higher temperatures. The oxygenator and circuit are primed via a port in a dependent part of the circuit slowly and with care to avoid splashing and turbulence. If possible the oxygenator and circuit are primed without filling the bubble column. If it is essential to prime including the bubble column the gas flow should be kept to a minimum and after a brief circulation the fluid should be drained from the column. Even when there has been no circulation with gas flow and all other precautions have been taken it is still possible to detect gaseous emboli in the patient's circulation at the start of bypass. For this reason we believe that nitrous oxide should, if it is being used as a component of the pre-bypass anaesthetic, be discontinued at least 10 minutes before bypass commences. The choice of priming fluids is the subject of Chapter 14. Our preference for adult patients is a crystalloid prime with added mannitol (0.5 g kg^{-1}) to increase the oncotic pressure to 360 mosmol.

11.2.2 Initiation of cardiopulmonary bypass

The speed with which cardiopulmonary bypass is instituted should be controlled to avoid precipitate falls in the PO_2 of the blood leaving the

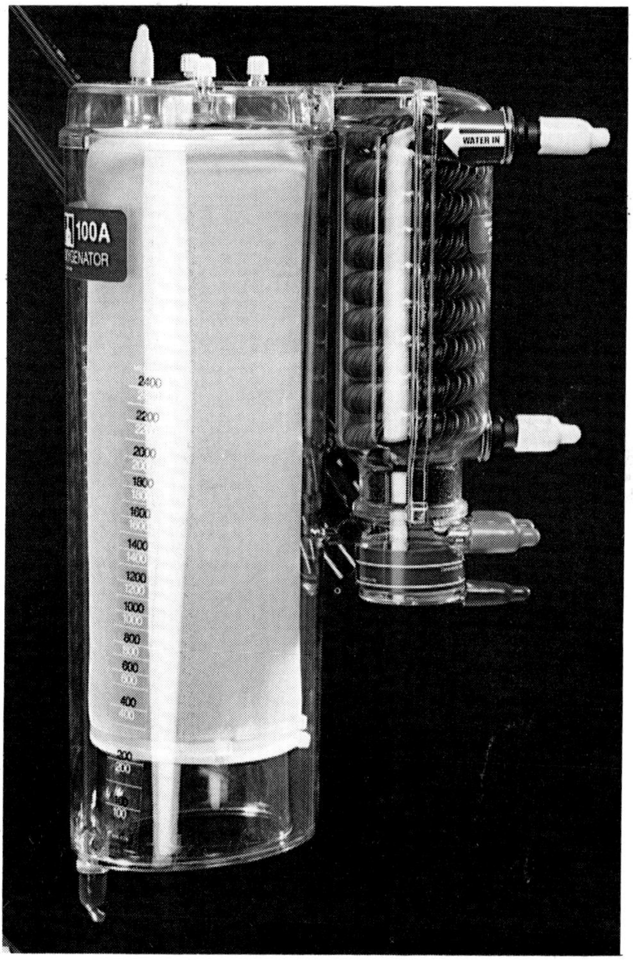

Fig. 11.4 The Shiley 100A bubble oxygenator.

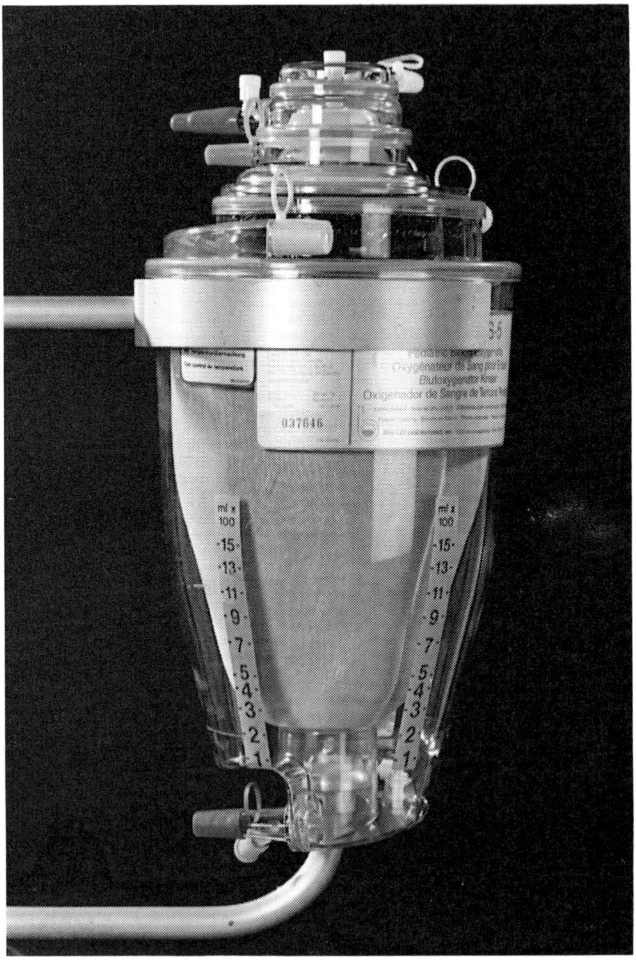

Fig. 11.5 The Bentley Bos-5 paediatric bubble oxygenator.

oxygenator. In virtually all bubble oxygenators a significant part of the gas exchange occurs in the film phase which is established in the defoamer. This film phase takes a minute or two to develop after bypass has started and the improvement in oxygenating capacity can be very marked with some sequential devices (Rygg, 1973).

11.2.3 Bubble oxygenation during established cardiopulmonary bypass

During established cardiopulmonary bypass the level in the arterial reservoir should be maintained to allow a reasonable reaction time for the perfusionist.

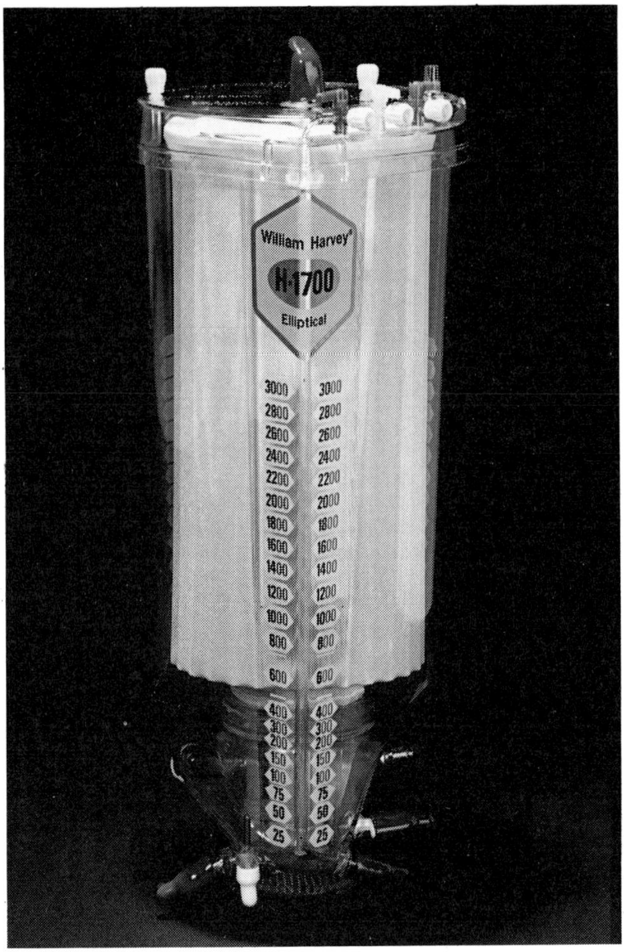

Fig. 11.6 Harvey-1700 bubble oxygenator.

The importance of an adequate arterial reservoir level in controlling the number of gaseous microemboli has been quantified by Pearson *et al.* (1980) (see Chapter 18). A greater volume in the arterial reservoir will increase the transit time of the blood and allow more time for gaseous microemboli to be absorbed or in the case of larger bubbles allow them to float away from the arterial outlet. A further reason for maintaining a reasonable level is to minimize any possibility of vortex formation and entrainment of gas. With rigid reservoirs some form of level alarm, possibly incorporating a switch to control the arterial pump, is mandatory. With collapsible reservoirs of the Rygg Polystan type the wall of the reservoir will be sucked onto the arterial outlet and effectively prevent massive air embolism.

11.2.4 Control of gas tensions during cardiopulmonary bypass

All extracorporeal circuits used during open-heart surgery are liable to contain gaseous microemboli in the perfusate. Perfusions should be conducted in a manner which will reduce the number of such microemboli to a minimum and provide an environment which will encourage the free gas to pass into solution. The subject of the causation of gaseous microemboli is covered extensively in Chapter 18, however as such emboli are invariable with bubble oxygenators it is worthwhile reiterating those points which govern the length of time a bubble will continue to exist.

Factors affecting the lifespan of gaseous microemboli include:

(a) Size of gaseous microemboli.
(b) Time delay source/tissues.
(c) Pressure of gas in bubble and dissolved gas tension.
(d) Characteristics of gases in bubble and solution.

(a) Bubble size

The smaller the bubble the less gas there is to absorb and there is a proportionately greater surface area and higher internal pressure in the bubble from surface tension effects.

(b) Time delay

Increasing circuit volume allows more time for the gas to absorb. This effect must partly explain the reduction in bubble counts across arterial line filters as with appropriate gas tensions no free gas appears in the filter even during prolonged perfusions. The experimental studies by Patterson *et al.* (1971) demonstrated the effectiveness of the device they used. Unfortunately their device had an internal volume of 400 ml in addition to the filter screen and they did not consider the effect of the time delay they were imposing which with the 1.5 l min^{-1} flow would amount to 16 s. It is therefore not surprising that they achieved a 95% reduction in bubble activity. To achieve a similar delay in an average clinical perfusion a volume of over one litre would be needed. In studies on clinical perfusion circuits it has been shown that part of the reduction in bubble activity across a 40 μm arterial line filter may be achieved by increasing the tubing length to impose a similar time delay on the arterial blood.

(c) Pressure of the gas in the bubble and dissolved gas tension

The major factor affecting the lifespan of a gaseous microembolus is the gradient for absorption of the gas in the bubble. The internal pressure of the gas in the bubble is forcing the gas into solution and this is opposed by the tension of the dissolved gas in the surrounding fluid. This balance will vary at differing points in the circulation and at various times during the perfusion.

The conditions during established bypass in the arterial line should be particularly favourable for absorption of gaseous microemboli. The pressure exerted on the gas in the bubble is atmospheric pressure plus the 'line' pressure and a smaller component as a result of surface tension. Due to the resistance of the arterial cannula the line pressure during an average perfusion is around 26 kPa and the total pressure exerted on the gas in the bubble is therefore over 126 kPa (see Equation b p. 172). This pressure tends to force the gas into solution and is opposed by the total dissolved gas tension. The total dissolved gas tension during a well-conducted bypass should be no more than 26 kPa. The only gases present in appreciable amounts will be oxygen and carbon dioxide. Studies using gas chromatography confirmed that even when nitrous oxide had formed part of the anaesthetic mixture immediately prior to bypass, after 10 minutes its partial pressure was less than 5 kPa and dissolved nitrogen could not be detected even though cardiotomy suction was in use. Therefore for all practical purposes the total dissolved gas tension on established bypass can be taken to be the sum of the partial pressures of oxygen and carbon dioxide if no other gas is used to ventilate the oxygenator. This emphasizes the importance of maintaining a physiological partial pressure of oxygen during perfusion. A PO_2 of 20 kPa is sufficient to saturate the haemoglobin and any rise in the PO_2 will only produce a minimal increase in the quantity of oxygen carried. In the early years of cardiopulmonary bypass a relationship between sudden postoperative death and very high levels of arterial PO_2 on bypass was observed. It was postulated that this was due to oxygen toxicity but that view is hardly tenable as the syndrome described bore no relationship to the recognized toxic effects of oxygen. A more rational explanation is that the 'hyperventilation' of the oxygenator produced more microbubbles which persisted due to the lowered gradient for absorption resulting from the high PO_2 and consequent high total dissolved gas tension. Under these circumstances the persistent bubbles would impact in the vascular system producing microembolic damage and causing the syndrome described by the authors. The idea of oxygen toxicity on bypass has even led to some misguided interest in ventilating bubble oxygenators with a mixture of oxygen and an 'inert gas' (Meager and Swan, 1971; Groom *et al.*, 1982). In the context of bubble oxygenators this is an unsound idea. A greater total gas flow will be needed which will cause more trauma and microbubble formation. In addition the inert gas will pass into solution raising the total dissolved gas tension and retarding the absorption of the free gas in the microbubbles. The force tending to cause the gas in a bubble to dissolve will vary during the bypass and at different points in the circulation. The worst case is that of a bubble from the priming fluid injected into the patient's aorta at the start of bypass. The balance of forces is shown in Equation a. The gas bubble arising from the operative site which is ejected from the heart when bypass is discontinued is in an identical pressure relationship. The position of these bubbles can be contrasted with the bubble in the arterial line during a well-conducted perfusion (Equation b). It is obvious that gaseous microemboli at the start and end of bypass will have a much longer life and greater capacity for causing damage.

(i) Equation a.

Bubble in patient's aorta at the beginning of bypass and after bypass has been discontinued.

$$\underset{\text{in bubble}}{\text{Pressure of gas}} - \underset{\text{tension}}{\text{total dissolved gas}} = \text{gradient for absorption}$$

$$(\text{AP} + \text{MPP} + \text{ST}) - (Pag + PO_2 + PCO_2) = \text{gradient for absorption}$$

$$(100 + 10 + 1.5) - (70 + 20 + 5) = 16.5 \text{ kPa}$$

(ii) Equation b.

Bubble in arterial line of heart–lung machine during established bypass.

$$\underset{\text{in bubble}}{\text{Pressure of gas}} - \underset{\text{tension}}{\text{total dissolved gas}} = \text{gradient for absorption}$$

$$(\text{AP} + \text{LP} + \text{ST}) - (PO_2 + PCO_2) = \text{gradient for absorption}$$

$$(100 + 26 + 1.5) - (20 + 6) \qquad = 101.5 \text{ kPa}$$

where:

AP = atmospheric pressure; MPP = mean perfusion pressure in patient; ST = surface tension effect (approx. for 40 μm bubble); *Pag* = partial pressure of anaesthetic agents; LP = line pressure. (Sum of gas tensions in arterial blood before and after bypass less than atmospheric due to venous admixture effect.)

(d) Effect of the characteristics of the gas in the bubble and in solution

The composition of the gas in the bubble will have a marked effect on the speed with which it passes into solution. Oxygen, because it combines with haemoglobin, behaves as a very soluble gas at physiological PO_2 levels. Carbon dioxide is intrinsically very soluble which makes it useful for flushing circuits prior to fluid priming. Nitrogen and other 'inert' gases (including helium, which has been specifically recommended as a diluent gas to allow control of the PO_2 in 'efficient' bubble oxygenators (Groom *et al.*, 1982)) are relatively insoluble. The gas trapped in the heart after cardiotomy will be air (80% nitrogen) and its low solubility coupled with the unfavourable pressure gradients after bypass (Equation a) will mean that bubbles from this source will have a long life. Carbon dioxide flooding of the operative site has been recommended to reduce the effects of this potential hazard (Burbank *et al.*, 1965). Direct evidence of gas embolism is rare apart from coronary air which can be inferred from sudden ischaemic ECG changes when coming off bypass (or later). In gross cases the air can be seen in the vessels. The duration of the ischaemic changes can be reduced by giving a vasopressor. The rise in arterial pressure will force the gas bubble further down the vascular tree and increase the rate of absorption.

Of the gases which may be dissolved in the patient's blood the most significant must be nitrous oxide as in comparative terms it is very soluble. In our unit we found that discontinuing nitrous oxide 10 minutes before going on bypass reduced the incidence of unexplained changes in the cerebral function monitor trace (Bethune, 1980). This effect of nitrous oxide is not surprising. If a patient is ventilated with a mixture containing 66% nitrous oxide a bubble of air or oxygen would be expected to triple in volume. This effect of nitrous oxide has been confirmed in relation to venous air embolism (Munson and Merrick, 1966).

11.3 LIMITATIONS ON THE USE OF BUBBLE OXYGENATORS

Bubble oxygenators are intrinsically not biocompatible. The blood/gas interface represents an unphysiological state. There are numerous studies which demonstrate this fact in the context of open-heart surgery. Even more convincing evidence of the effect of an isolated blood/gas interface can be found in studies on decompression sickness. The demonstration by Lee *et al.* (1961) and Lee and Hairston (1971) of a layer of electrokinetic force at the blood/gas interface explains many of the phenomena associated with bubble oxygenators in clinical practice. The electrokinetic forces at the blood/gas interface tend to orientate the proteins so that their hydrophilic groups are in the blood phase leaving the non-polar groups sticking out into the gaseous phase. This distortion disrupts the normal configuration of the proteins, alters their biological specificity and causes functional alteration. The denatured proteins resulting from the surface activity of the bubbles cause platelet aggregation and in addition some of the altered proteins acquire enhanced biological activity. In this way the surface activation at the blood/gas interface leads to activation of the complement system and possible release of kinins. Other factors causing damage to blood during clinical cardiopulmonary bypass are dealt with in Chapter 15, but it is the reaction of blood to free gas interface which is the principal limiting factor in the use of bubble oxygenation for longer perfusions.

11.4 THE FUTURE OF BUBBLE OXYGENATORS

If one accepts the fact that bubble oxygenation is less compatible with blood than membrane oxygenation some rationale has to be advanced to explain their continued use in large numbers.

The first point must be that for periods of cardiopulmonary bypass of less than two hours duration no clinically significant difference can be demonstrated between membrane and bubble oxygenation. Bubble oxygenators are easier to set up and debubble. If designed correctly, there is no major problem in controlling the gas tensions with acceptable accuracy. The essence of the bubble oxygenator is that the surface area available for oxygenation is variable dependent on the gas flow. Within limits this means that the oxygen content of the blood leaving the device can be regulated by adjusting the flow of oxygen ventilating the device. If the device has been designed to allow adequate CO_2 removal under all clinical situations the CO_2 level can be regulated by adding a small percentage of CO_2 to the oxygen supply. In the immediate future the recent development of commercially available devices which can control the oxygen flow to give a predetermined arterial oxygen content, derived from saturation or PO_2 measurement, will enable perfusionists to provide less traumatic oxygenation with bubble devices. An additional advantage of autoregulation will be in allowing easier comparison between devices of the damage to the blood components at identical levels of oxygenation.

REFERENCES

Andreasen, A. T. and Watson, F. (1952) Experimental cardiovascular surgery. *Br. J. Surg.*, **39**, 548.

Andreasen, A. T. and Watson, F. (1953) Experimental cardiovascular surgery: Discussion of results so far obtained and report on experiments concerning donor circulation *Br. J. Surg.*, **41**, 195.

Bethune, D. W. (1976) Organ damage after open heart surgery. (Letter) *Lancet*, **ii**, 1410.

Bethune, D. W. (1980) The life span of gaseous microemboli and organ damage. In *Psychic and Neurological Dysfunctions after Open-heart Surgery* (eds. F. Speidel and G. Rodewald), Georg Thieme Verlag, Stuttgart, pp. 92–9.

Bethune, D. W., Gill, R. D. and Wheeldon, D. R. (1975) Performance of heat exchangers used in whole body perfusion circuits. *Thorax*, **30**, 569–73.

Branthwaite, M. A. (1975) Prevention of neurological damage during open heart surgery. *Thorax*, **28**, 464.

Burbank, A., Ferguson, T. B., Burford, T. H. (1965) Carbon dioxide flooding of the chest in open heart surgery. *J. Thorac. Cardiovasc. Surg.*, **50**, 691.

Clark, R. E., Dietz, D. R. and Miller, J. G. (1976) Continuous detection of microemboli during cardiopulmonary bypass in animals and man. *Circulation*, **54**, 74.

DeWall, R. A., Warden, H. E., Gott, V. L., Read, R. C., Varco, R. L. and Lillehei, C. W. (1956) Total body perfusion for open cardiotomy utlizing the bubble oxygenator. *J. Thorac. Surg.*, **32**, 591.

Diesh, G., Flynn, P. J., Marable, S. A., Mulder, D. G., Schmutzer, K. J., Longmire, W. P. Jr. and Moloney, J. V. Jr. (1957) Comparison of low (azygos) and high flow principles of extracorporeal circulation employing a bubble oxygenator. *Surgery*, **42**, 67–72.

Gibbon, J. H. (1953) Application of a mechanical heart-lung apparatus to cardiac surgery. In *Recent Advances in Cardiovascular Physiology and Surgery*. University of Minnesota, Minneapolis, p. 107.

Gott, V. L., DeWall, R. A., Paneth, M., Zudhi, M. N., Weirich, W., Varco, R. L. and Lillehei, C. W. (1957) A self-contained disposable oxygenator of plastic sheet for intra-cardiac surgery. *Thorax*, **12**, 1–9.

Groom, R. C., Kramer, M. and Reed, C. C. (1982) Use of a sweep gas in bubble oxygenators to obtain independent control of blood carbon dioxide levels. *Proc. Am. Acad. Cardiovasc. Perf.*, **3**, 69–72.

Kirklin, J. W., Patrick, R. T. and Theye, R. A. (1957) Theory and practice in the use of a pump-oxygenator for open intracardiac surgery. *Thorax*, **12**, 93.

Landsteiner, K. (1901) Uber Agglutinationserscheinungen normalen menschlischen Blutes. *Wien Klin. Wchnschr.*, **14**, 1132.

Lee, W. H. and Hairston, P. (1971) Structural effects on blood proteins at the blood gas interface. *Fedn Proc. Fedn Am. Socs Exp Biol.*, **30**, 1615.

Lee, W. H., Krumhaar, D., Fonkalsrud, E. W., Schjeide, C. A. and Maloney, J. V. (1961) Denaturation of plasma proteins as a cause of morbidity and death after intracardiac operations. *Surgery*, **50**, 29.

McLean, J. (1916) The thromboplastic action of cephalin. *Am. J. Physiol.*, **41**, 250.

Meager, D. and Swan, H. J. C. (1971) Oxygenation of blood with low oxygen gas mixtures by means of a bubble oxygenator. *J. Thorac. Cardiovasc. Surg.*, **61**, 729.

Munson, E. S. and Merrick, H. C. (1966) Effects of nitrous oxide on venous air embolism. *Anesthesiology*, **27**, 783.

Patterson, R. H., Kessler, J. and Bergland, R. M. (1971) A filter to prevent cerebral damage during experimental cardiopulmonary bypass. *Surg. Gynecol. Obstet.*, **132**, 71.

Pearson, D. T., Carter, R. F., Hammo, M. B. and Waterhouse, P. S. (1980) Gaseous microemboli during open heart surgery. In *Towards Safer Cardiac Surgery* (ed. D. B. Longmore) MTP Press, Lancaster.

Rygg, I. H. (1973) *Studies in Extracorporeal Circulation*. Fadls Forlag, Copenhagen.

Rygg, I. H. and Kyvsgaard, E. (1956) A disposable polyethylene oxygenator system applied in a heart–lung machine. *Acta Chir. Scand.*, **112**, 433–7.

Tamiya, T., Kitagawa, S., Yamashiro, T., Takemasa, A., Sadamitsu, T., Nishizawa, T., Suzuki, I. and Shiramatsu, K. (1982) The TM bubble oxygenator: Development and clinical application. *Artificial Organs*, **6**, 198–204.

Warden, H. E., Cohen, M., Read, R. C. and Lillehei, C. W. (1954) Controlled cross-circulation for open intracardiac surgery. *J. Thorac. Surg.*, **28**, 331.

Warden, H. E., Read, R. C., DeWall, R. A., Aust, J. B., Cohen, M., Ziegler, N. R., Varco, R. L. and Lillehei, C. W. (1955) Direct vision intracardiac surgery by means of a reservoir of 'arterialized venous' blood. *J. Thorac. Surg.*, **30**, 649.

12
Membrane oxygenation

E. CONVERSE PEIRCE

12.1 INTRODUCTION

The primary purpose of this chapter is to explore the advantages and disadvantages of membrane devices in perfusion for current and future heart surgery. Fifteen or 20 years ago, when essentially all perfusions for heart operations employed an oxygenator with a direct blood to gas interface (bubble, disk, or screen), membrane lungs were of small capacity and rarely used clinically. At that time patients had all too frequent major complications, including brain damage and death, that could reasonably be related to embolic phenomena (antifoam, gas, fibrin, fat, etc.) or bleeding problems. These things were gradually identified as being (in many cases) the result of damage to protein and various blood cells by the raw blood to gas interface. It came to be an accepted belief, supported also by encouraging reports, that eventual wide use of the membrane lung (when at last a full capacity device) would dramatically moderate these problems and make perfusion for heart surgery enviably safe and sure.

Since that time excellent membrane devices have been built for full perfusion support, even at normal body temperature, and they have gradually come to be used in an appreciable number of clinical heart cases. These devices have also lived up to their expectations of less blood trauma. It has been possible, for example with extracorporeal membrane oxygenation (ECMO), to sustain life in the presence of lung failure for periods of several weeks (Peirce, 1981), something not possible with a bubble or other raw interface device (see Chapter 13). At the same time, the bubble oxygenator has also evolved to a safer device and has become dominant clinically. Perfusion practices have improved so that, for example, high gas to blood flow rates are now seldom used to enhance oxygen exchange and embolic problems in bubble oxygenation have been further reduced with appropriate microfiltration (Bartlett and Gazzaniga, 1981). In addition, the major contribution of suctioned shed blood to the overall problem has become widely appreciated and slow hesitant steps in containing this source of trouble have been introduced. The net result is that using bubble devices for perfusion has been progressively much safer and the advantage of using a membrane lung, for short-term perfusions where shed blood is saved, is less certain and more difficult to demonstrate. It is not surprising then that a considerable controversy has arisen with many maintaining that membrane devices are more expensive, require more time and effort, and, at best, offer only marginal superiority (Kayser, 1974). Failure to increase the clinical use of membrane lungs more rapidly, coupled with the discovery that ECMO is not a panacea for acute respiratory failure (Zapol *et al.*, 1979; Peirce, 1981) has had important commercial repercussions. Several good disposable membrane devices (e.g. Landé-Edwards and General Electric–Peirce) are no longer manufactured and development and introduction of new devices were for years markedly slowed.

It has been easy to believe that clinical perfusion is highly developed, eminently safe, and requiring only more and better trained perfusion personnel, and perhaps a few minor embellishments to be optimal. Unfortunately, clinical perfusions are still potentially very dangerous. A few moments distraction, the wrong reaction to some new situation, a sudden component malfunction – any such event may trigger a catastrophe in the form of a massive gas embolism. A recent retrospective survey by Stoney *et al.* (1980), of approximately 375 000 perfusions for heart surgery, recorded 429 instances of gas embolism (recognized and reported), an incidence of more than one case per 1000 perfusions. There were 92 deaths (21%) and 61 recognized instances of permanent neurological damage (14%). Similarly, the survey found a very high incidence of postoperative bleeding (more than 1 in 800 cases) with 34% mortality and 6% permanent injury. Blood damage by the oxygenator is almost certainly a major aetiologic factor. Unfortunately, it is frequently not perceived to be in the best interest of the surgical team, the hospital, the device manufacturer, etc. to search for, record, or publish the incidence of complications. Perfusion is still highly unphysiological. It regularly results in measurable blood damage and frequently in temporary organ dysfunction. For patients who end up not quite the same mentally (e.g. altered affect, emotionally unstable, with poorer memory), electing to have coronary artery bypass may have been a very bad bargain. Insofar as the problems are due to actual organic damage, and that is the most likely possibility (Tufo *et al.*, 1970; Dubin *et al.*, 1979), they should be largely preventable with more physiological perfusion. This chapter will attempt to marshal what is currently known of the differences between membrane and bubble devices (a task complicated by a shifting definition of what constitutes a membrane, see next section) with the belief that conversion to a more physiological and safer technique of oxygenation should have a very high order of priority even if this means a small additional expense and a little more effort. There will also be a number of other advantages (see Section 12.4).

12.2 HISTORY OF THE MEMBRANE LUNG*

Although artificial oxygenation was demonstrated by Hooke in 1667 and the concept of extracorporeal oxygenation was suggested by Le Gallois in 1812, development of oxygenators was slow until the first attempt at cardio-pulmonary bypass by Dennis *et al.* in 1951 using a modification of a filming device described by Gibbon in 1937. By 1955 prototypes of most of the various kinds of oxygenators had been tried clinically. Based on the observation in 1944 by Kolff and Berk that blood in the coil kidney became oxygenated during passage, Kolff designed the first membrane oxygenator, a very small capacity polyethylene coil that was, surprisingly, used successfully by Effler *et al.* (1956). Clowes *et al.* (1956) described the clinical use of a large sandwich type membrane lung employing at first very large surfaces of polyethylene and later more permeable teflon membranes. ('Oxygenator' is used more conventionally but 'lung' is more descriptive of function. Here the term of the developer will generally be followed.) In 1958 Clowes reported the use of this device in nearly 100 cases. Although manufactured briefly, the Clowes lung was bulky, hard to assemble, and prone to leak. It was never widely used but it inspired the development of many other oxygenators.

From the start, the membrane lung had an influence out of proportion to its clinical use. Clowes firmly believed it to be much less traumatic to blood and much safer, a concept that became firmly entrenched. The special mystique of the membrane lung was well expressed by Melrose in 1959: 'Of the artificial systems, the most attractive is that where, in imitation of the natural pulmonary anatomy, a membrane separates blood from gas.'

In early membrane devices using teflon, simplicity (crudeness of design) tended to produce a relative balance in oxygen and carbon dioxide exchange. The latter was determined almost entirely by the characteristics of the membrane and a reasonable blood PCO_2 and was low (Table 12.1). Oxygen being much less diffusible in the blood phase than carbon dioxide (O_2/CO_2 solubility ratio 1:25), but being available in the gas phase at a high pressure (close to 760 mmHg (100 kPa)), was readily diffusible through the membrane. Oxygen exchange was determined by the blood film characteristics (dimensions and uniformity) and, because of the usual crude design, was low enough to keep the two gases in balance. There was little advantage in building more efficient oxygen-exchange devices until more permeable membranes became available (Peirce and Peirce, 1963).

A smaller 'modified' Clowes lung using teflon was developed by Peirce and

* For additional historical details see Galletti and Brecher (1962), Peirce (1967), Drinker (1972), Nosé (1973) and Peirce (1973).

others between 1958 and 1968. It was used clinically, especially with hypothermia (Peirce, 1969). This lung was later modified to use a patterned membrane 'a copolymer of dimethyl silicone and polycarbonate' (Peirce and Dibelius, 1968; Peirce, 1970) and was manufactured for several years for clinical use (Kirsh *et al.*, 1973; Geelhoed *et al.*, 1975) by The General Electrical Co. This device incorporated a heat exchanger and, if two were used in parallel, had enough capacity for full flow normothermic perfusion (reference blood flow for single 3 m^2 unit about 3 l min^{-1} (Peirce, 1976). See Section 12.4.1.) It was also used for long-term ECMO for periods up to 21 days though proteinoid deposition on membranes and in ports was sometimes troublesome necessitating that lungs be changed at intervals of one to ten days (Peirce, 1977).

Kolobow and Bowman (1963) described a coiled silicone lung reminiscent of a Kolff kidney. For a long time clinical application was principally for extended ECMO (Kolobow *et al.*, 1971; White *et al.*, 1971; Zapol *et al.*, 1979) but the design has proven very durable and the device is being used increasingly for heart surgery (see Sci Med™ in Section 12.5.3).

The clinical use of a semidisposable, round, sandwich silicone lung was described by Bramson *et al.* in 1965 (Hallikainen Instruments, Richmond, CA). This superbly designed, full-capacity machine (reference blood flow more than 3 l min^{-1} (Bartlett and Gazzaniga, 1981) see Section 12.4.1) was used in hundreds of heart cases and, by Hill *et al.* (1968, 1972) in the first successful long-term ECMO patients. The use of this oxygenator has recently been reviewed by Bramsom *et al.* (1981). They report a clinical experience of more than 500 heart operations and 35 instances of use for acute respiratory insufficiency, the longest case being more than 20 days. A fully disposable modification, using microporous polypropylene, was later manufactured by Cutter Laboratories (Hill *et al.*, 1975) but has not apparently been marketed.

An additional Clowes-type lung using silicone membrane was developed by Landé. First reported by Landé in 1967 (Landé *et al.*, 1970), this was manufactured by Edwards Laboratories and was used in many countries for clincal heart surgery for nearly a decade, especially in children (Carleson *et al.*, 1973; Geirab and Semb, 1974; Wright *et al.*, 1975; Birnbaum *et al.*, 1979; Feuchel *et al.*, 1979). Though each unit was relatively small in capacity (reference blood flow of under 2 l min^{-1}) multiple parallel use was very satisfactory for adult heart surgery or prolonged ECMO (Landé *et al.*, 1970; Carleson *et al.*, 1973). It is most unfortunate that this excellent, well designed and popular device is no longer available.

Capillary configurations have included devices with blood outside the capillaries (see Table 12.2) and inside the capillaries. The latter type was studied by Dorson *et al.* (1968), De Filippi *et al.* (1968), and Marx (1970) who pulsed the blood and dispersed the gas in oil. Several commercial models were developed as the Dow-Cordis Oxygenator in the early 1970s. Although very compact and with excellent gas transfer properties these were ultimately unsatisfactory because of a tendency for the capillary outlets to become clogged by aggregates of platelets activated in their passage through the devices (Galletti *et al.*, 1971).

The development of 'expanded' or 'microporous' membranes has had an important effect on membrane device development. Known for many years and used widely for filters, their possible use in oxygenators was investigated by McCaughan *et al.* and reported in 1969. Further promising preclinical work was published by Eisman *et al.* (1972). In 1975 Bartlett *et al.* reported favourable haematological responses to prolonged perfusions with microporous membranes. The membrane devices so far mentioned are limited in their function by cardon dioxide transfer (Table 12.1) since to simulate the natural lung, the membrane should have high gas transmission and be 20 to 30 times more permeable to carbon dioxide than to oxygen. That is a major reason why developing large capacity membrane devices has been such a problem. Of the available materials, only methyl silicone has really worked and it has a CO_2/O_2 ratio of only about five to one. Relatively large areas of membrane are required. For example, 4.5 m^2 of 2–3 μm silicone is required for a reference blood flow of about 6 l min^{-1}. Microporous teflon and polypropylene have no inherent limit to carbon dioxide transfer (Table 12.1). The new 'vorticeal' microporous oxygenator (Extracorporeal inter-

Table 12.1 Membrane oxygenator materials Lung Max is the maximum oxygen exchange with a blood PCO_2 of 40 mm Hg (5.3 kPa). Teflon devices (and others with *low permeability* membrane) are little influenced by fluid phase resistance and so are 'membrane limited'. Fluid phase design is not very demanding. Devices with membranes of *intermediate permeability*, such as 'copolymer', are limited by both membrane and fluid phase resistance. In a copolymer lung with a blood film of 200 μm, the blood phase resistance for O_2 is about 35% of the total. Fluid phase design becomes important. Since microporous teflon, even as thick as 2 mm, provides minimal resistance to gas flow, devices using this material have gas exchange limited by fluid phase resistance (boundary layer effects plus diffusion distance). For this kind of membrane, design improvements can provide spectacular increases in gas exchange.

		Gas Transmission			
Membrane	*Thickness (μm)*	O_2	CO_2	CO_2/O_2	*Lung Max*
Cellophane	75	6	130	23	6
Polyethylene	20	8	30	3.7	2
Teflon	12	50	130	2.6	9
Copolymer	25	330	1600	4.8	85
Silicone	25	1200	6000	5	325
Microporous	50–200	NMV	NMV	NMV	NMV

Values in ml gas m^{-2} min^{-1} atm^{-1}
NMV = no meaningful value

pulse; see Section 12.5) has only 0.8 m^2 of a thicker membrane but has a greater oxygen exchange capacity (see Table 12.8). The availability of devices of relatively simple and inexpensive construction is now practicable. There are now several sandwich designs, a vorticeal type, and a capillary model, all utilizing microporous membranes, in commercial production and clinical use.

Many do not consider the microporous materials to be true membranes since they start out with blood and gas in direct contact. Very thin protein layers are quickly deposited, however, to form molecular membranes. Unlike most previous membrane devices, and perhaps more like the natural lung, some oxygenators utilizing microporous membranes (such as the Travenol TMO using 3–5 μm pore size teflon) are very sensitive to transmembrane pressure. Even with a controlled low blood phase pressure slow protein leakage makes such devices unsatisfactory for long-term perfusion. Special pump arrangements must be made to prevent pulmonary oedema, on the one hand, or aspiration of ventilating gas into the blood phase on the other. For heart surgery these problems are largely theoretical. The newest microporous oxygenators utilize either teflon or polypropylene with very much smaller pore sizes (in the Cobe CML the pore size is only 0.3 μm). The membranes are non-wettable and the pores so small that blood cannot be forced through under any clinical operating conditions. This makes it possible, as in the Sci Med oxygenators to utilize a single pump on the venous side that must operate at pressures sufficient to overcome both the arterial pressure and the oxygenator resistance.

Table 12.2 Some other membrane devices

Year	*Reported by*	*General Description*	*Clinical use*
1958	Thomas *et al.*	Rotating silicone drum – aerosol of oxygen and bicarbonate	Yes
1964	Crystal *et al.* (Waters Co.)	Tilting of large horizontal silicone envelopes	Yes
1968	Katsuhara *et al.*	Stationary, or moving, vertical silicone envelopes	Yes
1967	Illickal *et al.*	Hollow silicone disk, spinning in blood, carrying gas	No?
1974 1963	Hill *et al.* Bodell *et al.*	Agitated blood outside gas carrying capillaries	No
1969	Williams *et al.*	Blood flows through 'cloth' with hollow filaments carrying gas	No
1969	Drinker and Bartlett (see Drinker, 1972)	Oscillating torus (a doughnut-shaped hollow ring) carries blood	No?
1974	Schults *et al.*	Vorticeal dialyser with transmembrane catalysis of H_2O_2	No

Many other ingenious membrane lungs have been developed and some have been used clinically. Some are still waiting in the wings. An attempt is made in Table 12.2 briefly to describe some of these devices. Additional devices and more details are to be found in Drinker (1972) and Eberhart *et al.* (1978).

12.3 PATHOPHYSIOLOGY OF PERFUSION

That perfusion is unphysiological is attested by many reports during the past 25 years. Postoperative damage to kidney, lung, brain, and other vital organs has not regularly been recognized, however, in the clinical setting because damage is often difficult to detect and because it is not often searched for diligently or reported when found. Nevertheless, enough instances have been published to indicate that perfusion is associated with real clinical problems.

It would, of course be a mistake to assume that the oxygenator is the only problem. The magnitude and handling of the shed blood may be more important actually because it is damaged by tissue contact and by entrained air. Clinical oxygenator comparisons are likely not to be very discriminating if shed blood is not controlled or minimized. Another source of confusion in attempting to judge devices is the marked improvement in bubble and particulate traffic that occurs when a micro filter is used in the arterial line (Carleson *et al.*, 1973). Such a filter is probably very desirable for a bubble oxygenator but it makes it more difficult to ascertain the effect of the oxygenator.

Because of the many problems of discriminating between devices used clinically, *in vitro* blood cell trauma tests are advised (Peirce *et al.*, 1969, 1976; AAMI, 1982). Unfortunately, there are no well-standardized tests for protein denaturation or for the monitoring of gas or solid emboli.

12.3.1 Denaturation of proteins

Denaturation of albumin by a device much resembling a disk oxygenator was described by Bull in 1938. There should be no serious doubt that clinically significant protein damage occurs in all oxygenators. This involves first a thin protein layer, probably a monolayer (Vroman, 1971). The denatured protein is continually ploughed back into the bulk blood if the interface is moving blood to gas, as it is in most devices with no separation between blood and gas. The damaged proteins have reactive groups that may cause red cell agglutination with 'sludging' of blood, exhibit important vasoactive properties, or result in embolic plugging of capillaries and tissue damage in vital organs from protein aggregations or neutral fat released from lipoproteins (Owens *et al.*, 1960; Dobell *et al.*, 1965; Zapol *et al.*, 1969). Clotting factors may be altered, extracted, or prematurely activated leading to serious coagulation abnormalities (Fong *et al.*, 1974; Bartlett and Gazzaniga, 1981).

If the interface is solid, as it is in most membrane lungs, the thin denatured protein layer tends to remain in place. This alters the surface reactivity, 'passivating' it, and further protein damage is slowed. Study of these phenomena is difficult in whole blood because of the masking effect of free plasma haemoglobin. In clinical situations meaningful protein denaturation studies may be impossible. Standard clinical tests are relatively insensitive and the denatured proteins are rapidly lost by adherence to apparatus, precipitation, and filtration by the perfused subject's capillary beds. It is not surprising that recent clinical comparisons generally fail to show significant differences between membrane and bubble devices (see Tables 12.4 and 12.5).

Protein denaturation occurs in all perfusions and almost certainly causes some pathological changes but unless organ damage is very gross, the individual will survive, most damage will be repaired or compensated for, and only subtle evidences of injury, at most, will remain. Until we have good clinical tests that will quantitate the extent of denaturation and damage this will be an area of confusion and disagreement and it will not improve the situation to draw conclusions from batteries of insensitive and inappropriate 'standard' laboratory determinations (Peirce, 1980a).

12.3.2 Damage to formed elements of blood

Although there are still questions regarding its clinical importance, there has been abundant proof that all types of gas-exchange devices are damaging to the formed elements of the blood (Peirce *et al.*,1969; Unger *et al.*, 1976; Bartlett and Gazzaniga, 1981). The damage is greatest at the blood–gas interface, is most easily and predictably seen in the magnitude of the free plasma haemoglobin, and, as shown in Table 12.3, is about an order of

Table 12.3 *In vitro* red blood cell trauma test (From J. D. Mortensen (Utah Biomedical Test Laboratory), 1976). Evaluation of ASAIO blood damage test

Approximate mean plasma haemoglobin (mg/100 ml)			
Perfusion hours	2	4	6
Control* (C)	10	20	30
Bubble Oxy X	80	200	375
Bubble Oxy Y	40	225	450
Mean minus (C)	50	190	380
Membrane Oxy R	8	16	24
Membrane Oxy S	25	50	80
Mean minus (C)	6	13	22

* Control values are from an identical perfusion without an oxygenator.

magnitude greater for a bubble than a membrane device (Mortensen, 1977). These differences are easily seen in a bench test but the level of plasma haemoglobin is greatly moderated by the reticuloendothelial system when an animal or a patient is being perfused. Similarly, the debris from the red cell haemolysis, the red cell 'ghosts' are removed in the subject's various capillary beds. Conventional micropore filters will not remove particles as small as red cell ghosts which may contribute to organ damage (Bernstein *et al.*, 1965).

Because blood shed into the pericardium or pleura is very severely traumatized (Siderys *et al.*, 1975) and any suctioned blood is considerably damaged, it may not be possible to differentiate between modern bubble and membrane oxygenators in terms of haemolysis unless the suctioned blood is small in amount or processed to washed red blood cells, before it is returned to the patient (Siderys *et al.*, 1975). Table 12.4 shows some recent clinical bubble–membrane comparisons. In any instance where the haemolysis values are not significantly different, there must be a presumption that haemolysis in the shed blood is obscuring any device differences. Unfortunately, in very few instances has the volume of shed blood been reported or its haemolysis been separately determined (as recommended by Siderys *et al.*, 1975).

Platelet changes are a very sensitive indicator of perfusion damage. Large platelet changes occur even in the most atraumatic perfusions so that device comparison on the basis of platelet alterations always involves judging differences between two major events. The problem of platelet damage is complex because both loss of platelets and change in platelet function must be considered. A drop in platelet count may be the result of destruction, reversible adherence to some part of the device, or reversible sequestration within the patient (especially in liver or spleen). The functional changes may involve activation or inactivation, may be quite variable quantitatively, and may or may not be reversible. Clinical studies must deal realistically with the great biological variability of platelet numbers and function and any determination of numbers must also correct for dilution to be meaningful (Edmunds *et al.*, 1982). These caveats should be kept in mind when test results are compared. In the face of these obstacles, it is surprising how many clinical studies (Table 12.5) have shown membrane devices to be less traumatic than bubble devices. Several other platelet comparison studies, all favourable to the membrane, are shown in Table 12.6. In general, one can expect a somewhat smaller drop in platelet count when perfusion is initiated with a membrane device, and a more reversible situation with less platelet dysfunction and an early rebound in numbers.

12.3.3 White blood cells

White blood cells are also very sensitive during perfusion and may undergo many changes from outright destruction to alteration in function. As with

Table 12.4 Some recent comparisons of membrane and bubble oxygenators

Reference	*Type of study*	*Number of cases*	*Type of case*	*Average time (min)*	*Devices compared*	*Shed blood excluded*	*Filter*	
							Shed blood	*Artery*
Williams *et al.*, 1978	Prospective alternate	80	Adult all types	96 NS	Travenol Teflon (M) Harvey Hybrid (B)	No	Yes	Yes
Feuchel *et al.*, 1979	Retrospective	156 (M) 112 (B)	All: adults and children	Longer membrane	Landé-Edwards (M) Two types (B)	No	–	–
Hicks *et al.*, 1979	Prospective randomized	52	Adult: coronary bypass	96 NS	Travenol Teflon (M) Bentley 100 (B)	No	No	No
Sade *et al.*, 1981	Prospective randomized	60	All infants and children	98 NS	Sci Med^{TM} (M) Harvey Hybrid (B)	No	No	Yes
Clark *et al.*, 1979	Prospective randomized	40 each short and long	Adult: 50% each valves and coronary	109 NS	Travenol Teflon and Silicone (M) 4 types (B)	No	Yes	No
Hessel *et al.*, 1980	Prospective randomized	64	Adult: 50% not coronary	115 NS	Travenol TMO (M) Bentley 100 (B)	No	No	No
Cosgrove and Loop, 1981	Prospective randomized	80	Adult coronary bypass	129 NS	Travenol TMO (M) Travenol Variflow (B)	No	Yes	No
Van den Dungen *et al.*, 1982	Prospective	74	Adult coronary bypass	110 NS	Travenol TMO (M) Polystan (B)	No*	Yes	No

NS: Not significantly different; * Shed blood was measured.

Table 12.4 (continued)

Reference	*Blood damage*			*Organ dysfunction*				*Coagulation problems*	*Blood required*	*Hospital course*	*Comment and conclusions*
	Protein	*Red cell*	*Platelet*	*Brain*	*Heart*	*Kidney*	*Lung*				
Williams *et al.*, 1978	–	NS	NS	–	–	–	–	NS	NS	NS	O_2 exch. problem membrane (5) Prefer bubble oxygenator
Feuchel *et al.*, 1979	–	Less (M)	Less (M)	–	–	NS	–	–	Less (M)	NS	Prefer bubble oxygenator unless long perfusion
Hicks *et al.*, 1979	NS	Less (M) by 65%	NS	NS	NS	NS	NS	NS	NS	NS	Hgb in urine 19(B) 29(M) No choice between (M) and (B)
Sade *et al.*, 1981	NS	Less (M)	NS	NS	–	NS	NS	NS	NS	NS	NS even in long cases No choice between (M) and (B)
Clark *et al.*, 1979	Short: NS	NS	NS	–	–	–	–	NS	NS	NS	Best flow and lowest PVR (M)
	Long: NS	Less (M)	Less (M)					NS	Less (M)	NS	NS short but choice long perf.
Hessel *et al.*, 1980	NS	NS	Less (M)	NS	NS	NS	–	NS	NS	NS	NS even in long cases No choice between (M) and (B)
Cosgrove and Loop, 1981	–	NS	NS	–	–	–	–	NS	Less (M)	NS	NS in short cases Prefer membrane
Van den Dungen *et al.*, 1982	–	Less (M)	Less (M)	–	–	NS	–	NS	Less (M)	NS	Bilirubin 7 days greater (M) For future, believe in (M)

(M) membrane oxygenator; (B) bubble oxygenator; PVR peripheral vascular resistance.

Table 12.5 Comparison studies of membrane (M) versus bubble (B) oxygenators

Reference	*Clinical*	*What was compared*	*Result*
Rhodes *et al.*, 1974	Puppies	Pulmonary function	NS difference. (M) no advantage for short perfusions
Dutton *et al.*, 1974	Yes	Platelet emboli versus oxygenator and filter	Fewer emboli from (M) NS diff. if filter used
Siderys *et al.*, 1975	Yes	Haemolysis with and without shed blood	With no 'pericardial' blood, haemolysis less with (M)
Byrick and Noble, 1978	Yes	Postoperative pulmonary function	Suggest less pulmonary vascular injury with (M)
Brown, 1979	Dog	Heart function in isolated perfused heart	NS difference with 3 hours perfusion
Parker *et al.*, 1979	Yes	Blood loss during and after perfusion	NS difference in short clinical perfusions
Pranger *et al.*, 1980	Dog	(1) Muscle O_2 histograms (2) Platelet loss	(1) Histogram impaired in (B) (2) Less platelet loss in (M)
Dancy *et al.*, 1981	Yes	Postoperative pulmonary function	NS difference shunt fraction. Less WBC sequestration (M)
Peterson *et al.*, 1982	Dog	The fate of platelets tagged with ^{111}In	(1) Less destruction in (M) (2) Sig. deposition on both
Edmunds *et al.*, 1982	Yes	(1) Platelet counts (2) Pl. aggregation ADP	(1) NS if dilution considered (2) NS function

NS, No significant
ADP, Adenosine diphosphate

platelets there is almost always a very marked reduction in white blood cell counts (especially polymorphonuclear cells) at the very start of a perfusion. This reflects a combination of destruction and device/patient sequestration. There is then usually a rather prompt increase in numbers (which does not often occur with platelets) and at the end of a several hour perfusion the numbers may be significantly greater than at the start. Studies using cell morphology or labelling will show that the polymorphs at the end of perfusion are to a considerable extent new young cells and not those present at the start (Galletti, 1965; Peirce *et al.*, 1971).

The implication of this information is that clinical changes in mere white blood cell numbers may be very misleading. For this reason white cell changes are not listed in Table 12.4. As with red cell damage, *in vitro* studies are very helpful in discriminating between devices and show membrane oxygenators to be less damaging to white blood cells than bubble oxygenators (Mortenson, 1977). This may relate to the phenomena of complement activation, white cell activation and release of free radical species.

12.3.4 Embolic events

Extracorporeal perfusion may generate gas emboli and a wide variety of solid particles (Allardyce *et al.*, 1966; Carleson *et al.*, 1973; Dutton *et al.*, 1974, Bartlett and Gazzaniga, 1981). Gas bubbles are always present to some extent at priming (Bethune, 1976), are added in the natural course of events in some devices (Allardyce *et al.*, 1966), and may be accidentally introduced in a wide variety of ways during perfusion (Peirce, 1980b). Their detection and removal should always have a very high priority. Unfortunately, massive air embolism with a high morbidity and mortality, occurs in perhaps one clinical perfusion in 1000 (Stoney *et al.*, 1980). Of possibly greater importance is the constant traffic in gas bubbles which cannot be removed completely and may cause real, though presently undetectable, organ dysfunction or permanent damage (Carleson *et al.*, 1973). Membrane lungs, and/or suitable filters, should greatly moderate this problem though returned shed blood and other sources of gas bubbles may continue the risk.

Solid particles include denatured proteins, neutral fat released from lipoproteins, red cell ghosts, fibrin, red cell, white cell or platelet aggregates, small bits of tubing from the pumps, and various combinations. These are present in large numbers and are only partially removed by microfiltration. The current clinical filters usually leave many particles below 40 μm. As yet few units attempt to monitor particle (or bubble) traffic and, unless the clinical problems caused are very gross, clinicians are generally quite unaware of the situation. As with gas bubbles, membrane lungs should moderate, but cannot eliminate, the situation which must be considered for the present a standard risk of perfusion. It should be noted that this important area is generally excluded in making clinical device comparisons although it has been repeatedly demonstrated that fewer particles are present in the arterial line when a membrane oxygenator is used (Carleson *et al.*, 1973; Dutton *et al.*, 1974) (see Chapter 15).

12.3.5 Clinical oxygenator comparisons

This section will summarize remarks about clinical comparison made in Section 12.3. There have now been quite a number of comparative studies of a prospective nature (Table 12.4). Although there have been no dramatic differences in blood damage or blood loss, and no demonstrable differences in organ function, in short perfusions (especially where shed blood is returned or large in volume), superior results have usually been shown when the perfusions last more than two hours.

Under the circumstances one should be less influenced by the numerous non-significant (NS) entries in Table 12.4 than by the fact that whatever differences are shown favour the membrane over the bubble oxygenator. For further discussion see Peirce (1980a).

Table 12.5 abstracts an additional group of studies that have compared several more restricted aspects of membrane and bubble devices than the reports shown in Table 12.4. Some authors reported that there were no significant differences and some found only subtle distinctions but the differences which were found again favour the membrane oxygenator.

The new membrane devices have other interesting features which set them apart from bubble oxygenators (Table 12.6). Some offer independent control of blood gases and most should be satisfactory for prolonged perfusions.

Table 12.6 Membrane and bubble oxygenators; some desirable features

Feature	*Membrane*	*Bubble*
Low blood trauma		
Protein	Yes	No
Red blood cells	Yes	No
Platelets	Better	Worse
White blood cells	Better	Worse
Low embolic risk		
Gas bubbles	Yes	No
Solid particles	Yes	No
Control blood volume	Easier	Harder
Filtration	Some	No
Independent regulation		
PO_2, PCO_2 (and pH)	Some	No
Usable long term	Many	No

Several of the devices (Sci Med, Terumo Capiox) have a very controlled volume, especially helpful in long-term perfusions if the reservoir has no blood–gas interface. The higher resistance devices (notably the Sci Med units) also provide a considerable degree of filtration for both solid and gaseous emboli. To some extent the microporous devices provide gas venting also, but this is not a wholly reliable feature. For the most part, large gas bubbles entering in the blood also leave with it, though in the form of microbubbles.

12.4 ASSESSMENT OF MEMBRANE DEVICES

A partial compilation of factors to be considered in comparing membrane devices is shown in Table 12.7.

12.4.1 Capacity reference blood flow rate

Efforts to standardize the testing of oxygenators have been partially successful. Most, if not all, new oxygenators coming on the market are using the

Table 12.7 Important factors in assessing oxygenators

Factor	*What to look at*
Capacity	Reference blood flow
Safety	Low blood trauma
	Gas embolism
	Special features
Blood damage	*In vitro* data
Modulation	O_2 and CO_2 exchange
Special features	Pulsatile flow
	Safety alarm and shut off
Long-term use	Time dependent changes
	Safety features
Ease of use	Assembly time
	Complexity
Economics	Cost versus efficacy

recommended tests for gas exchange and blood damage and are submitting the data to the appropriate national organization. Unfortunately, these data are not being disclosed in any uniform or complete fashion to the perfusionist and the physician users. In consequence, comparison of devices is still an extremely difficult task. The question of gas exchange capacity is important. The proposed standards which greatly simplify the comparison of device size are the reference blood flow rates for oxygen and for carbon dioxide (see Table 12.8).

Oxygen reference blood flow rate is in $l\,min^{-1}$ and is that blood flow rate in a blood gas exchanger which produces an increase in oxygen content of $45\,ml\,l^{-1}$ when the blood at the inlet has a haemoglobin content of $12\,g\,100\,ml^{-1}$ and an oxygen saturation of 65%

Carbon dioxide reference blood flow rate is in $l\,min^{-1}$ and is that blood flow rate in a blood gas exchanger which reduces the carbon dioxide content by $38\,ml\,l^{-1}$ when the blood at the inlet has a PCO_2 of 45 mmHg (6.0 kPa).

When a single reference blood flow rate is given it should be the lower of the values for oxygen and carbon dioxide. The reference flow units will approximate those computed as the normothermic perfusion requirement when the respiratory quotient (RQ) is 0.8. For example, the predicted requirement for a full flow normothermic perfusion in a 70 kg adult would be about 6 l. Table 12.8 shows that most available membrane devices can meet this demand with some margin to spare but that several (e.g. Travenol Teflon device) are suitable only for hypothermic perfusion.

When making a comparison with bubble devices it is important to know that these will have a varied gas transfer rate depending on the ratio of gas flow to blood flow. But blood damage is also greater at higher gas flows and these higher gas flow rates may also be very dangerous since they cause more damage and increase the gas bubble traffic. See what gas flow rate is specified by the manufacturer for the reference blood flow rate(s) that are supplied. This information is essential for intelligent device comparison (see Section 12.4.4).

12.4.2 Safety

Blood damage should be very low with all current membrane devices and there should be very little difference in this respect. Methyl silicone, teflon and polypropylene are all classed as non-wettable. They all have a low level of interaction with the perfusing blood and hence produce smaller and fewer solid emboli. Platelets are activated but aggregates are small and the process appears to be reversible. Filters are not generally recommended in the arterial line of membrane devices, though they may be chosen in clinical practice for other reasons. Microporous devices may be superior to solid membrane devices because membrane areas are less for the same capacity. It must be appreciated that gas embolism may occur with membrane devices if priming is not correctly carried out, and if gas or air is introduced into the circuit during perfusion. Priming bubbles will, however, be very small, and, in any event, are completely avoidable with the manufacturer's recommended techniques. Serious bubbles are readily generated in any microporous device if negative blood phase pressures ever develop during operation. Special precautions must always be taken. Reservoirs for all types of devices should have low level alarms and shut offs (Stoney *et al.*, 1980). Membrane devices operating with both blood and gas in the reservoirs are no exceptions. With the oxygenator interposed between the reservoir and the patient there is more time to respond and this may be a very important safety feature. Large gas bubbles will be broken into very small ones in passage through the membrane device and this may be less dangerous. Single pump membrane devices are probably safer than those requiring two pumps and the trend is to the use of a single pump, though compatibility with pulsatile perfusion is an additional consideration.

Devices that incorporate a rigid reservoir cannot be used with a closed reservoir. This is very important in choosing an oxygenator for prolonged use and may become important if all shed blood can be discarded, processed to packed cells (Siderys *et al.*, 1975), or saved for later re-infusion (very desirable developments).

Not all membrane devices do well when perfusion is interrupted. If circulatory arrest is to be employed, this aspect should be considered. The older Teflon Travenol device, and possibly the two pump polypropylene unit, may be operated at low flow with the gas turned off during arrest because it employs a recirculation line. The Cobe CML unit apparently works well with arrest and the reservoir provides ample place for blood displacement. Each device should be checked for the need to maintain blood flow in the oxygenator if circulatory arrest is to be utilized.

12.4.3 Blood damage

Because data obtained from animal and clinical perfusions may be seriously deceptive, detailed information from bench tests (*in vitro*) is essential. Gas exchange data, for instance, may be obtained over a much wider range of conditions. Of more importance, blood damage data are not obscured by greater biological variability and by moderation due to such things as capillary filtration and activity of the reticuloendothelial system. The problems of substantial damage in the shed blood in a clinical perfusion have been mentioned.

12.4.4 Modulation of gas exchange and pH in oxygenators

Because of very different solubilities and diffusion rates ($CO_2/O_2 = \sim 25:1$), oxygen and carbon dioxide exchange are dependent on quite different factors in both bubble and membrane oxygenators. A desirable feature in a gas exchange device is the ability to vary gas exchange without changing blood flow rate. More or less oxygen may be needed as metabolism varies, for example with temperature, and control of the carbon dioxide exchange is the key to PCO_2 regulation and acid–base compensation. In a bubble device, at a constant blood flow, oxygen exchange varies with the surface area of the bubbles while carbon dioxide exchange is roughly proportional to the gas volume flow. If the bubbles are very small (large surface area to volume ratio), full oxygenation can be achieved with very little (or no) carbon dioxide exchange. If the bubbles are large (small surface area to volume ratio), carbon dioxide exchange can be effected with very little oxygen exchange. Systems have, therefore, been devised with small bubbles for oxygen and large bubbles for carbon dioxide exchange (Clark, 1958). In most bubble oxygenators the bubbles average a medium size and increases in gas flow enhance both oxygen and carbon dioxide exchange about equally. For this reason when changes in gas flow are used to vary oxygen exchange, it is not unusual to add carbon dioxide to the ventilating gas to suppress wide swings in the PCO_2 and pH. Now that it is well recognized that increasing gas flow in a bubble oxygenator also increases blood damage and the number of gaseous microbubbles liberated, options for gas exchange regulation have been reduced. The devices, for safety, are operated far below their maximum exchange capabilities at a gas to blood flow ratio of approximately one to one, or even lower ratios.

In a membrane device of adequate gas transfer capacity, such as those currently available, carbon dioxide exchange is readily varied without changing blood flow or increasing the risk of blood damage or embolization by simply changing gas flow. In a Cobe CML lung, for example, carbon dioxide exchange is approximately doubled by increasing gas flow threefold. For the highly permeable membranes now employed, oxygen exchange is largely a function of the blood phase geometry (effective diffusion distance) and nearly maximum oxygen exchange at a given blood flow is achieved at rather low gas flows. For this reason, the PCO_2 and pH may be controlled over a wide range without significantly affecting oxygenation. Several of the membrane devices have special means of specifically controlling oxygen transfer. This is done in the Travenol units by varying blood film dimensions with a pneumatic shim. In the extracorporeal device oxygen exchange may be controlled over a range of at least two to one by varying the blood flow pulse rate without changing the blood flow rate. Regulation of oxygen and carbon dioxide exchange independently (at a constant blood flow rate) is a very attractive and desirable feature of membrane oxygenators not shared by the commercial bubblers (Beall *et al.*, 1976).

12.4.5 Long-term perfusion (discussed in detail in Chapter 13)

Of all the oxygenator types, membrane devices are the only ones with acceptably low levels of blood trauma for long-term use (Hill *et al.*, 1968, 1972, 1978; White *et al.*, 1971; Peirce 1972, 1977, 1981; Geelhoed *et al.*, 1975; Kolobow *et al.*, 1975; Hoffmeister *et al.*, 1975; Bartlett *et al.*, 1975, 1976; Gille and Bagniewski, 1976; Birnbaum *et al.*, 1979; Zapol *et al.*, 1979; Bartlett and Gazzangia 1981). There is still a place for long-term extracorporeal oxygenation (ECMO) despite the 'negative' National Study results (Zapol *et al.*, 1979). For certain children with acute respiratory failure the results have been excellent with a better than 25% survival (Bartlett *et al.*, 1976). When severe respiratory failure and circulatory failure are both present, or there is a *specific therapy* available to treat the underlying disease, ECMO is a powerful technique (Hill, 1978; MacDonnell *et al.*, 1980; Peirce, 1981). Because additional testing information is needed before manufacturers may properly recommend devices for prolonged perfusion (Peirce *et al.*, 1976; AAMI, 1982), and because ECMO is not a sufficiently major use, most current membrane oxygenators do not carry a manufacturer's endorsement for this. Only the Sci Med units are recommended by the manufacturer for long-term perfusions.

12.4.6 Ease of use

Neither the complexity nor the assembly time should be very significant factors in choosing a membrane oxygenator now that most work well with available pumping systems and require only a single pump. The oxygenators that come complete with a hard shell reservoir and an integral heat exchanger should be extremely convenient and very little different from a bubbler in complexity and set up time. Priming may be slightly more difficult for the Terumo and the Sci Med devices because of special techniques recommended for removing bubbles but this should be only a very minor problem at most. The only membrane oxygenator requiring a major new piece of perfusion apparatus is the Extracorporeal membrane oxygenator.

12.5 AVAILABLE MEMBRANE DEVICES

Membrane oxygenators currently being marketed in the United States are described briefly in this section and listed in Table 12.8 (see also Figs 12.1–12.5). The omission of any other fully commercial devices that may now be available in other countries is regretted. Of the devices shown in Table 12.8, the majority have reached the market within the last three years. They are well designed and well tested. Their recent appearance strongly suggests great interest in their advantages to patients and the greater flexibility they add to perfusion. Some of these new devices have been under development for more than ten years; others are more recent in conception. It is recognized that additional membrane oxygenators continue to appear and that the information below will not long be comprehensive. (Recent additions include the Shiley membrane lung, and the Bard–Harvey capillary membrane oxygenator.)

12.5.1 Cobe Membrane Lung (Cobe Laboratories Inc., 1201 Oak Street, Lakewood, Colorado 80215) (Hlavinka, 1983; Cobe Laboratories 1983) (Some details of an adult model are shown in Table 12.8.)

The recently marketed Cobe (Model CML) membrane lung is one of a new generation of devices designed for full support at normal body temperature even at the 5300 ft (1615 m) altitude of Denver. The reference blood flow (see Section 12.4.1) is more than $6\,l\,min^{-1}$ and there is both an integral heat exchanger and a ‘hard shell’ reservoir that will hold up to 3600 ml. Blood is delivered by gravity to the reservoir and heat exchanger. It is then pumped by a single pump through the gas exchange portion of the device and returned to the patient’s arterial system. Using a fine pore microporous polypropylene membrane, even obstructive pressures will not drive blood through the membrane. Like other microporous devices using either teflon or polypropylene, this oxygenator is very atraumatic to blood. *In vitro* and *in vivo* data show low haemolysis levels and relatively minor platelet and white blood cell interactions. Carbon dioxide exchange is readily varied by adjusting the gas flow. There is no special provision for varying oxygen exchange, however, so models of smaller size and variable prime may be expected to follow.

Table 12.8 Membrane devices – a comparison

Source and designation configuration	*Membrane material*	*Pore size membrane (μ2m)*	*Membrane (m^2)*	*Number of pumps, position in circuit*	*Priming volume (ml†)*	*Integral heat exchanger*	*Reference flow ($l\,min^{-1}$)* O_2	CO_2	*Oxygenator special features*
Sci Med™ spiral coil	Methyl silicone	—	0.4–4.5 (6 sizes)	One on the venous side	100/m^2 +100	Yes, 3 largest	1.3/m^2	1.3/m^2	Special priming advised to avoid bubbles
Travenol TMO	Teflon	3 to 5	1.12	Two: Ven+Art	225E	No	2E	3E	Uses a pneumatic shim to vary oxygen transfer
Travenol TMO sandwich	Poly-propylene	0.2 by 3	2.25	Two: Ven+Art	450	No	4E	6E	Uses a pneumatic shim to vary oxygen transfer
Travenol LPM-50 sandwich	Poly-propylene	0.2 by 3	2.25	One on the arterial side	450	Yes	?	?	Uses a pneumatic shim Integral reservoir
Cobe CML sandwich	Poly-propylene	0.3	2.5	One on the venous side	1165	Yes	6*	6*	Integral 3.6 l reservoir
Extracorporeal interpulse	Teflon	0.8	0.8	One on the venous side	920	Yes	6*	6*	May be used to give pulsatile flow
Terumo Capiox capillary	Poly-propylene	0.7	1.6–5.4 (4 sizes)	One on the venous side	200 to 700	Yes	6*	6*	Extremely compact

* By definition of reference blood flow, 6 l min^{-1} is the maximum. This underestimates the true gas exchange capacity by about 15–20%.
† Blood volumes are not always directly comparable. Some are for the oxygenator alone. Others include minimum reservoir volume and/or heat exchanger volume.
E, ?: Estimates or open question. Data not available from Travenol at the time of writing.

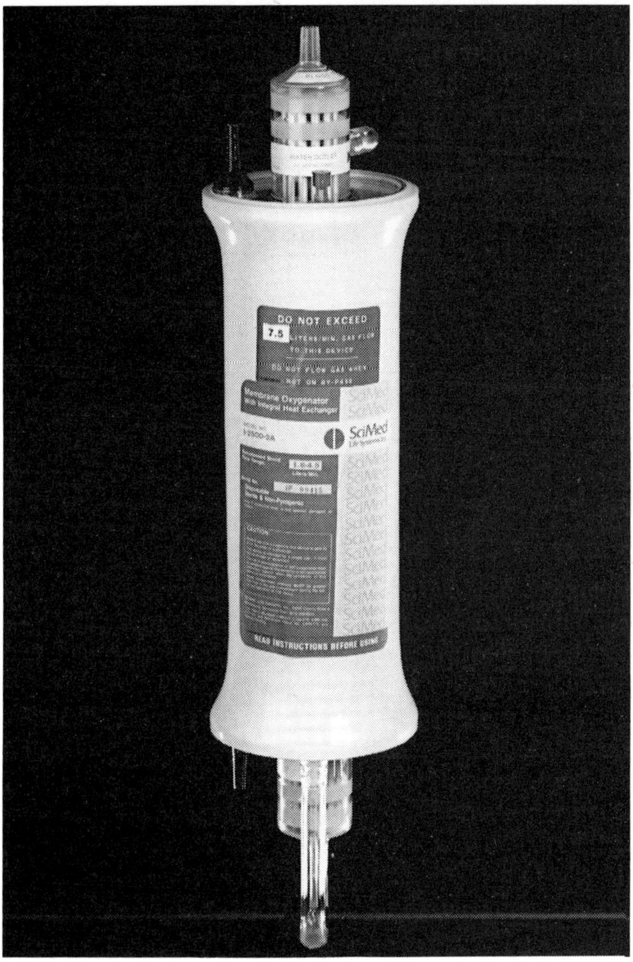

Fig. 12.1 The Sci Med membrane oxygenator.

12.5.2 Extracorporeal membrane oxygenator (Extracorporeal Inc., Royal and Ross Roads, King of Prussia, Pa. 19406) (Badolato, 1983; Extracorporeal Inc., 1982). (One adult model called Interpulse, see Table 12.8.)

This interesting new membrane device is the result of 10 years of research in the UK. This device overcomes the boundary layer problem by rapid reversal of blood flow in relatively wide low resistance blood channels as originally demonstrated by Bellhouse *et al.* (1973) and Bellhouse (1976). Baffles in the blood channels cause the blood to mix by forming vortices (whirlpools) when

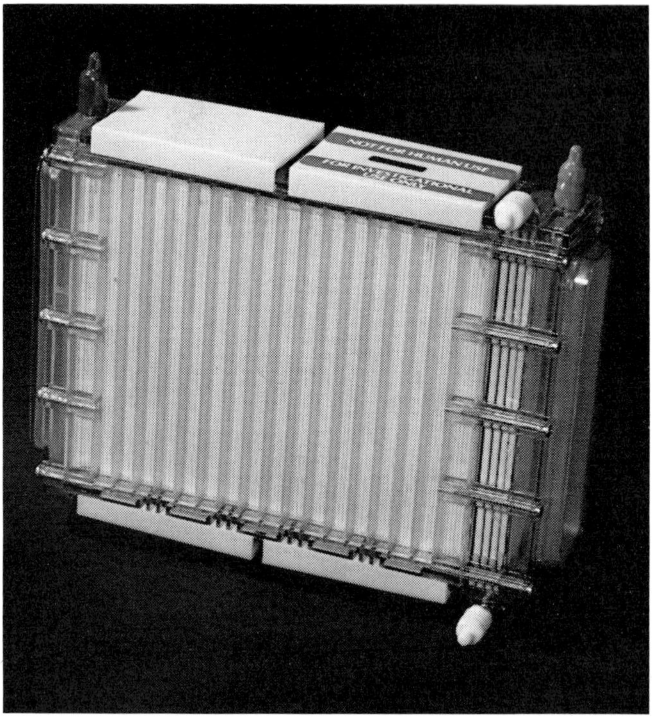

Fig. 12.2 The membrane section of the Extracorporeal interpulse membrane oxygenator.

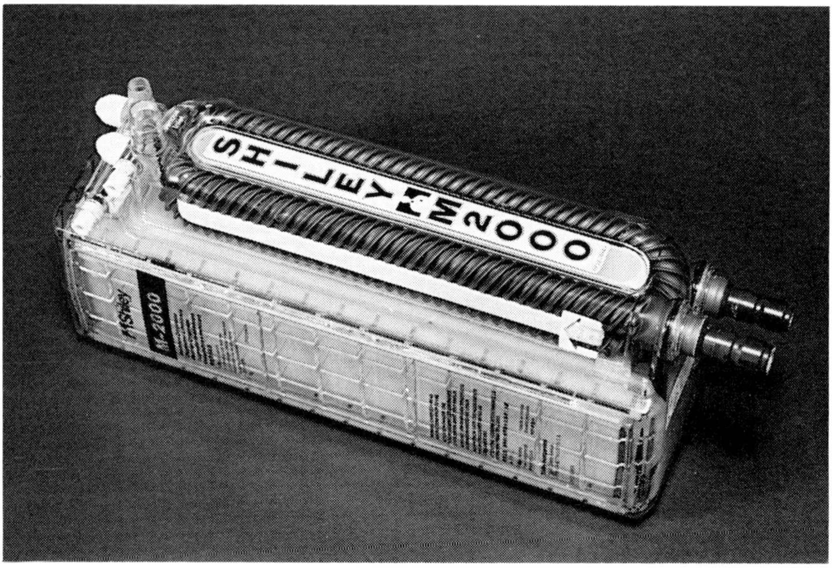

Fig. 12.3 Shiley M-2000 membrane oxygenator.

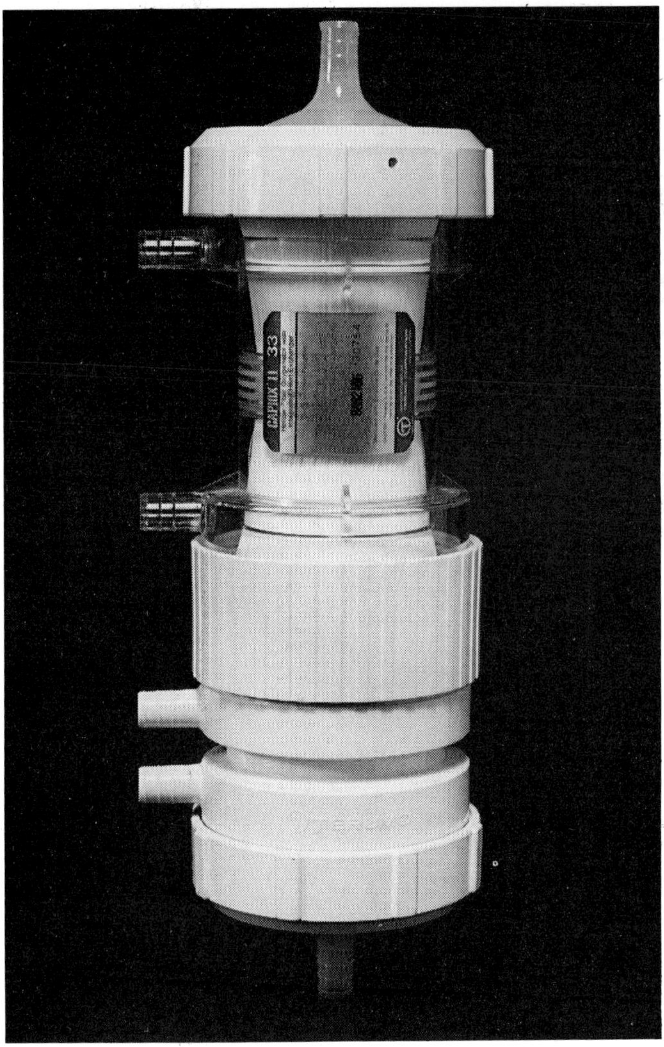

Fig. 12.4 Terumo-Capiox hollow-fibre membrane oxygenator.

the flow is reversed or 'pulsed'. This markedly enhances gas exchange, especially oxygen, so that the functional membrane area of only 0.8 m^2 of microporous teflon (pores 0.3 μm) is the equal of perhaps 5 m^2 in other microporous devices. Despite many attractive features, the device has been less successful than envisaged, though recent modifications may combine the low surface area/high efficiency concept in a much more compact form.

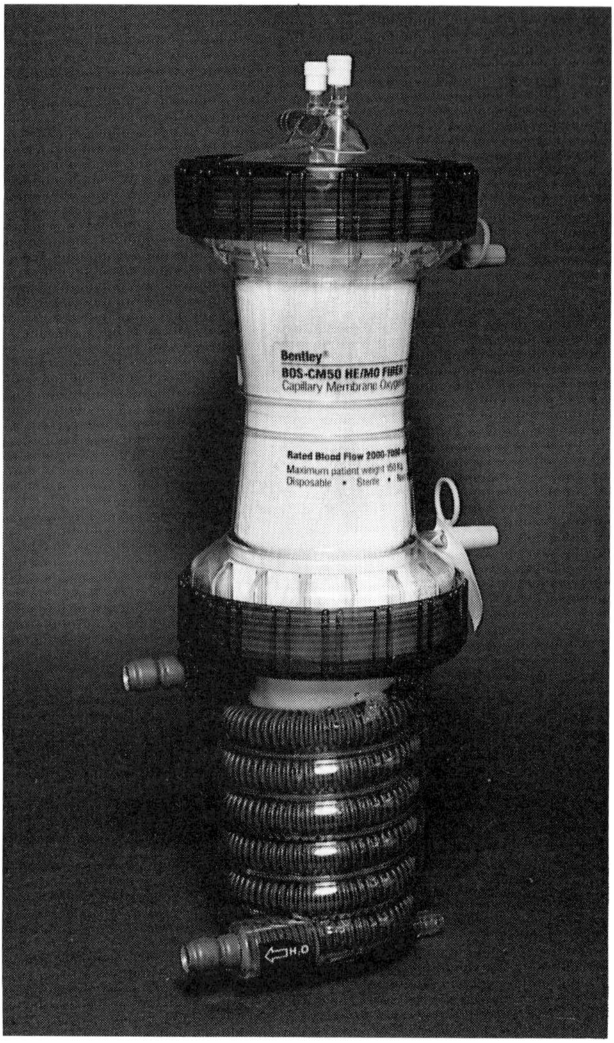

Fig. 12.5 Bentley hollow-fibre membrane oxygenator.

12.5.3 Sci Med membrane oxygenators (Sci Med Life Systems Inc., 13 000 Country Road 6, Minneapolis, Minnesota 55 441) (Anderson, 1983; Sci Med, 1983). (These are available in 6 sizes (plus an even smaller one for organ perfusion) see Table 12.8.)

Sci Med spiral coil oxygenators have been on the market longer than any of the other currently commercial membrane devices and they can truly be said to have stood the test of time. Developed on a design, reminiscent of the Kolff kidney, and originally described by Kolobow and Bowman (1963) at the National Institutes of Health, they are now produced in a wide range of sizes with a dacron-reinforced methyl silicone membrane. Until the advent of microporous materials, silicone 'rubber' was the optimum material for membrane devices and it is still competitive. The membrane is rough on one side which provides considerable blood mixing and reduces the boundary layer effects. The coils are tightly rolled so that the blood film space is very thin. This enhances gas exchange and reduces the priming volume. Even though this is a high resistance device, it is commonly operated with a single pump on the venous side. Often called Kolobow or Bowman lungs, the Sci Med oxygenators are (as the only survivors of a larger group) the standard for long-term perfusion and are the only devices on the market in the United States which are specifically recommended by the manufacturer for that purpose. The sizes available are suitable for cardiac procedures in all weights of patients and the device has been very well adapted to heart surgery (Helton *et al.*, 1978). It is important to choose the appropriate size as it is difficult to modulate the oxygen exchange once a perfusion is started unless a recirculation line is provided or there is provision for adding an inert gas (Riley and Pfaender, 1980). The exchange of carbon dioxide is, of course, readily controlled by varying the gas flow rate.

The recommended priming procedure, to avoid retained gas nuclei which may embolize, entails the use of carbon dioxide and adds a few minutes. This is a very minor negative point and will not pose any problems to the careful perfusionist. Further refinements of this group of oxygenators are under way at the present time.

12.5.4. Terumo Capiox oxygenators (Terumo Corporation, Japan. In the United States, 120 New England Ave, Piscataway, NJ 08 854) (Marsh, 1983; Terumo Corp., 1982). (Currently four sizes, the three larger with integral heat exchangers, see Table 12.8.)

A capillary oxygenator using microporous polypropylene has recently been developed in Japan (Tsuji *et al.*, 1981). A 1981 clinical article by Suma *et al.* reports the clinical performance of a 3.3 m^2 prototype in 100 open-heart procedures. Perfusion duration was up to 496 min (74 ±66 SD) and the weight 4.8–78 kg. The performance of the oxygenators was excellent. They have been tested at the Cleveland Clinic by Valdés *et al.* (1981) with satisfactory results and are now, with an added integral heat exchanger, in clinical use.

The hollow fibres are 20 cm long, have an inside diameter of 200 μm, and a wall thickness of 25 μm. The pore size averages 0.7 μm (700 Å). Three models with instrinsic tubular stainless-steel heat exchangers (placed before the oxygenator) have 1.6, 3.3 and 5.4 m^2 of active surface (about 1.1×10^4 capillaries m^{-2}). The exchange of oxygen and carbon dioxide is well balanced and the rated blood flow is about 1.4 l min^{-1} m^{-2} (well in excess of 6 l min^{-1} for the largest units). The priming volume is about 130 ml m^{-2} so these devices are extremely compact. The oxygenators operate with a single venous side pump (of any standard cardiac type). Some positive pressure must be maintained at all times, as in other microporous devices, and care must be taken to dislodge bubbles (by tapping) during priming but there are no other special precautions. Carbon dioxide exchange can be modulated by varying the gas flow but, since there is no special method for adjusting oxygen exchange, units of different oxygen exchange capacities are available. There is a very low platelet activation and outlet obstruction has not occurred as in the earlier Dow capillary devices, though maintenance of the activated clotting time (ACT) above 480 sec is advised. Haemolysis is very low and there should not be much, if any, decrease in function with time during prolonged perfusions. The newly developed Bard–Harvey oxygenator is a capillary membrane device with less restriction to blood flow, low flow resistance, and the potential for compatibility with single pump pulsatile perfusion.

12.5.5 **Travemol membrane oxygenators** (Travenol Laboratories, Inc., Round Lake, Ill. 60 073) (Pearson, 1983). (Currently two paediatric and two adult models, see Table 12.8.)

A paediatric device utilizing microporous teflon was introduced by Travenol Laboratories in 1971 and has had encouraging reports despite a somewhat larger priming volume than a paediatric bubble device (Hardesty *et al.*, 1980). Karlson *et al.* (1974) reported enthusiastically on the larger (2.25 m^2) model for adult clinical use. Since that time the membrane has been changed to polypropylene with reduction of the pores from 3–5 μm to 1–2 μm in diameter. The smaller pore size has virtually eliminated the occurrence of 'pulmonary oedema' resulting from the gradual outflow of water and protein through the membrane. This has rendered the device function much more stable and made perfusions of many hours feasible. Both teflon and polypropylene paediatric oxygenators are still available at the time of writing but the adult teflon unit has been discontinued. The membranes are reinforced with polyvinyl-coated fibre glass and there is a fine nylon screen in the blood phase, probably to decrease boundary layer effects. Blood phase dimensions can be decreased to improve oxygen transfer by means of an inflatable shim. The device is held in a rigid steel frame (as is the separate heat exchanger) to prevent leakage of blood.

The details of clinical use of the Travenol (TMO) microporous oxygenator have been discussed recently by Cosgrove and Loop (1981) who report satisfactory performance in more than 4000 cases at the Cleveland Clinic.

Special servo connected pumps or a proper balancing of the pumps are required as it is essential that the pressure in the blood phases is always slightly positive. This is brought about by using a recirculation line and running the venous pump about 10% faster than the arterial pump. Without this positive pressure, of course, gas could pass freely through the membrane into the blood phase. The gas phase is specially vented to air to prevent any possibility of an increased gas phase pressure as this would be very dangerous. The microporous membrane assists with gas venting during priming but does not eliminate the need for a bubble trap. Oxygenation is adjusted by changing the shim pressure and carbon dioxide exchange is increased or decreased by varying the gas flow. This provides considerable functional flexibility.

Recently, a new Travenol device with the same microporous polypropylene membrane (designated the LPM–50) has been marketed. This incorporates an integral heat exchanger and a reservoir. Blood flows through the device by gravity and is returned to the patient by an arterial pump. This device will be easier to use and since it has a higher gas exchange capacity (probably similar to the other high-capacity devices listed in Table 12.8), will be more suitable for normothermic perfusions.

REFERENCES

AAMI (1982) *Draft Standard for Blood Gas Exchange Devices.* Association for the Advancement of Medical Instrumentation, Arlington, Va.

Allardyce, D. B., Yoshida, S. H., Ashmore, P. G. (1966) The importance of microembolism in the pathogenesis of organ dysfunction caused by prolonged use of the pump oxygenator. *J. Thorac. Cardiovasc. Surg.*, **52**, 706.

Anderson, A. (1983) Personal communication. Sci Med Life Systems Inc.

Badolato, T. (1983) Personal communication. Extracorporeal Inc.

Bartlett, R. H., Drinker, P. A., Burns, N. E., Fong, S. W. and Hyans, T. (1972) The toroidal membrane oxygenator: Design, performance and prolonged bypass testing of a clinical model. *Trans. Am. Soc. Artif. Int. Organs*, **18**, 369–73.

Bartlett, R. H., Fong, S. W., Woldanski, C., Hung, E., Styler, D., and MacArthur, C. (1975) Hematologic responses to prolonged extracorporeal circulation (ECC) with microporous membrane devices. *Trans. Am. Soc. Artif. Intern. Organs*, **21**, 250–6.

Bartlett, R. H. and Gazzaniga, A. B. (1981) Physiology and pathophysiology of extracorporeal circulation. In *Techniques in Extracorporeal Circulation* (ed. M. I. Ionescu), 2nd edn, Butterworths, London, pp. 3–43.

Bartlett, R. H., Jeffries, M. R., Haidue, N. and Gazzaniga, A. B. (1976) Extracorporeal membrane oxygenation (ECMO) cardiopulmonary support in infancy. *Trans. Am. Soc. Artif. Int. Organs*, **22**, 80–93.

Beall, A. C. Jr, Solis, R. T., Kakvan, M., Morris, G. C. Jr, Noon, G. P. and DeBakey, M. E. (1976) Clinical experience with the Teflo disposable membrane oxygenator. *Ann. Thorac. Surg.*, **21**, 144–50.

Bellhouse, B. J. (1976) Design of the Oxford membrane oxygenator and its performance during prolonged support of newborn lambs. *Membrane Lungs for Acute*

Respiratory Failure (eds W. M. Zapol and J. Qvist), Academic Press, New York, p. 197.

Bellhouse, B. J., Bellhouse, F. H., Curl, F. H., MacMillan, C. M., Grunning, T. I., Spratt, A. I., MacMurray, E. H. and Nelems, J. M. A. (1973) A high efficiency membrane oxygenator and pulsatile pumping system and its application to animal trials. *Trans. Am. Soc. Artif. Int. Organs*, **19**, 72–9.

Bernstein, E. F., Castaneda, A. R. and Varco, R. L. (1965) Some biologic limitations to prolonged blood pumping. *Trans. Am. Soc. Artif. Int. Organs*, **11**, 118–21.

Bethune, D. W. (1976) Organ damage after open heart surgery. *Lancet*, **ii**, 1410–1.

Birnbaum, D., Thom, R. and Bücherl, E. S. (1979) Choice of the most suitable oxygenator for long-term pulmonary support. *World J. Surg.*, 3, 353–9.

Bodell, B. R., Head, J. M., Head, L. R., Formolo, A. J. and Head, J. R. (1963) A capillary membrane oxygenator. *J. Thorac. Cardiovasc. Surg.*, **46**, 639–50.

Bramson, M. L., Osborn, J. J. and Gerbode, F. (1981) The membrane lung. In *Techniques in Extracorporeal Circulation* (ed. M. I. Ionescu), 2nd edn, Butterworths, London, pp. 65–82.

Bramson, M. L., Osborn, J. J., Main, F. B., O'Brien, M. F., Wright, J. S. and Gerbode, F. (1965) A new disposable membrane oxygenator with integral heat exchanger. *J. Thorac. Cardiovasc. Surg.*, **50**, 391–400.

Brown, A. H. (1979) Membrane and bubble oxygenators compared by preservation of myocardial function. *J. Cardiovasc. Surg.*, **20**, 233–40.

Bull, H. B. (1938) Studies of surface denaturation of egg albumin. *J. Biol. Chem.*, **123**, 17.

Byrick, R. J. and Noble, W. H. (1978) Postperfusion lung syndrome. Comparison of Travenol bubble and membrane oxygenators. *J. Thorac. Cardiovasc. Surg.*, **76**, 685–93.

Carleson, R. G., Landé, A. J., Landis, B., Rogoz, B., Baxter, J., Patterson, R. H. Jr, Stenzel, K. and Lillehei, C. W. (1973) The Landé–Edwards membrane oxygenator during heart surgery: oxygen transfer microembolism counts, and Bender-Gestalt visual motor scores. *J. Thorac. Cardiovasc. Surg.*, **66**, 894–905.

Clark, L. C. Jr (1958) Optimal flow rate in perfusion. In *Extracorporeal Circulation* (ed. J. G. Allen), Thomas, Springfield, Ill., pp. 150–63.

Clark, R. E., Beauchamp, R. A., Magrath, R. A., Brooks, J. D., Ferguson, T. B. and Weldon, C. S. (1979) Comparison of bubble and membrane oxygenators in short and long perfusions. *J. Thorac. Cardiovasc. Surg.*, **78**, 655–66.

Clowes, G. H. A. Jr, Hopkins, A. L. and Neville, W. E. (1956) An artificial lung dependent upon the diffusion of oxygen and carbon dioxide through plastic membranes. *J. Thorac. Surg.*, **32**, 630–7.

Clowes, G. H. A. Jr, and Neville, W. (1958) Membrane oxygenator. In *Extracorporeal Circulation* (ed. J. G. Allen), Thomas, Springfield, Ill., pp. 81–100.

Cobe Laboratories (1983) *Membrane Lung (CML): Performance Characteristics.*

Cosgrove, D. M. and Loop, F. D. (1981) Clinical use of Travenol TMO membrane oxygenator. In *Techniques in Extracorporeal Circulation* (ed. M. I. Ionescu), Butterworths, London, pp. 85–99.

Crystal, D. K., Day, S. W., Wagner, C. L., Martinis, A. J., Owen, J. J. and Walker, P. E. (1964) A gravity-flow membrane oxygenator. *Arch. Surg.*, **88**, 122–7.

Dancy, C. M., Townsend, E. R., Boylett, A., Chan, S. L., Parker-Williams, E. J. and Parker, J. (1981) Pulmonary dysfunction associated with cardiopulmonary bypass: A comparison of bubble and membrane oxygenators. *Circulation*, **64**(2), 54–7.

De Filippi, R. P., Tompkins, F. C., Porter, J. H., Timmins, R. S. and Buckley, M. J

(1968) The capillary membrane oxygenator; *in vitro* and *in vivo* gas exchange measurements. *Trans. Am. Soc. Artif. Int. Organs*, **14**, 236–41.

Dennis, C., Spring, D. S., Nelson, G. E., Karlson, K. E., Nelson, R. M., Thomas, J. V., Eder, W. P. and Varco, R. L. (1951) Development of pump oxygenator to replace the heart and lungs; an apparatus applicable to human patients and application in one case. *Ann. Surg.*, **134**, 709–21.

Dobell, A. R. C., Galva, R., Sarkozy, E., Mitri, M. and Murphy, D. R. (1965) Biologic evaluation of blood after prolonged recirculation through film and membrane oxygenators. *Ann. Surg.*, **161**, 617–22.

Dorson, W. Jr, Balker, E. and Hall, H. (1968) A shell and tube oxygenator. *Trans. Am. Soc. Artif. Int. Organs*, **14**, 242–9.

Drinker, P. A. (1972) Progress in membrane oxygenator design. *Anesthesiology*, **37**, 242–60.

Dubin, W. R., Field, H. L. and Gastfriend, D. R. (1979) Postcardiotomy delirium. A critical review. *J. Thorac. Cardiovasc. Surg.*, **77**, 586–94.

Dutton, R. C., Edmunds, L. H. Jr, Hutchinson, J. C. and Roe, B. B. (1974) Platelet aggregate emboli produced in patients during cardiopulmonary bypass with membrane and bubble oxygenators and blood filters. *J. Thorac. Cardiovasc. Surg.*, **67**, 258–65.

Eberhart, R. C., Dengle, S. K. and Curtis, R. M. (1978) Mathematical and experimental methods for design and evaluation of membrane oxygenators. *Artif. Organs*, **2**, 19–33.

Edmunds, L. H. Jr, Ellison, N., Colman, R. W., Niewiarowski, S., Rao, A. K., Addonizio, V. P. Jr, Stephenson, L. W. and Edie, R. N. (1982) Platelet function during cardiac operation: comparison of membrane and bubble oxygenators. *J. Thorac. Cardiovasc. Surg.*, **803**, 805–12.

Effler, D. B., Kolff, W. J., Groves, L. K. and Sones, F. N. Jr (1956) Disposable membrane oxygenator and its use in experimental surgery. *J. Thorac. Surg.*, **32**, 620.

Eisman, B., Birnbaum, D., Leonard, R. and Martinez, E. J. (1972) A new gas permeable membrane for oxygenators, *Surg. Gynecol. Obstet.*, **135**, 732–6.

Extracorporeal Inc (1982) *Interpulse Membrane Oxygenation System: Instructions for Use.*

Extracorporeal Inc. (1983) *Interpulse Clinical Fact Book.*

Feuchel, G., Seybold-Epting, W., Schmidt, K., Stunkat, R. and Hoffmeister, H. E. (1979) Clinical comparison between membrane and bubble oxygenators in cardiopulmonary bypass. *J. Cardiovasc. Surg. (Torino)*, **20**, 419–22.

Fong, S. W., Burns, N. E., Williams, G., Woldanski, C., Gazzaniga, A. B. and Bartlett, R. H. (1974) Changes in coagulation and platelet function during prolonged extracorporeal circulation (ECC) in sheep and man. *Trans. Am. Soc. Artif. Int. Organs*, **20**, 239–47.

Galletti, P. M. (1965) Laboratory experience with 24 hours partial heart–lung bypass. *J. Surg. Res.*, **5**, 97.

Galletti, P. M. and Brecher, G. A. (1962) *Heart–Lung Bypass*. Grune and Stratton, New York, pp. 108–20.

Galletti, P. M., Richardson, P. D. and Snider, M. T. (1971) *Blood Oxygenator Testing and Evaluation, Part I. Evaluation Techniques*, National Institute of Health Report No. NIH–69–2047–1.

Geelhoed, G. W., Adkins, P. C., Corso, P. J. and Joseph, W. L. (1975) Clinical effects of membrane lung support for acute respiratory failure. *Ann. Thorac. Surg.*, **20**, 177–87.

Geirab, O. and Semb, G. (1974) Cardiopulmonary bypass using the Landé–Edwards membrane oxygenator and the Rygg–Kyvsgard perfusion apparatus. *Scand. J. Cardiovasc. Surg.*, **8**, 184.

Gibbon, J. H. Jr (1937) Artificial maintenance of circulation during experimental occlusion of pulmonary artery. *Arch. Surg.*, **34**, 1105–31.

Gille, J. P. and Bagniewski, A. (1976) Ten years of use of extracorporeal membrane oxygenation (ECMO) in treatment of acute respiratory insufficiency (ARI). *Trans. Am. Soc. Artif. Int. Organs*, **22**, 102–8.

Hardesty, R. L., Deeb, G. M., Griffith, B. P. and Borovetz, H. S. (1980) Clinical experience with pediatric microporous oxygenator for profound hypothermia. *Arch. Surg.*, **115**, 1355–8.

Helton, W. C. Johnson, F. W., Howe J. B., Freedman, F. B., Lindsay, W. G. and Nicoloff, D. M. (1978) Development of a practical membrane lung system. *Ann. Thorac. Surg.*, **26**, 54–61.

Hessel, E. A., II, Johnson, D. D., Ivey, T. D. and Miller, D. W. Jr (1980) Membrane versus bubble oxygenator for cardiac operations. A prospective randomized study. *J. Thorac. Cardiovasc. Surg.*, **80**, 111–22.

Hicks, G. L., Zwart, H. H. J. and DeWall, R. A. (1979) Membrane versus bubble oxygenators: A prospective study of 52 patients. *Arch. Surg.*, **114**, 1285–7.

Hill, J. D. (1978) Membrane oxygenators: An editorial introduction. *Artif. Organs*, **2**, 4–5.

Hill, J. D., Bramson, M. L., Hackel, A., Deal, C. W., Sanchez, P. A., Osborn, J. J. and Gerbode, F. (1968) Laboratory and clinical studies during prolonged partial extracorporeal circulation using the Bramson membrane lung. *Circulation*, 37(suppl. 2), 139–45.

Hill, D. G., de Lanerolle, P., Kosek, J. C., Aguilar, M. J. and Hill, J. D. (1975) The pulmonary pathophysiology of membrane and bubble oxygenators. *Trans. Am. Soc. Artif. Int. Organs*, **21**, 165–70.

Hill, J. D., Iatridis, A., O'Keefe, R. and Kitrilakis, S. (1974) Technique for achieving high gas exchange rates in membrane oxygenation. *Trans. Am. Soc. Artif. Int. Organs*, **20**, 249–52.

Hill, J. D., O'Brien, T. G., Murray, J. J., Dontigny, L., Bramson, M. L., Osborn, J. J. and Gerbode, F. (1972) Prolonged extracorporeal oxygenation for acute post-traumatic respiratory failure (shock-lung syndrome): Use of the Bramson Membrane Lung. *New Engl. J. Med.*, **286**, 629–34.

Hlavinka, D. (1983) Personal communication. Cobe Laboratories Inc.

Hoffmeister H. E., Schorer, R. and Stunkat, R. (1975) Klinische Verwendung von Membran-Oxygenatoren für länger dauernde extakorporale Zirkulation. *Thoraxchirurgie*, **23**, 49–57.

Hooke, R. (1667) An account of an experiment made by Hooke, of preserving animals alive by blowing through their lungs and bellows. *Phil. Trans. Royal Soc. London*, **2**, 539–40. (From Comroe, J. H. Jr (1977) *Am. Rev. Resp. Dis.*, **115**, 343.

Illickal, M. M., Brown, G. E., Van de Water, J. M., Lee, J. M., Pall, D. B. and Maloney, J. V. Jr (1967) Boundary layer phenomena in membrane oxygenators. *Surg. Forum*, **18**, 134.

Karlson, K. E., Murphy, W. R., Kakvan, M., Anthony, P., Cooper, G. N. Jr, Richardson, P. D. and Galletti, P. M. (1974) Total cardiopulmonary bypass with a new microporous teflon membrane oxygenator. *Surgery*, **76**, 935–45.

Katsuhara, K., Yokosuka, T. and Sakakibara, S. (1968) The swing-type membrane oxygenator: Gas exchange performance of the swing motion system. *J. Surg. Res.*, **8**, 245–52.

Kayser, K. L. (1974) Blood gas interface oxygenators versus membrane oxygenators: what are the proved differences? *Ann. Thorac. Surg.*, **17**, 459–63.

Kirsh, M. M., Rhodes, E. L., O'Rourke, P. T., Prager, R., Kirkland, J., Waldman, J. and Sloan, H. (1973) Comparison in children of the Peirce–General Electric membrane oxygenator with a bubble oxygenator. *Mt Sinai J. Med.*, **40**, 146–52.

Kolff, W. J. and Berk, H. T. J. (1944) Artificial kidney: dialyzer with great area. *Acta Med. Scand.*, **117**, 121–34.

Kolobow, T. and Bowman, R. L. (1963) Construction and evaluation of an alveolar membrane artificial heart–lung. *Trans. Am. Soc. Artif. Int. Organs.*, **9**, 238–43.

Kolobow, T., Spragg, R. C., Pierce, J. F. and Zapol, W. M. (1971) Extended term (to 16 days) partial extracorporeal gas exchange with the spiral membrane lung in unanesthetized lambs. *Trans. Am. Soc. Artif. Int. Organs*, **17**, 350–4.

Kolobow, T., Stool, E. W., Sacks, K. L. and Vurek, G. G. (1975) Acute respiratory failure: Survival following ten days support with a membrane lung. *J. Thorac. Cardiovasc. Surg.*, **69**, 947–53.

Landé, A. J., Edwards, L., Bloch, J. H., Carleson, R. G., Subramanian, V., Ascheim, R. S., Scheidt, S., Fillmore, S., Killip, T. and Lillehei, C. W. (1970) Prolonged cardio-pulmonary support with a practical membrane oxygenator. *Trans. Am. Soc. Artif. Int. Organs*, **16**, 352–6.

Lee, W. H. Jr, Brady, M. P., Rowe, J. and Miller, W. C. Jr. (1970) Effects of extracorporeal circulation upon behavior, personality, and brain function: Part II, hemodynamic, metabolic and psychometric correlations. *Ann. Surg.*, **173**, 1013–23.

Le Gallois, J. J. C. (1812) *Expériences sur le Principe de la Vie.* D'Hautel.

McCaughan, J. S. Jr, Weeder, R. R., Schuder, J. C. and Blakemore, W. S. (1969) Evaluation of new non-wettable microporous membranes with high permeability coefficients for possible use in a membrane oxygenator. *J. Thorac. Cardiovasc. Surg.*, **40**, 574.

MacDonnell, K. F., Moon, H. S., Seker, T. S. and Ahluwalia, M. P. (1980) Extracorporeal membrane oxygenator: Support in a case of severe status asthmaticus. *Ann. Thorac. Surg.*, **31**, 171–5.

Marsh, D. (1983) Personal communication. Terumo Corp.

Marx, G. H. (1970) A capillary membrane-oxygenator utilizing gas dispersed in oil. *Trans. Am. Soc. Artif. Int. Organs*, **16**, 381–3.

Melrose, D. S. (1959) Pumping and oxygenating systems. *Br. J. Anesth.*, **31**, 393–400.

Mortensen, J. D. (1977) Evaluations of tests for blood damage produced by oxygenators. *Trans. Am. Soc. Artif. Int. Organs*, **23**, 747–54.

Nosé, Y. (1973) *Manual on Artificial Organs.* Vol. II. *The Oxygenator.* Chapter 6, Membrane Oxygenator, Mosby, St. Louis, pp. 127–61.

Owens, G., Adams, J. E. and Scott, H. W. Jr (1960) Embolic fat as a measure of adequacy of various oxygenators. *J. Appl. Physiol.*, **15**, 999–1000.

Parker, J. L., Hackett, J. E., Clark, D., Crane, T. N. and Reed, C. C. (1979) Membrane versus bubble oxygenators: a clinical comparison of postoperative blood loss. *Bull. Texas Heart Inst.*, **6**, 78–84.

Pearson, D. (1983) Personal communication. Travenol Laboratories.

Peirce, E. C. II (1967) The membrane lung; its excuse, present status, and promise. *Mt Sinai J. Med.*, **34**, 437–68.

Peirce, E. C. II (1969) *Extracorporeal Circulation for Open-Heart Surgery*, Thomas, Springfield, Ill.

Peirce, E. C., II (1970) A comparison of the Landé–Edwards, the Peirce, and the

General Electric–Peirce membrane lungs. *Trans. Am. Soc. Artif. Int. Organs*, **16**, 358–64.

Peirce, E. C., II (1972) The role of the artificial lung in the treatment of respiratory insufficiency: a perspective. *Chest (Suppl. 2)*, **62**, 107–17.

Peirce, E. C., II (1973) The theory and function of the membrane lung. *Mt Sinai J. Med.*, **40**, 119–34.

Peirce, E. C., II (1974) Is the blood–gas interface of clinical importance. *Ann. Thorac. Surg.*, **17**, 526–9.

Peirce, E. C., II (1976) Artificial lungs. *Proc. Int. Conf., Systems, Man and Cybernetics Society*, The Institute of Electrical and Electronics Engineers, Inc., Washington, DC, pp. 201–7.

Peirce, E. C., II (1977) Extracorporeal membrane oxygenation for acute respiratory insufficiency: Current status. In *Mechanical Support for the Failing Heart and Lungs* (ed. D. Bregman), Appleton-Century-Crofts, New York, Chapter 6, pp. 144–63.

Peirce, E. C., II (1980a) The membrane versus bubble oxygenator controversy. *Ann. Thorac. Surg.*, **29**, 497–9.

Peirce, E. C., II (1980b) Cerebral gas embolism (arterial) with special reference to iatrogenic accidents. *Hyperbaric Oxygen Rev.*, **1**, 161–84.

Peirce, E. C., II (1981) Is extracorporeal membrane oxygenation a viable technique? *An. Thorac. Surg.*, **31**, 102–4.

Peirce, E. C., II, Bartlett, R. H., De Fillipi, R. H., Keller, R. P., Landé, A. J., Martinez, J., Richardson, P. D. and Kennedy, J. H. (1976) Draft proposal: standards for blood gas exchangers. *Trans. Am. Soc. Artif. Int. Organs*, **22**, 734–40.

Peirce, E. C., II, Corrigan, J. J., Kent, B. B., Cate, C. L., Johnson, R. L. and Reves, A. E. (1969) Comparative trauma to blood in the disc oxygenator and membrane lung. *Trans. Am. Soc. Artif. Int. Organs*, **15**, 33–9.

Peirce, E. C., II and Dibelius, N. R. (1968) The membrane lung: studies with a new high permeability co-polymer membrane. *Trans. Am. Soc. Artif. Int. Organs*, **14**, 220–6.

Peirce, E. C., II and Peirce, G. (1963) The membrane lung: The influence of membrane characteristics and lung design on gas exchange. *J. Surg. Res.*, **3**, 67–76.

Peirce, E. C., II, Rogers, W. K., Dabbs, C. H. and Rawson, F. L. (1960) Clinical experience with membrane lung used in conjunction with hypothermia. *J. Tenn. Med. Assoc.*, **54**, 39–45.

Peirce, E. C., II, Thebaut, A. L., Kent, B. B., Kirkland, J. S., Goetter, W. E. and Wright, B. G. (1971) Technique of extended perfusion using a membrane lung. *Ann. Thorac. Surg.*, **12**, 451–70.

Peterson, K. A., Dewanjee, M. K. and Kaye, M. P. (1982) Fate of ^{111}indium labelled platelets during cardiopulmonary bypass performed with membrane and bubble oxygenators. *J. Thorac. Cardiovasc. Surg.*, **84**, 39–43.

Pranger, R. L., Mook, P. H., Elstradt, J. M., Kessler, M., Lübbers, D. M. and Wildevuur, C. R. H. (1980) Improved tissue perfusion (pO_2 histograms) in extracorporeal circulation using membrane instead of bubble oxygenators. *J. Thorac. Cardiovasc. Surg.*, **79**, 513–22.

Rhodes, E. L., Kirsh, M. M., Howatt, W., O'Rourke, P. T., Straker, J. and Sloan, H. (1974) A comparison of pulmonary function in puppies undergoing total cardiopulmonary bypass with bubble or membrane oxygenators. *J. Thorac. Cardiovasc. Surg.*, **68**, 658–63.

Riley, J. B. and Pfaender, L. M. (1980) Blood oxygenation control by vacuum drawn mixture of room air and oxygen in a membrane oxygenator. *J. Extra-Corporeal Tech.*, **12**, 40–5.

Sade, R. M., Bartels, D. M., Dearing, J. P., Campbell, R. N. and Loadholt, C. B. (1981) A prospective randomized study of membrane versus bubble oxygenators in children. *Ann. Thorac. Surg.*, **32**, 105–6.

SciMed Life Systems Inc. (1983) *Data and Instruction Manual* and *Operator's Manual.*

Schults, M. C., Updike, S. J., Treichel, P. M. and Treichel, I. W. (1974) High efficiency Oxford type oxygenator based on hemodialysis and transmembrane catalysis of hydrogen peroxide. *Trans. Am. Soc. Artif., Int., Organs*, **20**, 186–291.

Siderys, H., Herod, G. T., Halbrook, H., Pittman, J. N., Rubush, J. L., Kasebaker, V. and Berry, G. R. Jr (1975) A comparison of membrane and bubble oxygenation as used in cardiopulmonary bypass in patients. The importance of pericardial blood as a source of hemolysis. *J. Thorac. Cardiovasc. Surg.*, **69**, 708–12.

Stoney, W. S., Alford, W. C. Jr, Burrus, G. R., Glassford, D. M. Jr and Thomas, C. S. Jr (1980) Air embolism and other accidents using pump oxygenators. *Ann. Thorac. Surg.*, **29**, 336–40.

Suma, K., Tsuji, T., Takeuchi, Y., Inoue, K., Shiroma, K., Yoshikawa, T. and Narumi, J. (1981) Clinical performance of microporous polypropylene hollow-fiber oxygenator. *Ann. Thorac. Surg.*, **32**, 558–62.

Terumo Corp. (1982) Descriptive data on Capiox.

Thomas, J. A., Vaysse, J., d'Allaines, C., Laurent, D., Chevrier, J. L., Ricordeau, G., Jaulmes, B., du Bouchet, N., Mirabel, J., Latscha, B. I., Arfel, G., Vallon, M. and d'Allaines, J. (1958) Le coeur-poumon à membrane pulmonaire artificielle: premiers résultats chirurgicaux. *Arch. Mal Coeur*, **51**, 801.

Tsuji, T., Suma, K., Tanashita, K., Fukasawa, H., Kanno, M., Hasegawa, H. and Takahashi, A. (1981) Development and clinical evaluation of hollow fiber membrane oxygenator. *Trans. Am. Soc. Artif. Int. Organs*, **27**, 280–4.

Tufo, H. M., Ostfeld, A. M. and Shekelle, R. (1970) Central nervous system dysfunction following open heart surgery. *J. Am. Med. Assoc.*, **212**, 1333–40.

Unger, F., Domanig, E., Rastl, P. and Salem, G. (1976) Traumatische Hämolyse verschiedener Herz-Lungen-Maschinen und Oxygenatorentypen. *Thoraxchirurgie*, **24**, 59–65.

Valdés, F., Haraski, H., Meserko, J., Kambic, H., Malchesky, P., Golding, L. and Nosé, Y. (1981) Ex vivo evaluation of a new capillary membrane oxygenator. *Trans. Am. Soc. Artif. Int. Organs*, **27**, 270–5.

Van den Dungen, J. J., Korliczek, G. F., Brenken, U., van der Heide, J. W. H. and Wildevuur, C. R. H. (1982) Clinical study of blood trauma during perfusion with membrane and bubble oxygenators. *J. Thorac. Cardiovasc. Surg.*, **83**, 108–16.

Vroman, L. (1971) Summation: protein at the interface. *Conference on Mechanical Surface and Gas Layer Effects on Moving Blood, Fed. Proc.*, **30**, 1703.

White, J. J., Andrews, H. B., Risemberg, H., Mazur, D. and Haller, J. A. Jr (1971) Prolonged respiratory support in newborn infants with a membrane oxygenator. *Surgery*, **70**, 288–96.

Williams, D. R., Tyers, F. O., Williams, E. H., Kurusz, M., Shaffer, C. W., Pierce, W. S. and Waldhausen, J. A. (1978) Similarity of laboratory and clinical results obtained with microporous teflon membrane oxygenator and bubble-film hybrid oxygenator. *Ann. Thorac. Surg.*, **25**, 30–5.

Williams, T. L., Bosher, L. H. and Nakamuro, T. (1969) A hollow filament fabric blood oxygenator. *Proceedings Artificial Heart Conference*, National Heart Institute (eds F. W. Hastings and L. T. Harmison), US Govt Printing Office, Washington, DC, p. 365.

Wright, J. S., Fish, G. C., Torda, T. A., Stacey, R. B. and Hicks, R. G. (1975) Some advantages of the membrane oxygenator for open heart surgery. *J. Thorac. Cardiovasc. Surg.*, **69**, 884–90.

Zapol, W. M., Levy, R. I., Kolobow, T., Spragg, R. and Bowman, R. T. (1969) *In vitro* denaturation of plasma alpha lipoproteins by bubble oxygenation in the dog. *Curr. Topics Surg. Res.*, **1**, 449–67.

Zapol, W. M., Snider, M. T., Hill, J. D., Fallat, R. J., Bartlett, R. H., Edmunds, H., Morris, A. H., Peirce, E. C., II, Thomas, A. H., Proctor, H. J., Drinker, P. A., Pratt, P. C., Bagniewski, A. and Miller, R. G. (1979) Extracorporeal membrane oxygenation in severe acute respiratory failure: A randomized prospective study. *J. Am. Med. Assoc.*, **242**, 2193–6.

13

Extracorporeal membrane oxygenation

J. DONALD HILL and EVANGELOS IATRIDIS

13.1 INTRODUCTION AND SUMMARY

The adult respiratory distress syndrome (ARDS) became a clinical entity in medicine during the late 1950s and early 1960s with the development and widespread use of intensive care facilities for seriously ill medical and surgical patients. The early success reached in treating these seriously ill patients was achieved by bringing together expertise in pulmonary and cardiac pathophysiology coupled with the availability of respiratory ventilators. Many of these patients went on to develop ARDS, whereas ten years earlier they would have succumbed to their initial illness. This event in the early 1960s resulted in over two decades of intensive investigation and application of many new interventions to understand, diagnose, prevent and treat ARDS resulting from a variety of causes.

One such intervention proposed was extracorporeal membrane oxygenation (ECMO). The principle was simple and not original. If a patient was dying due to a pathological process in the lungs, which prevented sufficient oxygen and carbon dioxide traversing the alveolar membrane, the employment of an artificial and extracorporeal gas exchange device would sustain the patient until such time as the lungs recovered. For this premise to succeed two things had to be true and/or possible. (1) The lungs had to have the capacity to recover with time; (2) ECMO had to be done safely and efficiently without significant secondary complications. Now, two decades later, we know that ECMO can, under most specified circumstances, be done safely. However, the inability of the lung to recover with time has been a major limiting factor in the widespread successful use of this therapy. ECMO in the treatment of ARDS has some specifically defined applications where it has proved to be a significant adjunct to conventional therapy. However, considering the magnitude of the problem, and the number of deaths per year attributed to ARDS, ECMO now, and in this coming decade, will not have a significant impact on this syndrome. However, in the neonate with respiratory distress syndrome, ECMO has been successful and will continue to play a significant role in this syndrome in the coming years.

13.2 THE EQUIPMENT

The first successful prototype of a membrane oxygenator was developed by Clowes (1958). The Bramson membrane oxygenator was the first successful device commercially available and used in any significant numbers (Bramson *et al.*, 1965). Until recently, the development of membrane oxygenators has been hindered by their inability to compete with the simplicity and economics of bubble oxygenators. Most investigators and clinicians readily acknowledged that on a theoretical basis membrane oxygenators were superior to conventional oxygenators. However, for the length of perfusion necessary in routine open-heart surgery, disposable simple and economical bubble oxygenators were performing well. Furthermore, no investigator in controlled randomized studies could demonstrate the superiority of the membrane oxygenator for use in routine open-heart surgery. Conversely, no one could demonstrate that bubble oxygenators could be used successfully for long-term respiratory support, as membrane oxygenators had been successfully used in animal experiments. Now this is changing. There are a number of commercially available membrane oxygenators that are used in routine open-heart surgery and are possible devices for use in ECMO. Each has its individual advantages and disadvantages but all have been demonstrated to be effective and safe in routine open-heart surgery, and are being developed further for use in chronic membrane oxygenation.

The two most important features that a membrane oxygenator should have for use in ECMO are continued efficiency and safety during long-term use and acceptably low thrombogenic characteristics. At this point all patients undergoing ECMO must still receive heparin to prevent thrombogenesis in the extracorporeal circuit (Hill *et al.*, 1974a).

13.3 THE ADULT RESPIRATORY DISTRESS SYNDROME

ARDS became a clinically significant entity in the early 1960s with the development of intensive care units, which arose with the complications associated with the immediate postoperative care of open-heart surgical patients. The aetiology, pathogenesis and therapy of this syndrome were not understood in the early 1960s. The introduction of positive and expiratory pressure ventilation (PEEP) by Hill *et al.* (1965) was the first significant mechanical intervention other than ventilators which improved serious respiratory hypoxia in postoperative open-heart surgical patients. Later in 1967, pulmonary clinicians successfully applied PEEP therapy to patients with ARDS arising from other causes. Since that time, an enormous amount of scientific literature has been published on the aetiology, prevention and treatment of this syndrome. Now this complication is seen much less commonly in medical and surgical ICUs. Therefore, potential candidates for ECMO are also less frequently seen. However, when identified, they are more seriously ill because improved conventional respiratory therapy has failed to bring them under control.

The first attempts to treat ARDS with ECMO took place in the late 1960s. Success came in 1971 when Hill treated a patient dying with ARDS associated with trauma (Hill *et al.*, 1972). In the following three years sporadic success was seen but there was still a lingering doubt as to whether ECMO *per se* was superior to conventional therapy. What was needed was a controlled, randomized study of conventional therapy and ECMO. This was organized in 1973 and completed in 1977. Nine different centres and approximately 100 patients entered the trial (Collaborative program, 1974). The results indicated that there was no statistical difference between patients treated with conventional therapy or ECMO (Zapol *et al.*, 1979). However, at the end of the study one thing was recognized which had been suspected for some time. Using the entrance criteria chosen the mortality rate with either therapy was over 90%. For ECMO to be successful it would have to used as intervention early in the course of the disease before the architecture of the lung had been destroyed and while reversibility was possible (Pratt *et al.*, 1979). The observation and scientific documentation of this principle have established early intervention as the key to the successful application of ECMO. If one is going to allow the lungs to recover, and reverse the pathological process, intervention must take place early. Once the architecture of the lung has been destroyed no amount of time on ECMO will bring about reversal. Therefore, by the late 1970s two things were clear: the lung did not have the intrinsic capacity to repair itself in most instances, as did, for example, the kidney; and secondly, that despite some limitations of the technology *per se*, ECMO could most often be carried out safely without serious complications.

13.4 CURRENT INDICATIONS AND CONTRAINDICATIONS

The important questions in selecting any patient for ECMO intervention are: how long has the patient been sick? and is pulmonary fibrosis present in the lung? (Hill *et al.*, 1974b). As a general guideline effective intervention must take place in the first five days since thereafter reversibility is unlikely. If one has taken a lung biopsy, which usually requires an open technique, the absence of pulmonary fibrosis is an indication that reversibility may be possible (Hill *et al.*, 1976).

The selection of cases for ECMO therefore, has fallen more into the sphere of time, pathology and clinical syndromes rather than specific physiological studies of gas exchange in the lungs. Gas exchange and pulmonary mechanics are merely a reflection of the severity of the pathology and how threatening the hypoxia is rather than any indication for ECMO *per se*. The ideal patient for ECMO is one who has severe and life-threatening hypoxia of very short duration. This is an area in which ECMO has been dramatically successful. Faced with a patient with acute and lethal hypoxia, ECMO can dramatically change the course of events to allow one to get control of ventilatory function. At the other end of the spectrum are the patients who develop respiratory failure and in whom ECMO has not been successful. Key examples of this are viral and aspiration pneumonia. Except for isolated successes ECMO has largely been unsuccessful in these two syndromes. The best candidates for ECMO are those with acute shock lung, trauma and opportunistic infections. Certain patients with congenital heart disease who develop respiratory failure during surgical correction are also good candidates because the pathology is largely congestive, not destructive and ECMO can successfully support these patients for 2 to 3 days until their own lungs recover.

There are some specific contraindications to ECMO. Foremost among these, of course, is the risk of bleeding. Despite many advances in the membrane device technology the large surface area involved still requires heparin anticoagulation to block thrombogenesis. This, of course, may have a detrimental effect on the patients if they are already bleeding or at a significant risk from further bleeding (e.g. subdural haematoma).

Other contraindications to ECMO include: significant and irreversible left heart failure, septic schock, CNS damage, pre-existing degenerative diseases, late stages of malignancy and the presence of an untreated and possibly untreatable large broncho-pleural fistula. Fractures, or multiple traumas in the absence of bleeding risk, are not contraindications to ECMO. Age *per se* is not a contraindication to instituting ECMO.

In unselected cases, as was the case in the large co-operative study, the retrieval rate is 10–15% in ARDS. If discrimination is used in the selection of patients who have possible reversible lung disease the success rate can be increased to 30–40%.

13.5 METHODS

There are three basic cannulation techniques used in ECMO: veno-arterial, veno-venous, and mixed veno-arterial–veno-venous. It should be stated at the outset that the veno-venous is presently the technique of choice.

13.5.1 Veno-arterial bypass

Veno-arterial bypass, using the groin vessels, is the most obvious approach for chronic extracorporeal oxygenation. It carries with it certain disadvantages and is not at this time the method of choice in ARDS. The venous cannula (32 French) is positioned in the right atrium after being introduced into the right common femoral vein. The arterial cannula is introduced into the right common femoral artery. The distal common femoral artery is perfused by way of a side-arm off the main arterial perfusion line. This bypass technique will capture 80% of the cardiac output and return it oxygenated to the systemic circulation. The pulmonary artery pressure is significantly decreased and the ventilatory pressures and FIO_2 on the ventilator can be significantly decreased.

The disadvantages of this technique are that the oxygenated blood introduced into the common femoral artery does not always reach the arch of the aorta and the coronary arteries and the brain may continue to be perfused with hypoxic blood. This is partially overcome by introducing a long cannula into the arch of the aorta for perfusion. This, however, introduces a greater potential risk of thromboembolism. Removing these cannulae has, on occasion, been difficult due to the friction between the cannula and the common femoral, external iliac and the common iliac arteries. A second risk of this approach is the stasis which develops in the pulmonary circulation and in the left atrium. Of the cardiac output 80% is being bypassed and this low flow in the presence of oedema and inflammatory reaction taking place in the lung may result in primary thrombosis in the pulmonary arterial and venous circulation (Ratliff *et al.*, 1975). In addition, decreasing the pulmonary artery pressure was thought, at first, to be advantageous, but it is now considered more important to maintain pulmonary artery pressure to ensure the continued perfusion of the lung nutrients and oxygen to aid in healing and prevent further deterioration. One further disadvantage of veno-arterial bypass is that on many occasions it will result in non-pulsatile flow in the systemic circulation.

13.5.2 Veno-venous bypass

Veno-venous bypass was the first method used in the treatment of ARDS with ECMO. It was then largely abandoned because one could only remove 40–45% of the cardiac output with venous cannulation of the inferior vena cava, and it was felt that a higher bypass flow was necessary. Now with better knowledge of the shortcomings of veno-arterial bypass and improvements in cannulation techniques veno-venous bypass is the method of choice. Initially the technique involved passing a 32 French cannula into the inferior vena cava by way of the right common femoral vein. The tip of the cannula was positioned just below the entrance of the inferior vena cava into the right atrium. Oxygenated blood was returned to the patient by way of a cannula positioned in the superior vena cava via the right internal jugular vein. This system was simple and easy to manage. However, it provided insufficient bypass flows to allow one adequately to oxygenate the patient, and thus lacked the ability to allow a reduction in inflation pressure and FIO_2 on the ventilator. If one advanced the efferent venous cannula further up into the right atrium to obtain a larger bypass flow, cross circulation from the efferent cannula developed.

This problem has now been eliminated by passing the afferent cannula, returning oxygenated blood to the patient, down into the right ventricle. This is easily and effectively done using fluoroscopic control and a pre-curved, wire-re-inforced cannula. The tricuspid valve effectively separates the two circulations and the venous efferent cannula can be passed directly into the right atrium and 80% of the venous return goes through the extracorporeal circuit. Oxygenated blood passes through the pulmonary circulation in sufficient quantities to allow the ventilator to have both its pressure and FIO_2 reduced. There is no problem with oxygenation of the aortic arch as occurs in veno-arterial bypass. In addition, the pressures in the pulmonary artery are kept elevated to perfuse the diseased lung sufficiently. Leaving the perfusion cannula in the right ventricle has not produced any significant cardiac arrhythmias or damage to the right ventricular or septal muscle. Pulsatile flow is obtained and the whole management of the patient is simplified.

13.5.3 Mixed veno-arterial–veno-venous bypass

This is merely a combination of the above two systems in which part of the oxygenated blood is returned to the femoral artery. It is a more complicated system to run, carries higher potential risks of thromboembolic problems, but has the advantage of allowing the adjustment of pulmonary artery saturation and pressure. This cannulation technique is not one to be advised until experience has been gained in the simpler approaches.

13.6 FUTURE PROSPECTS FOR ECMO AND ARDS

Continued improved success in the treatment of ARDS will probably arise more from increased understanding of prevention and pathophysiology than from improved techniques in ECMO. The fundamental problems still exist irrespective of which particular therapy is chosen. The lung is not particularly resilient in recovering from serious damage. In addition improved results will come only from therapy which alters the course of the pathology. Earlier hopes that eliminating the potential damaging effects of high FIO_2s and high airway pressures would significantly change the course of pathological events have not been confirmed. It is more probable that a better understanding of the sequence of pathophysiological events taking place will lead to more specific therapy designed to reduce pulmonary destruction and therefore prevent irreversible damage. However, there will probably always be a place for ECMO in certain situations, particularly in acute situations where a patient is faced with imminent death if hypoxia is not corrected. The successful development of an antithrombogenic membrane surface is the single most important advance necessary in this technology to allow ECMO to be performed with little risk. This would allow the clinician to initiate therapy very early and possibly avert the dismal course of events that are presently common place in ARDS. Of secondary importance in this situation is the development of more efficient membrane oxygenators with low priming volumes and reduced membrane surface areas.

A last and seemingly unimportant aspect of success in ECMO is the experience of the team using the therapy. Most centres are faced with the possibility of using ECMO only a few times a year. The infrequency of experience makes it difficult to develop an expertise which promotes success.

13.7 NEONATAL RESPIRATORY DISTRESS SYNDROME

The success associated with ECMO in this syndrome has been quite different from that experienced in ARDS. The reason for this is clear. Neonates have truly reversible pulmonary pathology whereas adults do not. Dr Robert Bartlett is the leader and individual responsible for the successful development of ECMO in neonates (Bartlett *et al.*, 1977, 1980, 1982). In the mid 1970s in association with neonatologists treating respiratory distress in neonates, he indentified patients expected to die despite conventional therapy and placed them on ECMO. Three clinical syndromes have now been indentified in which ECMO can significantly alter prognosis. These are (1) meconium aspiration syndrome, (2) congenital diaphragmatic hernia, and (3) persistent foetal circulation. If one moves quickly before the lung is significantly damaged a successful outcome can be obtained in 35–50% of these patients. More importantly, once treated these patients can go on to develop normal pulmonary function and growth without any of the complications associated with their initial disease or treatment.

The indications for the use of ECMO in neonates is in any newborn who becomes moribund due to pulmonary hypoxaemia with hypotension and acidosis. Under these circumstances when conventional intervention techniques are persistently unsuccessful ECMO should be initiated without delay.

Contraindications to ECMO include an intracranial bleed or neurological deficit, multiple congenital anomalies, renal failure or a weight less than 1300 g.

Veno-arterial bypass cannulation technique has been very successful in neonates. One reason for this is that the technique involves returning the arterial blood to the right internal carotid artery. This prevents the aortic arch hypoxia which is so common in adults with femoral artery return. Neonates tolerate temporary and permanent occlusion of their right common carotid artery which makes this technique possible. The venous inflow line is introduced into the right internal jugular vein and advanced to the right atrium. Neonates also tolerate the permanent occlusion of this vessel. The technique then becomes quite simple even though one is dealing with a tiny infant. Once bypass has been initiated the remaining major complication is intracranial haemorrhage which, of course, is a major cause of death in this group of patients even without ECMO.

Despite the success of Bartlett and other centres (Krummel *et al.*, 1982) using this therapy in the treatment of neonates, who otherwise would die, the approach has not been widely accepted by paediatric clinicians as a whole. Once again, one of the major problems is the absence of a large controlled clinical study which would demonstrate its distinct superiority over conventional therapy. As more and more centres develop this technique such studies will become available and the more specific characterization of the therapy and its specific application identified. In the meantime the major challenge of the technology is to be able to use it on smaller infants and to be able to have antithrombogenic surfaces and control the risk of haemorrhage more precisely.

13.8 CO_2 REMOVAL APPROACH IN ARDS

It is necessary to mention this alternative and intriguing approach to the treatment of ARDS. In recent years there has developed an interest in a simplified form of ECMO in which the prime objective is only to remove carbon dioxide in the treatment of ARDS. This allows a dramatic reduction in the ventilatory parameters which result in less damage to the lung one is trying to heal (Barthelemy *et al.*, 1982; Kolobow *et al.*, 1983; Gattinoni *et al.*, 1980).

REFERENCES

Barthelemy, R., Puel, P., Enjalbert, A. *et al.* (1982) CO_2 removal through a microporous membrane lung. *Int. J. Artif. Organs*, **5**, 149.

Bartlett, R. H., Andrews, A. F., Toomasian, C. C. P. *et al.* (1982) Extracorporeal membrane oxygenation for newborn respiratory failure: Forty-five cases. *Surgery*, **92**, 425.

Bartlett, R. H., Gazzaniga, A. B., Huxtable, R. F. *et al.* (1977) Extracorporeal circulation (ECMO) in neonatal respiratory failure. *J. Thorac. Cardiovasc. Surg.*, **74**, 826.

Bartlett, R. H., Gazzaniga, A. B., Wetmore, N. E. *et al.* (1980) Extracorporeal membrane oxygenation (ECMO) in the treatment of cardiac and respiratory failure in children. *Trans. Am. Soc. Artif. Int. Organs*, **26**, 587.

Bramson, M. L., Osborn, J. J., Main, F. B., O'Brien, M. F., Wright, J. S. and Gerbode, F. (1965) New disposable membrane oxygenator with integral heat exchanger. *J. Thorac. Cardiovasc. Surg.*, **50**, 391.

Clowes, G. H. A. Jr and Neville, W. E. (1958) in *The Membrane Oxygenator in Extracorporeal Circulation* (ed. J. G. Alles), Charles C. Thomas, Springfield, Ill.

Collaborative program (1974) Protocol for extracorporeal support for respiratory insufficiency. National Heart and Lung Institute, Division of Lung Diseases, 15 May.

Gattinoni, L., Angostoni, A., Pesenti, A. *et al.* (1980) Treatment of acute respiratory failure with low-frequency positive-pressure ventilation and extracorporeal removal of CO_2. *Lancet*, **ii**, 292.

Hill, J. D., Dontigny, L., deLeval, M. R. *et al.* (1974a) A simple method of heparin management during prolonged extracorporeal circulation. *Ann. Thorac. Surg.*, **17**, 129.

Hill, J. D., Main, F. B., Osborn, J. J. *et al.* (1965) Correct use of respirators in the postoperative cardiac patient. *Arch. Surg.*, **91**, 775.

Hill, J. D., O'Brien, T. G., Murray, J. J., Dontigny, L., Branson, M. L., Osborn, J. J. and Gerbode, F. (1972) Prolonged extracorporeal oxygenation for acute post-traumatic respiratory failure (shock-lung syndrome). *New Engl. J. Med.*, **286**, 629.

Hill, J. D., Ratliff, J. L., Fallat, R. J. *et al.* (1974b) Prognostic factors in the treatment of acute respiratory insufficiency with long-term extracorporeal oxygenation. *J. Thorac. Cardiovasc. Surg.*, **68**, 905.

Hill, J. D., Ratliff, J. L., Parrott, J. C. *et al.* (1976) Pulmonary pathology in acute respiratory insufficiency: Lung biopsy as a diagnostic tool. *J. Thorac. Cardiovasc. Surg.*, **71**, 64.

Kolobow, T., Gattinoni, L., Pesenti, A. *et al.* (1983) The past, present and future of the membrane artificial lung. In *The Past, Present and Future of Artificial Organs* (eds E. Piskin and T. M. S. Chang), Meteksan Publishing Co., Ankara.

Krummel, T. M., Greenfield, L. J., Kirkpatrick, B. V. *et al.* (1982) Clinical use of an extracorporeal membrane oxygenator in neonatal pulmonary failure. *J. Pediatr. Surg.*, **17**, 525.

Pratt, P. C., Vollmer, R. T., Shelburn, J. D. *et al.* (1979) Pulmonary morphology in a multihospital collaborative extracorporeal membrane oxygenation project: I. Light microscopy. *Am. J. Pathol.*, **95**, 191–214.

Ratliff, J. L., Hill, J. D., Fallat, R. J. *et al.* (1975) Complications associated with membrane lung support by venoarterial perfusion. *Ann. Thorac. Surg.*, **19**, 537.

Zapol, W. M., Snider, M. T., Hill, J. D. *et al.* (1979) Extracorporeal membrane oxygenation in severe acute respiratory failure – A randomized prospective study. *J. Am. Med. Assoc.*, **242**, 2193.

14
Choice of priming fluids

M. A. TOBIAS

14.1 INTRODUCTION

In 1964, the South Central Association of Blood Banks met in Oklahoma City to discuss which priming fluids were most suitable for cardiopulmonary bypass (Zuhdi *et al.*, 1964). The topic was 'Blood, mannitol, dextran, water and confusion' and in spite of the many pertinent publications appearing since then, there still remains no consensus as to what constitutes the ideal prime.

It is the purpose of this chapter to:

(1) Outline the rationale behind the shift away from whole blood towards the utilization of clear fluid primes in the extracorporeal circuit.
(2) Illustrate the behaviour of crystalloid and colloid solutions in the circulation with reference to changes in haematocrit, viscosity and hydrostatic, crystalloid and colloid osmotic pressures.
(3) Review the literature concerning associated clinical research and indicate future lines of development.

The associated topics of haemofiltration and salvage of blood following haemodilution will be discussed in detail in Chapter 17.

14.2 HISTORY

During the early period of open-heart surgery, heart-lung machines were primed with fresh heparinized homologous blood. The original film oxygenators required large priming volumes (3–5 litres), and the problem of providing an adequate supply of fresh donor blood soon forced clinicians to switch to routinely collected banked blood, in spite of fears that this might provoke citrate intoxication (Zuhdi *et al.*, 1960). These fears proved groundless and it is instructive to recall that in those early days of open-heart surgery, it was also considered a fundamental error to administer more than the barest minimum of clear fluids intra-operatively. Even the volume of heparinized saline required to flush the pressure catheter was suspected of causing the pulmonary oedema sometimes observed (Trede, 1969).

The disadvantages of perfusing patients with large volumes of genetically heterogenous blood soon became manifest. These included the 'homologous blood syndrome' (Dow *et al.*, 1960), where plasma migrated from the intravascular compartment in an unpredicatable fashion, causing a shock-like state with pooling of blood in the splanchnic circulation. Hepatic congestion and portal hypertension ensued, accompanied by increasing metabolic acidosis, coagulopathy and renal failure. Obstruction of the pulmonary vascular bed with platelet aggregates (McNamara *et al.*, 1972) and immunologically triggered opening of pulmonary shunts (Melrose *et al.*, 1965), helped to produce postoperative pulmonary congestion and hypoxia ('perfusion lung').

A significant reduction in pulmonary surfactant activity followed whole blood perfusion, accompanied by reduced lung compliance, increased surface tension and microscopic changes akin to those seen in infantile respiratory distress syndrome (Gardner *et al.*, 1962). Gadboys, Slonim and Litwak (1962) postulated that the homologous blood syndrome was precipitated by incompatibility reactions occurring not only between recipient and donor blood, but also between individual pooled donor elements.

Circulation of total blood primes through the early oxygenator/roller pump systems also produced damage to red blood corpuscles (haemolysis) and to plasma proteins (denaturation) and made extravagant demands upon transfusion services. Viral hepatitis remained a serious late complication even after screening donors for the presence of Australia antigen. The reported incidence following transfusion varies between 0.16% and 6% (Doenicke *et al.*, 1977) and has not been reduced by the introduction of frozen washed cells (Götz *et al.*, 1975).

14.3 HAEMODILUTION

In an attempt to conserve blood, Panico and Neptune (1959) designed a pump oxygenator in which a largely saline prime layered on top of the patient's blood. This development introduced the concept of haemodilution and promoted experimental and clinical work at various centres (Cooley *et al.*, 1962, Greer *et al.*, 1962). Only partial haemodilution was possible with most early large-volume oxygenators in order to guarantee delivery of a solution of adequate oxygen-carrying capacity to the patient. Litwak *et al.* (1965) utilized partial ACD blood/albumin/crystalloid primes and noted a reduction in pulmonary and coagulation complications, plus a linear increase in urine production with increasing haemodilution. Long *et al.* (1961) used dextran or albumin to improve the flow characteristics of blood and avoid the capillary blockage produced by intravascular aggregates (sludging). Experimentation with total non-haemic primes followed; Zuhdi's group (1961) used low volume primes of 5% dextrose in water and perfused at low flow rates (20 ml kg^{-1} min^{-1}) to minimize mechanical damage to erythrocytes. More recently higher volume primes utilizing more physiological flow rates have been employed. Some authors have advocated electrolyte solutions only (Laver and Buckley 1972; Lilleaasen *et al.*, 1978) and others crystalloid–colloid mixtures (Lee *et al.*, 1975; Zubiate *et al.*, 1974) sometimes supplementing with autologous blood transfusion post-bypass (Hardesty *et al.*, 1968). Universal agreement exists that high-volume dilution reduces intraoperative and postoperative blood requirements. Verska *et al.* (1974) were able to show a total peri-operative blood requirement of 1500 ml using a non-haemic prime compared with 3500 ml using a partial blood prime. Hallowell *et al.* (1972) demonstrated that a further reduction averaging 860 ml per case could be achieved by employing autologous blood transfusion. Platelet counts were consistently higher and there was less postoperative bleeding in patients treated with total haemodilution and autologous blood transfusion compared with patients receiving part-blood primes (Lilleaasen, 1977).

Haemodilution was also shown to produce a remarkable absence of metabolic acidosis interpreted as an index of good tissue perfusion with concomitant absence of peripheral vasoconstriction or cyanosis, stable electrolyte pattern, excellent urinary output and minimal renal problems (Roe *et al.*, 1964).

Finally, haemodilution has been shown to minimize the increase in pulmonary compliance in dogs seen during whole-blood perfusion (Camishion *et al.*, 1968) to reduce post-perfusion pulmonary complications in humans (Hepps *et al.*, 1963), and to oppose the adverse effects of hypothermia on cerebral cortical flow (Utley *et al.*, 1981).

14.4 RHEOLOGY

14.4.1 Viscosity function

The viscosity of blood depends mainly upon its haematocrit and the latter drops markedly when using non-haemic primes during cardiopulmonary bypass. Systemic vascular resistance varies with viscosity and arteriolar vasodilation (Smith and Crowell, 1967). Calculations for changes in systemic vascular resistance usually ignore the effect of viscosity on the assumption that this remains constant. However, the fall in blood pressure frequently seen when going on bypass using crystalloid primes has been shown by Gordon *et al.* (1975) to be substantially due to the acute reduction in viscosity produced by haemodilution (Fig. 14.1).

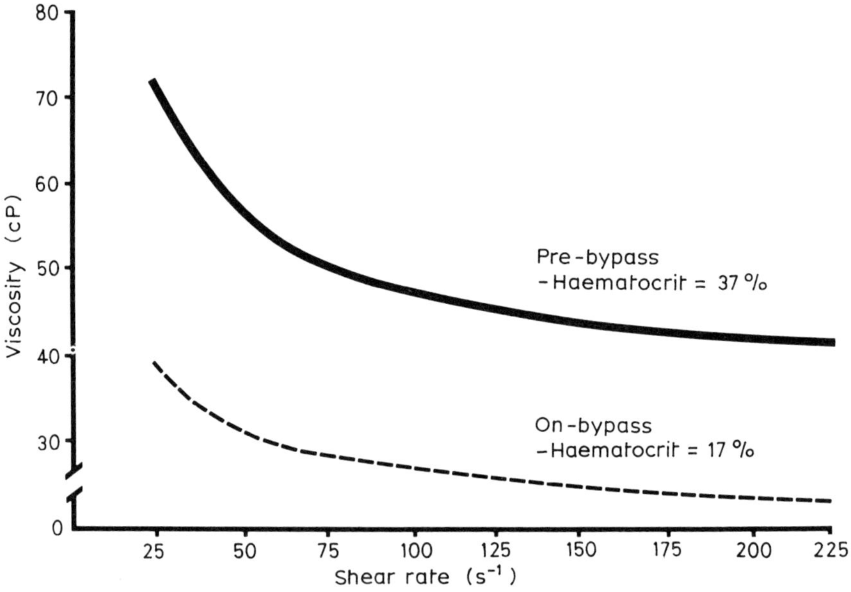

Fig. 14.1 Viscosity versus shear rate measured before and after the initiation of cardiopulmonary bypass. (Redrawn with permission from Gordon *et al.* (1975).)

Other factors contributing to the occurrence of hypotension at the commencement of bypass include:

(1) Reflex vasodilation of capacitance and resistance vessels during partial bypass, possibly caused by triggering of the baroreceptor system due to pulse generation by the beating heart during continuous fluid infusion from the arterial line (Boulanger, 1977).
(2) Alteration in baroreceptor perception as blood flow changes from a pulsatile to a non-pulsatile mode (Dunn *et al.*, 1974).
(3) Dilution of circulating catecholamines by the extracorporeal priming volume (Balasaraswathi *et al.*, 1980).

14.4.2 Optimum haematocrit

Patients respond to acute normovolaemic haemodilution (such as that produced by autologous blood removal before bypass) by increasing cardiac output involving two mechanisms; (a) augumentation of venous return (increased preload) (Guyton and Richardson, 1961); (b) smaller end-systolic volume (reduced afterload) (Murray *et al.*, 1969). Blood pressure and heart rate remain stable. Because cardiac output rises faster than oxygen content falls, oxygen availability actually increases as haematocrit is reduced towards 30% (Thorén, 1977) as shown in Fig. 14.2.

Oxygen availability falls steeply below a haematocrit of 20% when two further compensatory mechanisms are brought into play (Messmer, 1977):

(1) Enhanced oxygen extraction by lowering the venous PO_2 at tissue level;
(2) Displacement of the oxygen dissociation curve to the right.

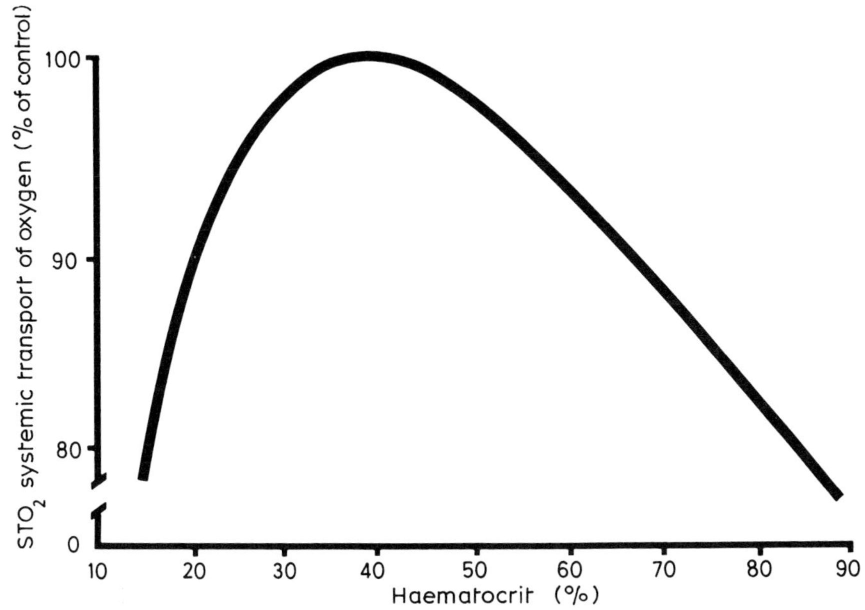

Fig. 14.2 Total systemic transport of O_2 versus haematocrit. Values are relative to a control haematocrit of 45%.

During cardiopulmonary bypass, oxygen transfer from heart-lung machine to the tissues is a product of flow rate, oxygen saturation and haemoglobin concentration. Kawashima *et al.* (1974), perfusing dogs at 80 ml kg^{-1} min^{-1}, at normothermia showed that once the haematocrit fell below 20% there was only partial compensation for the decline in oxygen flux, and a progressive decrease in total body oxygen consumption occurred (Fig. 14.3).

However, induced hypothermia is an important protective mechanism during haemodilution. Gott *et al.* (1962) have shown that oxygen requirements decline progressively with cooling to 50% of normal at 30°C and 20% at 20°C. In addition, oxygen solubility in plasma increases as temperature decreases.

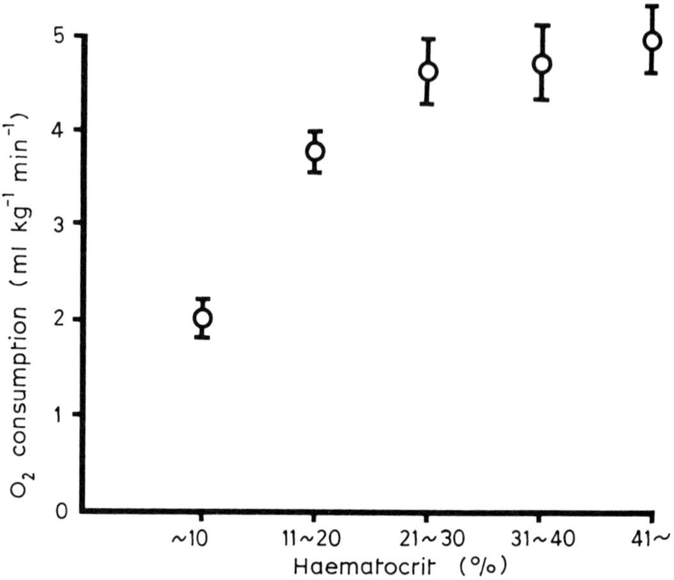

Fig. 14.3 Relationship between O_2 consumption and haematocrit. (Reproduced from Kawashima *et al.* (1974) with permission.)

Viscosity also rises with fall in temperature (Table 14.1) which helps to compensate for the initial viscosity change produced by clear perfusion primes. Clowes (1972) has shown that oxygen consumption falls and base deficit rises at perfusion rates below 2 l m^{-2} min^{-1} but flow rates above this value do not confer any further benefit (Fig. 14.4).

Table 14.1 Change in viscosity with temperature at a velocity gradient of 213 s^{-1}

	Viscosity, cP		
Fluid	*37°C*	*32°C*	*27°C*
Plasma	1.4	1.7	2.0
Blood–haematocrit = 20%	2.5	2.8	3.1
haematocrit = 40%	3.8	4.3	4.8
haematocrit = 60%	6.5	7.1	7.9

It can be concluded that the employment of moderate hypothermia (30°C) and high flow rates will ensure adequate tissue oxygen delivery down to a haematocrit of 20% or even less for short periods. Supportive evidence comes from Kessler and Messmer's (1975) work demonstrating adequate tissue PO_2 values in haemodiluted dogs.

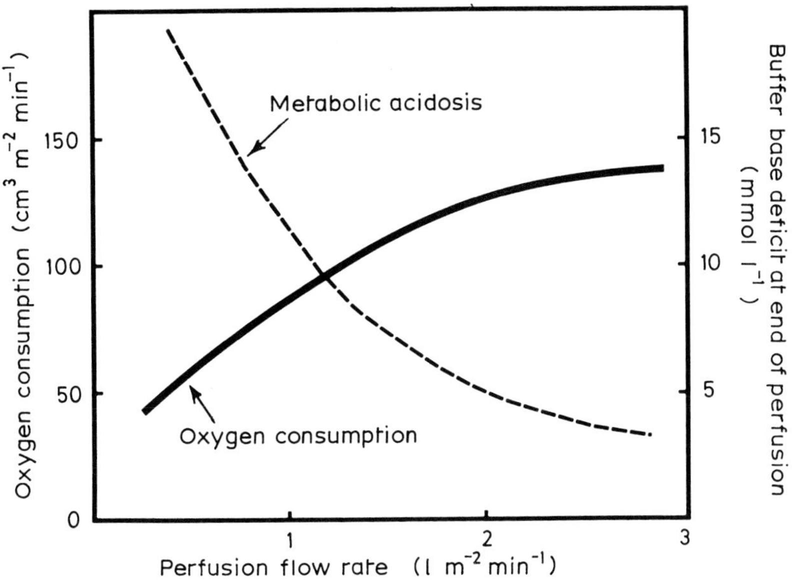

Fig. 14.4 The relationship between perfusion flow rate, total body oxygen consumption and the development of metabolic acidosis durng normothermic (34–37°C) cardiopulmonary bypass. Both oxygen consumption and base deficit reach an asymptotic level at about 2 l m^{-2} min^{-1}. Note the reciprocal relationship between the two. (From Clowes (1972) with permission.)

14.4.3 Yield stress, haemodilution and the coronary circulation

Various authors (Leaf, 1973; Kloner *et al.*, 1974) have shown that a 'no reflow' phenomenon occurs after a period of coronary occlusion whereby normal perfusion to areas of the heart cannot resume due to a local increase in viscosity consequent upon haemoconcentration. Buckberg and Brazier (1975) and Kleinman *et al.* (1978) have shown that under conditions of normothermia and moderate haemodilution (around 30% haematocrit) the flow increase required to maintain normal oxygen delivery to the subendocardium is not achieved, suggesting that some patients with severe coronary occlusion or aortic stenosis may suffer impaired sub-endocardial oxygenation at haemotacrits below 30% when the heart is beating.

14.5 OSMOMETRY

A fluid is isotonic if it causes neither contraction nor expansion of red blood cells suspended in it. Normal serum osmolality is 285±5 mosmol kg^{-1} and solutions of such dissimilar chemical composition as Ringer-lactate and 5%

dextrose have the same particle concentration and are said to be isotonic (Bevan, 1978a). The osmolality of body fluids is primarily dependent on the high concentration of small ions and may be considered as 'crystalloid osmolality'. Body fluids also contain a small number of large particles, mainly proteins, which contribute only about 0.5% to the total osmolality of plasma as show in Fig. 14.5. However, this colloid component is important in the distribution of water between the body fluid compartments because of the limited colloid permeability of biological membranes. Consequently osmotic forces influencing the movement of water will be generated wherever colloid concentration gradients exist.

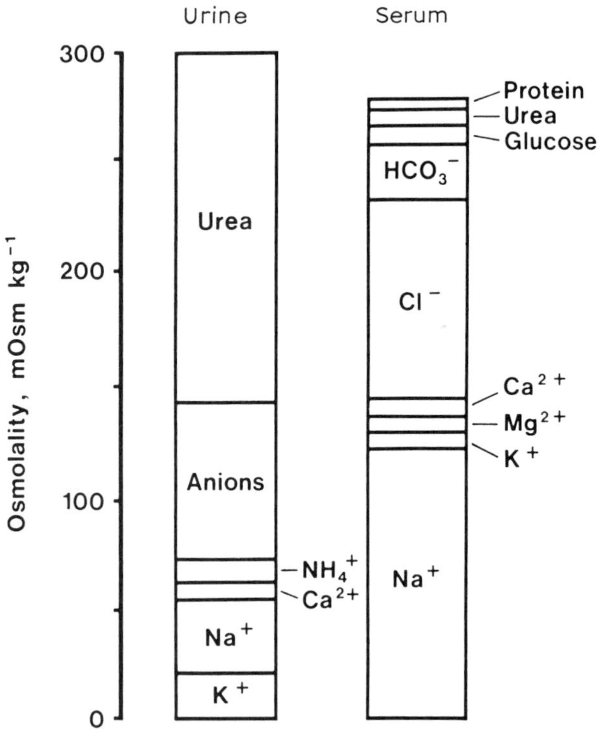

Fig. 14.5 The osmotic constituents of urine and normal serum of a healthy subject.

Using crystalloid primes, it was discovered early in the use of haemodilution that additional perfusate had to be added during bypass. In addition, at termination of bypass it was necessary to re-infuse the patient with a large portion of the diluted prime in order to restore normal cardiovascular dynamics (Edie *et al.*, 1981). This is because large volumes of crystalloid prime resulting in low colloid oncotic pressures lead to diffusion of perfusate into the interstitial fluid during bypass with subsequent re-entry into the intravascular space postoperatively. Neville *et al.* (1966) showed that low haematocrits occurring after the third postoperative day were due to dilutional hypervolaemia and not to a decreased red cell mass. This phenomenon was best treated with fluid restriction and diuretics, rather than blood transfusion.

During crystalloid haemodilution, Beattie *et al.* (1974) have shown that albumin enters the intravascular space at the rate of 0.2 g min^{-1}. This would represent a transfer of 16 g albumin during an average pump run, or approximately 40% of the rapidly exchangeable albumin pool. The maintenance of osmolal constancy is regulated primarily by the hypothalamus which adjusts the secretion of antidiuretic hormone (ADH) to modify renal excretion of water (Bevan, 1978b). Crystalloid haemodilution during cardiopulmonary bypass in children was noted by Deverall *et al.* (1973) to produce plasma hypotonicity postoperatively. This was not influenced by adjusting the osmolal concentration of the prime, nor by severely restricting postoperative water intake. The lack of water diuresis during the first 48 hours following surgery might have been related to unappropriately high ADH levels commented upon by Philbin *et al.* (1979) during crystalloid haemodilution and non-pulsatile flow. ADH release may be caused by the sudden reduction in blood pressure at the aortic baroreceptors (Kleeman and Cutler, 1963) and left atrium (Götz *et al.*, 1975) at the commencement of bypass, using low-viscosity primes.

14.6 CRYSTALLOIDS

14.6.1 5% Dextrose

5% Dextrose is readily available, cheap and has been studied extensively. It is slightly hypotonic, and becomes steadily more so as the dextrose is metabolized, leaving the patient with a sizeable water-load to excrete. The large dilutional effect on plasma bicarbonate produces a marked systemic metabolic acidosis (Ing *et al.*, 1977) with hyponatraemia and hypochloraemia. Hewitt *et al.* (1972) have commented on raised serum glucose and insulin levels during non-pulsatile perfusions with moderate hypothermia even with non-glucose clear primes. Both the peripheral utilization of glucose and pancreatic endocrine response are impaired (Landymore *et al.*, 1979), and addition of exogenous glucose can lead to very high serum glucose levels during bypass, which in diabetic patients may provoke hyperosmotic hyperglycaemic non-ketotic coma (Mills *et al.*, 1973). There is an extensive literature which suggests that glucose, in combination with insulin and potassium may be beneficial to the ischaemic myocardium (Kones, 1975; Brachfeld, 1973). On the other hand, Hearse *et al.* (1978)

Table 14.2 Comparison of crystalloid fluids used for priming in the UK

	5% Dextrose	*Hartmanns*	*'Plasmolyte 148'*	*10% Mannitol*
Cations (mmol/l)				
Na^+	0	131	140	0
K^+	0	5	5	0
Ca^{++}	0	2	0	0
Mg^{++}	0	0	1.5	0
Anions (mmol/l)				
Cl^-	0	111	98	0
Lactate	0	29	0	0
Acetate	0	0	27	0
Gluconate	0	0	23	0
Osmolality (mosmol/kg)	278	278	294	549
pH	4	5–7	4–6	4.5–7
NHS Cost/litre	88p	91p	£1.33p	£2.90p

have demonstrated a damaging effect on heart muscle by a combination of metabolic and osmotic factors when glucose is included in cardioplegic solutions.

14.6.2 Balanced salt solutions

These were introduced in an attempt to present the patient with a perfusate similar in ion concentration to his or her own serum. Lactate-containing solutions are initially slightly acid until the liver converts lactate into bicarbonate, eventually producing a metabolic alkalosis. 'Plasmolyte-148' possesses a slight advantage over Hartmann's Ringer–lactate in that it contains 1.5 $mmol\,l^{-1}$ of magnesium and presents alternative pathways for bicarbonate production, using acetate and gluconate.

Ringer–lactate when given to a diabetic patient causes an acute increase in blood sugar concentration over and above the normal hyperglycaemic response to surgery (Thomas and Alberti, 1978). This is probably related to a failure to dispose of lactate peripherally so that it is more readily converted into glucose. Neither Ringers (non-lactated) nor normal saline possess these disadvantages, although large volumes of the latter may provoke hyperchloraemic acidosis.

The delivery of a large solute load to the distal renal tubules occurring with balanced-salt primes produces exchange of sodium for potassium with excretion of the latter ion in the urine (Dieter *et al.*, 1970). Other factors producing hypokalaemia include hyperglycaemia (Barnard *et al.*, 1959), noradrenaline release during acidosis (De Wall *et al.*, 1956), previous diuretic therapy (Lockey *et al.*, 1966) and changes in phosphate metabolism (Vasko *et al.*, 1973). Administration of extra potassium into the extracorporeal circuit results in improved vascular tone with increases in both venous and arterial pressures. High potassium replacement to achieve serum K^+ levels in the range 5–5.5 mmol l^{-1} have been shown by Babka and Pifarré (1976) to promote spontaneous defibrillation and reduce the incidence of postoperative ventricular dysrhythmias. When using crystalloid primes Westhorpe *et al.* (1978) have shown calcium supplements to be unnecessary and the post-bypass administration of calcium chloride should not exceed 10 mg kg^{-1} if hypercalcaemia is to be avoided. Holden *et al.* (1972) and Khan *et al.* (1973) have stressed the importance of magnesium supplementation during open-heart surgery.

14.6.3 Mannitol

Mannitol is a non-metabolizable 6-carbon polyhydric alcohol. Intravenous infusion of this hypertonic low-molecular-weight crystalloid initially withdraws fluid across the capillary into the plasma. It quickly diffuses into interstitial fluid and increases the volume of the whole extracellular phase by withdrawing water from body cells. Mannitol is readily filtered into the tubular lumen and this strongly hygroscopic solute provokes a brisk water diuresis (Dagher *et al.*, 1966) even in the presence of high ADH levels.

Mannitol is only a transient plasma expander, and Das *et al.* (1969) found that osmolal equilibration between prime and patient's extracellular fluid occurred within ten minutes of commencing perfusion. A prime adjusted to 340–360 mosmol usually produces a final patient/prime value of approximately 300–310 mosmol. Renal plasma flow is linearly related to serum osmolality (Navar *et al.*, 1966), and urine flow on bypass is greater than with isotonic primes. Nevertheless, total urine and solute excretion diminish over the next 24 hours and the final output is similar to patients receiving isotonic primes.

Initially, mannitol-induced transfer of fluid from the intracellular to extracellular fluid space may cause interstitial pulmonary oedema and impair oxygenation (Edde and Smalley, 1979), and rapid infusion produces hypotension by vasodilation in skeletal muscles (Coté *et al.*, 1979). Mannitol's influence on the heart is controversial. Willerson *et al.* (1975) reported increased coronary flow and improved cardiac function in patients in whom serum osmolality was increased to a mean of 309 ± 3 mosmol. On the other hand using mannitol-containing cardioplegia solution with a much higher osmolality, Hearse *et al.* (1978) described a deleterious effect caused by excessive cellular dehydration. Recently, it has been suggested that the composition of cardioplegic solutions may be less important than the provision of an isoncotic hyperosmolar prime during the reperfusion period for improving post-ischaemic ventricular performance (Christlieb and Clarke, 1982).

14.7 COLLOID OSMOTIC PRESSURE

Colloid osmotic pressure is derived almost exclusively from the plasma proteins, especially albumin and fibrinogen. Starling (1896) formulated an equation which relates the transcapillary movement of water to the balance of osmotic and hydrostatic forces as shown in Table 14.3. For practical

Table 14.3 Transcapillary movement of water

$$V = Kf((Pc - P_{If}) - (\pi_p - \pi_{If}))$$

V	=	rate of liquid movement
Kf	=	capillary filtration coefficient
Pc	=	pulmonary capillary wedge pressure (≃ + 7 mmHg (0.13 kPa))
P_{If}	=	interstitial fluid hydrostatic pressure (≃ − 6 mmHg (− 0.8 kPa))
π_p	=	plasma colloid osmotic pressure (≃ + 22 mmHg (2.9 kPa))
π_{If}	=	interstitial fluid colloid osmotic pressure (≃ + 1 mmHg (0.13 kPa))

purposes the occurrence of pulmonary oedema can be regarded as depending primarily on the difference between colloid oncotic pressure and pulmonary capillary wedge pressure (COP−PCWP gradient) (Bevan, 1980). Guyton and Lindsey (1959) have shown that when protein concentration is normal, the critical mean left atrial pressure for transudation of plasma into the pulmonary parenchyma is 24 mmHg (3.2 kPa). Schüpbach *et al.* (1978) have shown in rabbits that reduction of COP below the normal level of 24 mmHg (3.2 kPa) is compensated by increased tissue lymph flow which removes interstitial protein and limits interstitial oedema down to a critical pressure of 16 mmHg (2.1 kPa) on cardiopulmonary bypass, this representing a plasma protein concentration of $42\,g\,l^{-1}$ ($30\,g\,l^{-1}$ albumin). Reduction of COP below this level causes progressive increases in pulmonary (Lowenstein *et al.*, 1975), myocardial (Laks *et al.*, 1977), intestinal wall (Hewson, 1978) and peripheral (Sanchez De Leon *et al.*, 1982) accumulation of extracellular water, capable of interfering with respiration, ventricular function, intestinal motility and wound healing during the postoperative period (Fig. 14.6).

Laver and Buckley (1972) showed that marked decreases in COP could be tolerated without occurrence of pulmonary oedema provided left atrial pressure remained low. On the other hand, Hewson (1978) has demonstrated a significant correlation between increasing hydrostatic pressure on bypass and deteriorating alveolar-arterial oxygen gradients in patients with low colloid oncotic pressures. A high COP inhibits renal ultrafiltration during hypotension and urine flow is diminished (Brenner and Humes, 1977). A low COP as a consequence of excessive haemodilution below a haematocrit of 20% will reduce perfusate buffering capacity and cause increasing metabolic acidosis requiring the addition of buffer base (bicarbonate or Tris (hydroxymethyl) amino methane – THAM) to the prime.

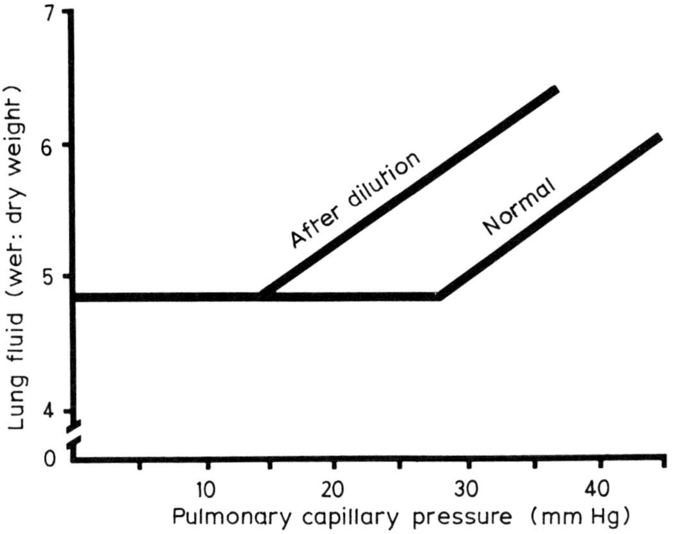

Fig. 14.6 The effect of increasing pulmonary capillary pressure on the appearance of pulmonary oedema (wet/dry lung ratio) in the isolated sheep's lung, perfused with whole blood and blood diluted 50% with isotonic saline. (Reproduced from Bevan (1980) with permission.)

14.8 PLASMA EXPANDERS

A prerequisite for the selection of an appropriate volaemic colloid is that it should be metabolized or excreted completely in the body after fulfilling its function. A balance is achieved between the intravascular and extravascular compartments following colloid infusion characterized by an increased circulating plasma volume, diffusion of smaller particles beyond the blood vessels, and excretion of low-molecular-weight fractions by the kidneys. Part of the colloid solution returns to the bloodstream via the lymphatics while some is stored in the reticuloendothelial system, mainly the liver, to be gradually released and excreted (Rudowski, 1980). The physical properties of some colloid solutions are summarized in Table 14.4.

14.8.1 Plasma preparations

The use of fresh plasma, human dried plasma and cooled stored plasma for the maintenance of colloid osmotic pressure on cardiopulmonary bypass cannot be justified because of the risk of hepatitis transfer. Plasma protein fraction contains approximately $50\,g\,l^{-1}$ pasteurized protein (mainly albumin) and requires four blood donors to provide one unit. Fortunately, plasma collected from time-expired blood is used but it is still rather

Table 14.4 Comparison of some plasma expanders. (From Mishler, J. M., 1984.)

	Colloid osmotic pressure, (mm Hg)	*Osmolity (m osmol kg^{-1})*	*Relative Viscocity at 37°C, (cP)*	*Plasma ½ life concentration (h)*	*NHS cost per litre (1986)*
Plasma protein fraction	16	285	1.3	15	£62.40
Urea-linked gelatin	27	310	1.8	2.5	£7.62
Modified fluid gelatin	34	310	1.9	2.5	£5.74
Dextran 70/ saline	28	308	3.5	25.5	£7.64
Dextran 40/ saline	17	308	5.2	2.5	£12.08
Hetastarch	29	310	5.0	25.5	£33.44

expensive. The commercial equivalent, 5% albumin, costs the NHS about £70 per litre; 20% ('salt poor') albumin is even dearer (£375 per litre). One gram of albumin retains 18 ml water in the intravascular compartment (Gruber, 1969) and the half-life in the circulation is about 15 hours (Farrow 1967). Rapid infusion of plasma protein fraction may cause vasodilation and a drop in blood pressure (Bland *et al.*, 1973). It would seem prudent to choose plasma protein fraction as the non-blood colloid component of priming fluid for children, because they possess a much smaller pool of readily exchangeable albumin than adults.

14.8.2 Dextrans

Dextrans are high-molecular-weight polysaccharides constructed of glucose molecules. The colloid-osmotic effectivity is based on the fact that each gram of dextran binds 20–25 ml water. The volume effect of dextran 70 ('Macrodex') is initially slightly greater than the amount infused, whereas dextran 40 ('Rheomacrodex') has a more pronounced effect, drawing in almost twice its own volume, but its action is less sustained because of more rapid renal excretion. The renal tubular concentration of dextran 40 may rise so quickly that the urine becomes viscous and of low volume, an effect which can be reversed completely in patients with normal renal function by adequate hydration and the concurrent administration of mannitol (Bergentz *et al.*, 1965). However, high dosage can be followed by tubular blockage and acute renal failure in some patients with pre-existing renal insufficiency (Matheson, 1966). At doses exceeding 1.5 g kg^{-1}, dextrans may cause impairment of haemostasis by the formation of a film on the surfaces of platelets and vascular endothelium (Hässig and Stampfli, 1969). This dose should be further reduced in the presence of heparin because of its synergism with dextran (Åberg *et al.*, 1977). Anaphylactoid reactions to dextrans have been reported and are usually apparent within ten minutes of starting infusion. The comparative incidence of reactions to synthetic colloids were compared by Ring and Messmer (1977) during 200,906 infusions carried out in a multi-centre prospective trial (Fig. 14.7).

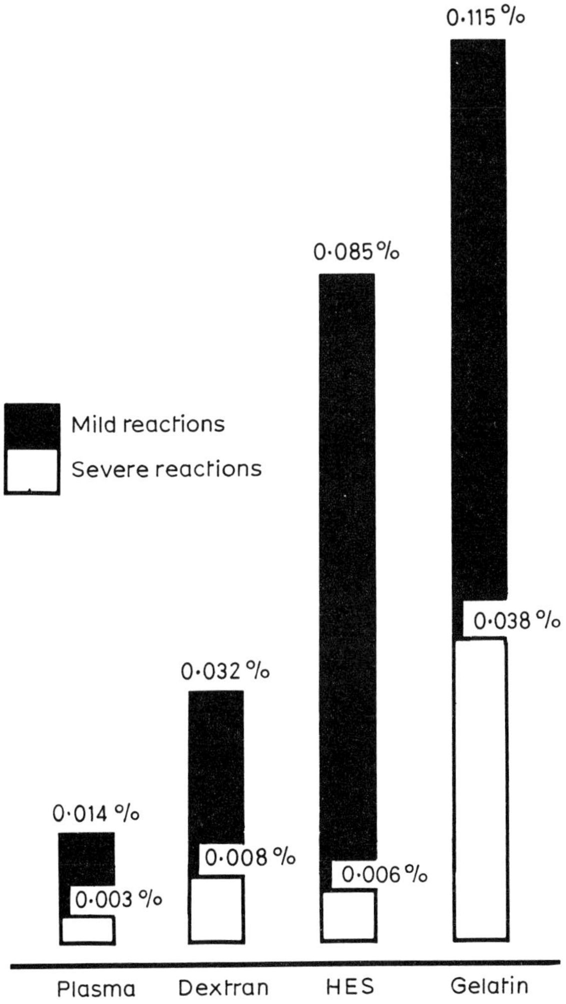

Fig. 14.7 The frequency of adverse reactions to four colloid solutions (after Ring and Messmer, 1977).

14.8.3 Gelatins

Gelatins are manufactured from bovine collagen and possess a molecular weight of approximately 35 000. The main portion of a gelatin solution therefore undergoes renal excretion within a few hours, which accounts for its relatively poor colloid osmotic effect and short half-life (see Table 14.4). Urea-linked gelatin ('Haemaccel'), has been studied during cardiopulmonary bypass (Moyes, 1974; Merakillio, 1976), and using this as the sole prime, De Vries *et al.* (1978) found in dogs that calcium and potassium levels rose markedly and metabolic changes occurred suggestive of impaired tissue oxygenation. The modified fluid gelatin 'Gelofusine' has a longer half-life and lower calcium content than 'Haemaccel'.

It is known that gelatins enhance erythrocyte aggregation (Werner, 1974) and allergic reaction with urea-linked gelatins are commoner than with any other synthetic colloids. On the credit side, the gelatins enhance diuresis and are pharmacologically inert. The possession of a neutral pH (7.3) plus some buffering capacity helps reduce electrostatic forces on erythrocytes thus reducing haemolysis (Mullerworth *et al.*, 1973).

14.8.4 Hetastarch

The original hydroxyethylated polymers of starch are similar to dextran 70 in viscosity, plasma expansion, maintenance of blood pressure and side-effects. Adding 20 ml kg^{-1} hetastarch ('Hespan') to a crystalloid prime reduces intra-operative pulmonary and systemic interstitial fluid accumulation and the observed transient fall in platelet count has no clinical consequence at this dosage (Sade *et al.*, 1985).

Hetastarch's high cost compared with other synthetic colloids has to be balanced by its much longer circulatory half-life of 26 hours (Metcalf *et al.*, 1970). By reducing the average molecular weight and degree of hydroxylation, one can shorten half-life to only 2.7 hours (Mishler *et al.*, 1979) and have no apparent effects on renal or biochemical indices. Reports of the use of such solutions in the extracorporeal circulation have not yet appeared.

14.9 OXYGEN CARRIERS

14.9.1 Blood

It may be necessary to add blood (whole or concentrated), to the perfusion circuit to maintain an optimum haematocrit (>20%) or following bypass to replace losses. The rapid infusion of large volumes of stored citrated blood may reduce the level of circulating ionized calcium, so prophylactic administration of 2 ml of calcium chloride per unit is advisable. In infants, whose liver capacity to handle a citrate load is limited, it is preferable to use fresh heparinized blood.

As shown in Table 14.5, stored blood becomes a progressively more unphysiological fluid with age. Continuing anaerobic glycolysis reduces pH and high potassium concentrations occur due to failure of erythrocyte membrane transport mechanisms (Leveen *et al.*, 1959). Subsequent metabolism of citrate to bicarbonate produces a metabolic alkalosis, maximal on the third post-transfusion day. The capacity of erythrocytes to release oxygen deteriorates with storage by losing 2,3-diphosphoglycerate (Bunn and Jandl, 1970) and it may take at least 4 hours in circulation before stored red cells recover normal function (Beutler and Wood, 1969). Platelet survival is

Table 14.5 Changes in citrated blood during storage at 4±1°C

	Storage period (days)			
Blood constituent	*0*	*7*	*14*	*21*
Haemoglobin mg/100 ml	0–10	25	50	100
pH	7.00	6.85	6.77	6.68
Glucose mg/100 ml	350	300	245	210
Lactic acid mg/100 ml	20	70	120	140
Inorganic phosphate mg/100 ml	1.8	4.5	6.6	9.0
Sodium mmol/l	150	148	145	142
Potassium mmol/l	3–4	12	24	32
Ammonia μg/100 ml	50	260	470	680

drastically reduced after 48 hours storage, and thrombocytopenia can be expected in patients who receive more than 8 units within a short time period (de Leval *et al.*, 1981). Other problems accruing from the use of stored blood have previously been mentioned in the historical introduction to this chapter.

14.9.2 Heterologous stroma – free haemoglobin (SFHS)

Haemolysates from outdated human blood can be prepared essentially free of stromal lipid contaminants. The resulting haemoglobin solution is capable of carrying oxygen but suffers two disadvantages:

(1) Increased oxygen affinity compared with intra-erythrocyte Hb, interfering with oxygen unloading at tissue level.
(2) Small molecular size causing rapid trans-capillary leakage and renal clearance with nephrotoxic effects occurring at high doses ($>3\ g\ kg^{-1}$).

Various attempts have been made to overcome these drawbacks;

(1) Cross-linking Hb molecules, or complexing them to other colloids

(dextran, albumin) improves intravascular persistence at the expense of a further increase in oxygen affinity.

(2) Attaching pyridoxyl phosphate to SFHS reduces oxygen affinity significantly and enhances oxygen tissue delivery at the expense of a short intravascular half-life (Table 14.6). However, the intravascular half-life may be prolonged greatly by intermolecular crosslinking of the pyridoxylated compound without jeopardizing oxygen affinity. Further progress awaits more information concerning interference with renal function, coagulation and metabolism before it becomes feasible for use in human extracorporeal systems (Messmer *et al.*, 1978; Jesch *et al.*, 1981).

14.9.3 Perfluorochemicals (PFCs)

These extremely stable compounds, comprising hydrocarbon molecules protected by a uniform shield of fluorine atoms are efficient carriers of respiratory gases dissolved in physical solution. Unfortunately, they are immiscible with blood, possess a detrimental effect on the vascular tree and interfere with electrolyte concentrations, metabolites and hormones and hence require to be emulsified for intravenous use. This is accomplished by mechanical homogenization. The 0.1 μ fluorocarbon particles are stabilized and dispersed in a modified Krebs–Ringer bicarbonate solution (Beisbarth and Suyama, 1981). The non-ionic surfactant, 'Pluronic F-68', a synthetic copolymer with hydrophilic and lipophilic properties is used to stabilize the emulsion. It contributes some colloid oncotic pressure plus intrinsic O_2- and CO_2-carrying properties, and is totally excreted, unchanged (Vasko *et al.*, 1972).

Table 14.7 summarizes the compositions of some currently available fluorocarbons. FC 43 is easily emulsified but undergoes prolonged and extensive storage in the reticuloendothelial system, hence is used as an oxygen carrier during biological investigations. Fluosol DA 35% has a viscosity similar to whole blood plus a high oxygen-binding capacity and is intended for application in the heart-lung machine. Fluosol DA 20% has a similar viscosity to plasma and is designed for blood replacement in shock therapy, and it is the effects of this latter emulsion upon humans which has been most extensively investigated (mainly in Jehovah's Witnesses) (Frey *et al.* 1981).

(a) Gas transport properties of perfluorochemicals

The volume of oxygen dissolved in PFC emulsions changes linearly with PO_2 according to Henry's Law (Fig. 14.8). It is therefore essential to provide an oxygen-enriched atmosphere. However, uptake and release of O_2 and CO_2 occurs about twice as fast as with haemoglobin.

Perfluorochemicals are eliminated via the lungs in proportion to their

Table 14.6 Artificial oxygen carriers

Source	*Chemical name*	*Comments*	*Half-life in plasma*
Haemoglobin	Stroma free Hb	High O_2 affinity	90 min
	X-linked Hb	Very high O_2 affinity	
	Albumin Hb	Very high O_2 affinity	Variable: 12h–3 days
	Dextran Hb	Very high O_2 affinity	
	Pyridoxal phosphate Hb	Low/normal O_2 affinity	90 min
Fluorochemicals	FC 43 (perfluorotributylamine)	Stable emulsion	
		Long half-life in body	
		Animal experiments	
	Fluosol DA (perfluorotripropylamine plus perfluorodecalin)	Variable emulsion stability	1 to 4 days
		Not retained in tissues	
		Human trials	

Table 14.7 Compositions and storage properties of fluorocarbons

<table>
<tr><th></th><th></th><th>Fluosol FC 43</th><th>Fluosol DA 35%</th><th>Fluosol DA 207</th></tr>
<tr><td>PFC (g%)</td><td>FC 43</td><td>20</td><td>—</td><td>—</td></tr>
<tr><td></td><td>FTPA</td><td>—</td><td>10.5</td><td>6.0</td></tr>
<tr><td></td><td>FDC</td><td>—</td><td>24.5</td><td>14.0</td></tr>
<tr><td>Emulsifier (g%)</td><td>Pluronic F68</td><td>2.56</td><td colspan="2">2.7</td></tr>
<tr><td></td><td>Egg yolk phospholipid</td><td>—</td><td colspan="2">0.4</td></tr>
<tr><td></td><td>Glycerol</td><td>—</td><td colspan="2">0.8</td></tr>
<tr><td>Oncotic agent (g%)</td><td>Hydroxyethyl starch (HES)</td><td>3.0</td><td colspan="2">3.0</td></tr>
<tr><td>Crystalloids (mmol/l)</td><td>Glucose</td><td>10</td><td>9.1</td><td>10</td></tr>
<tr><td></td><td>Na^+</td><td>128</td><td>117</td><td>128</td></tr>
<tr><td></td><td>K^+</td><td>4.6</td><td>4.2</td><td>4.6</td></tr>
<tr><td></td><td>Mg^{2+}</td><td>2.1</td><td>1.9</td><td>2.1</td></tr>
<tr><td></td><td>Ca^{2+}</td><td>2.5</td><td>2.3</td><td>2.5</td></tr>
<tr><td></td><td>Cl^-</td><td>112</td><td>102.5</td><td>112</td></tr>
<tr><td></td><td>HCO_3^-</td><td>25</td><td>23</td><td>25</td></tr>
<tr><td>Osmolarity (mosm/l)</td><td></td><td>290–300</td><td colspan="2">410 (320 without glycerol)</td></tr>
<tr><td>Colloid osmotic pressure (mm H_2O)</td><td></td><td>380–395</td><td colspan="2">380–395</td></tr>
<tr><td>Storage</td><td></td><td>Stable at room temperature for two years: or three years at 2–10°C</td><td colspan="2">Unstable at room temperature: particle size increases by 100 per cent per month. Emulsion is therefore frozen at −5°C to separate from artificial plasma</td></tr>
</table>

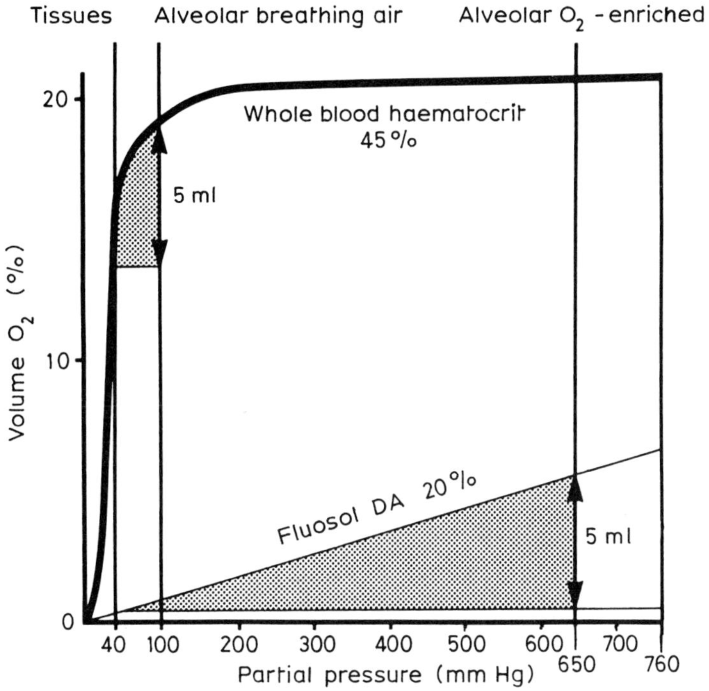

Fig. 14.8 Oxygen dissociation curves for whole blood (haematocrit 45%) and Fluosol DA ('fluocrit' 20%). Emulsification of PFCs limits their ability to dissolve oxygen and other gases. (Reproduced from Wickham and Hardy (1982) with permission.)

vapour pressures, the half-life in the circulation varying from around 5 hours for Fluosal DA to 42 hours for FC 43. Analogous to plasma lipids, there is no measurable renal excretion. PFC particles are reversibly removed from the circulation and stored in the reticuloendothelial system, but apart from some vacuolation, tissue reactions do not occur because of PFC's chemical inertness. Macrophages are probably involved in the transport of PFC from main storage sites to the lungs. There is insignificant biotransformation, and long-term studies have not revealed any lasting histological damage to any tissue in the presence of PFC (Wickham and Hardy, 1982).

14.10 CONCLUSIONS

Despite the enormous literature on extracorporeal circulation it would be rash to assert that we have any true understanding of what constitutes the optimum biochemical state under these conditions. Logic rebels at the notion that the 'normal' blood values necessarily have any relevance to a patient who is anaesthetized, paralysed, cooled and artificially perfused. The main criterion of adequacy should be the clinical and biochemical state of the patient after the operation (Harris *et al.*, 1970).

By this standard, haemodilution utilizing mainly crystalloid primes, with little regard for the preservation of normal levels of colloid oncotic pressure or plasma viscosity has stood the test of time in most cardiac surgical units (Tobias and Fryer, 1981).

Cheapness and absence of toxicity of balanced salt solutions have, to date, proscribed large-scale colloid supplementation, either on the grounds of cost (plasma protein fraction) or possible side-effects (dextrans, gelatins, *Letastarch*). A mass of theoretical and clinical evidence, however, indicates some solid advantages accruing from the partial replacement of crystalloids by cheap synthetic colloids, provided patients have pre-existing normal renal function, are well hydrated pre- and postoperatively, and heparin dosage is carefully controlled by serial estimations of activated clotting times.

Artificial oxygen carriers represent the most exciting new development in the field of extracorporeal perfusion (Jones, 1983). The most promising group, the perfluorochemicals, presently possesses two important disadvantages:

(1) Instability except when stored at very low temperatures.
(2) The necessity to ventilate with 100% oxygen to maximize their oxygen-carrying capabilities.

Further research is proceeding in an effort to solve these problems and the clinical potential of these emulsions should be realised in the near future.

REFERENCES

Åberg, M., Hedner, U. and Bergentz, S-E. (1977) The effect of dextran on hemostasis and coagulation with special regard to factor VIII. In *Dextran – 30 years. Acta. Univ. Uppsala Symp. Uppsala* (ed. D. H. Lewis), Vol. 3. Almqvist and Wiksell, Stockholm, pp. 23–30.

Babka, R. and Pifarré, R. (1976) Potassium replacement during cardiopulmonary bypass. *J. Thorac. Cardiovasc. Surg.*, 73, 212–15.

Balasaraswathi, K., Glisson, S. N., El-Etr, A. A. and Azad, C. (1980) Effect of priming volume on serum catecholamines during cardiopulmonary bypass. *Can. Anaesth. Soc. J.*, 27, 135–9.

Barnard, C. N., De Wall, R. A., Varco, R. L. and Lillehei, C. W. (1959) Pre and post-operative care of patients undergoing open cardiac surgery. *Dis. Chest*, 35, 194–211.

Beattie, H. W., Evans, G., Garnett, E. S., Regoezci, E., Webber, C. E. and Wong, K-L. (1974) Albumin and water fluxes during cardiopulmonary bypass. *J. Thorac. Cardiovasc. Surg.*, 67, 926–31.

Beisbarth, H. and Suyama, T. (1981) Perfluorochemicals (PFCs) – technological and experimental aspects. In *Oxygen Carrying Colloidal Blood Substitutes* (ed. R.

Frey, H. Beisbarth and K. Stosseck), W. Zuckschwerdt Verlag, Munich, pp. 3–12.
Bergentz, S-E., Falkheden, T. and Olsson, S. (1965) Diuresis and urinary viscosity in dehydrated patients: influence of Dextran 40 000, with and without mannitol. *Ann. Surg.*, **161**, 582–6.
Beutler, E. and Wood, L. (1969). The *in-vivo* regeneration of red cell 2,3-diphosphoglyceric acid (DPG) after transfusion of stored blood. *J. Lab. Clin. Med.*, **74**, 300–3.
Bevan, D. R. (1978a) Osmometry. 1. Terminology and principles of measurement. *Anaesthetics*, **33**, 794–800.
Bevan, D. R. (1978b) Osmometry. 2. Osmoregulation. *Anaesthetics*, **33**, 801–8.
Bevan, D. R. (1980) Colloid osmotic pressure. *Anaesthetics*, **35**, 263–70.
Bland, J. H. L., Laver, M. B. and Lowenstein, E. (1973) Vasodilator effect of commercial 5% plasma protein fraction solutions. *J. Am. Med. Assoc.* **224**, 1721–4.
Boulanger, M. (1977) Levels of circulating nonepinephrine and epinephrine before, during and after cardiopulmonary bypass in man. *Survey Anesthesiol.*, **21**, 48–53.
Brachfeld, N. (1973) The glucose–insulin–potassium (GIK) regimen in the treatment of myocardial ischemia. *Circulation*, **48**, 459–62.
Brenner, B. M. and Humes, H. D. (1977) Mechanics of glomerular ultrafiltration. *N. Engl. J. Med.*, **297**, 148–54.
Buckberg, G. D. and Brazier, J. (1975) Coronary blood flow and cardiac function during hemodilution. In *Intentional Hemodilution. Bibliotheca Haematologica* (eds K. Messmer and H. Schmid-Schonbein), Vol. 41, S. Karger, Basel, pp. 173–89.
Bunn. H. F. and Jandl, J. H. (1970) Control of hemoglobin function within the red cell. *N. Engl. J. Med.*, **282**, 1414–21.
Camishion, R. C., Fraimow, W., Kelsey, D. M., Tokunaga, K., Davies, A. L., Joshi, P., Cathcart, R. T. and Pierucci, L. (1968) Effect of partial and total cardiopulmonary bypass with whole blood or hemodilution priming on pulmonary surfactant activity. *J. Surg. Res.*, **8**, 1–6.
Christlieb, I. Y. and Clark, R. E. (1982) Adequacy of the perfusate: Its influence on successful myocardial protection. *J. Thorac. Cardiovasc. Surg.*, **84**, 689–95.
Clowes, G. H. A. Jr (1972) The physiologic basis of cardiac surgery. In *Cardiac Surgery* (ed. J. C. Norman) 2nd edn, Appleton-Century-Crofts, New York, pp. 13–66.
Cooley, D. A., Beall, A. C. Jr and Grondin, P. (1962) Open-heart operations with disposable oxygenators, 5% dextrose prime and normothermia. *Surgery*, **52**, 713–19.
Coté, C. J., Greenhow, D. E. and Marshall, B. E. (1979) The hypotensive response to rapid intravenous administration of hypertonic solutions in man and in the rabbit. *Anesthesiology*, **50**, 30–5.
Dagher, F. J., Lyons, J. H., Ball, M. R. and Moore, F. D. (1966) Hemorrhage in normal man: II. Effects of mannitol on plasma volume and body water dynamics following acute blood loss. *Ann. Surg.*, **163**, 505–22.
Das, J. B., Eraklis, A. J. and Jones, J. E. (1969) Water and solute excretion following cardiopulmonary bypass with hemodilution. The effects of the osmolarity of the perfusion prime. *J. Thorac. Cardiovasc. Surg.*, **58**, 789–94.
De Leval, M. R., Hill, J. D. and Mielke, C. H. (1981) Haematological aspects of

extracorporeal circulation. In *Techniques in Extracorporeal Circulation* (ed. M. I. Ionescu) 2nd edn, Butterworth, London, pp. 371–89.

Deverall, P. B., Muss, D. C., McCartney, F. J. and Settle, J. D. (1973) Osmolal balance after open intracardiac operations in children. *Thorax*, **28**, 756–61.

De Vries, H. W., Zimmerman, A. N. E. and Goslinga, H. (1978) Haemodynamic and metabolic consequences of haemodilution with different diluents. *Tijdschr. Diergeneesk.*, **103**, 1057–63.

De Wall, R. A., Warden, H. E., Gott, V. L., Read, R. C. and Lillehei, C. W. (1956) Total body perfusion for open cardiotomy utilizing the bubble oxygenator. *J. Thorac. Surg.*, **32**, 591–603.

Dieter, R. A. Jr, Neville, W. E. and Pifarré, R. (1970) Serum electrolyte changes after cardiopulmonary by-pass with Ringer's lactate solution used for hemodilution. *J. Thorac. Cardiovasc. Surg.*, **59**, 168–77.

Doenicke, A., Grote, B. and Lorenz, W. (1977) Blood and blood substitutes. *Br. J. Anaesth.*, **49**, 681–8.

Dow, J. W., Dickson III, J. F., Hamer, N. A. and Gadboys, H. L. (1960) Anaphylactoid shock due to homologous blood exchange in the dog. *J. Thorac. Cardiovasc. Surg.*, **39**, 449–56.

Dunn, J., Kirsch, M. M., Harness, J., Carroll, M., Straker, J. and Sloan, H. (1974) Hemodynamic, metabolic and hematologic effects of pulsatile cardiopulmonary bypass. *J. Thorac. Cardiovasc. Surg.*, **68**, 138–47.

Edde, R. R. and Smalley, S. (1979) Defect in oxygenation associated with mannitol. *Anesth. Analg.*, **58**, 145–6.

Edie, R. N., Haubert, S. M. and Malm, J. R. (1981) The use of haemodilution and a non-haemic prime for cardiopulmonary bypass. In *Techniques in Extracorporeal Circulation* (ed. M. I. Ionescu) 2nd edn, Butterworth, London, pp. 179–98.

Farrow, S. P. (1967) Effects of infusion of various colloid solutions upon the circulatory volumes of rabbits. *MSc. Thesis*, University of Birmingham, England, pp. 1–109.

Frey, R., Beisbarth, H. and Stosseck, K. (1981) *Oxygen Carrying Colloidal Blood Substitutes*, W. Zuckschwerdt Verlag, Berlin, pp. 147–242.

Gadboys, H. L., Slonim, R. and Litwak, R. S. (1962) Homologous blood syndrome: 1. Preliminary observations on its relationship to clinical cardio-pulmonary bypass. *Ann. Surg.*, **156**, 793–804.

Gardner, R. E., Finlay, T. N. and Tooley, W. H. (1962) The effect of cardiopulmonary bypass on surface activity of lung extracts. *Bull. Soc. Int. Chir.*, **21**, 542–51.

Goetz, K. L., Bond, G. C. and Bloxham, D. D. (1975) Atrial receptors and renal function. *Physiol. Rev.*, **55**, 157–205.

Gordon, R. J., Ravin, M., Rawitscher, R. E. and Daicoff, G. R. (1975) Changes in arterial pressure, viscosity and resistance during cardiopulmonary bypass. *J. Thorac. Cardiovasc. Surg.*, **69**, 552–61.

Gott, V. L., Bartlett, M., Long, D. M., Lillehei, C. W. and Johnson, J. A. (1962) Mycardial energy substrates in the dog heart during potassium and hypothermic arrest. *J. Appl. Physiol.*, **17**, 815–19.

Götz, E., Thoma, H. and Schäfer, A. (1975) Hepatitis in Abhangigkeit von der transfundierten Konservenzahl. *Anesthesiol. Wiederb.*, **90**, 346–48.

Greer, A. E., Carey, J. M. and Zudhi, N. (1962) Haemodilution principle of hypothermic perfusion: a concept obviating blood priming. *J. Thorac. Cardiovasc. Surg.*, **43**, 640–8.

Gruber, U. F. (1969) *Blood Replacement*, Springer-Verlag, Berlin, p. 48.

Gruber, U. F. (1969) *Blood Replacement*, Springer-Verlag, Berlin, p. 103.
Guyton, A. C. and Lindsey, A. W. (1959) Effect of elevated left atrial pressure and decreased plasma protein concentration on the development of pulmonary oedema. *Circ. Res.*, 7, 649–57.
Guyton, A. C. and Richardson, T. Q. (1961) Effect of hematocrit on venous return. *Circ. Res.*, **9**, 157–64.
Hallowell, P., Bland, J. H. L., Buckley, M. J. and Lowenstein, E. (1972) Transfusion of fresh autologous blood in open-heart surgery. *J. Thorac. Cardiovasc. Surg.*, **64**, 941–8.
Hardesty, R. L., Bayer, W. L. and Bahnson, H. T. (1968) A technique for the use of autologous fresh blood during open-heart surgery. *J. Thorac. Cardiovasc. Surg.*, **56**, 683–8.
Harris, E. A., Seelye, E. R. and Barratt-Boyes, B. G. (1970) Respiratory and metabolic acid–base changes during cardiopulmonary bypass in man. *Br. J. Anaesth.*, **42**, 912–22.
Hässig, A. and Stampfli, K. (1969) Plasma substitutes, past and present. In *Modified Gelatins as Plasma Substitutes. Bibliotheca Haematologica* (eds P. Lundsgaard-Hansen, A. Hässig and H. Nitschmann) S. Karger, Basel, Vol. 33, pp 1–7.
Hearse, D. J., Stewart, D. A. and Braimbridge, M. V. (1978) Myocardial protection during ischemic cardiac arrest. Possible deleterious effects of glucose and mannitol in coronary perfusates. *J. Thorac. Cardiovasc. Surg.*, **76**, 16–23.
Hepps, S. A., Roe, B. R., Wright, R. R. and Gardner, R. E. (1963) Amelioration of the pulmonary postperfusion syndrome with hemodilution and low molecular weight dextran. *Surgery*, **54**, 32–43.
Hewitt, R. L, Woo, R. D., Ryen, J. R. and Drapanas, T. (1972) Plasma insulin and glucose relationships during cardiopulmonary bypass. *Surgery*, **71**, 905–12.
Hewson, J. R. (1978) Perfusion characteristics during cardiopulmonary bypass and subsequent changes in alveolar–arterial oxygen tension gradients. *Anesth. Analg.*, **57**, 298–302.
Holden, M. P., Ionescu, M. S. and Wooler, G. H. (1972) Magnesium in patients undergoing open-heart surgery. *Thorax*, **27**, 212–18.
Ing, T. S., Wu, C., Rosenberg, J. C., Ng, P. S. Y., Su, W-S., Bernard, A. A. and Wilson, R. F. (1977) Cerebrospinal fluid changes in experimental cardiopulmonary bypass using hemodilution with glucose water. *Neurology*, **27**, 85–9.
Jesch, F., Peter, K. and Messmer, K. (1981) Stromafree hemoglobin solutions – actual state. In *Oxygen Carrying Colloidal Blood Substitutes* (eds R. Frey, H. Beisbarth and K. Stosseck), W. Zuckschwerdt Verlag, Munich, pp. 13–18.
Jones, P. M. (1983) Artificial blood. *Br. Med. J.*, **286**, 246–7.
Kawashima, Y., Yamamoto, Z. and Manabe, H. (1974) Safe limits of hemodilution in cardiopulmonary bypass. *Surgery*, **76**, 391–7.
Kessler, M. and Messmer, K. (1975) Tissue oxygenation during hemodilution. In *Intentional Hemodilution. Bibliotheca Haematologica* (eds K. Messmer and H. Schmid-Schonbein), S. Karger, Basel, Vol. 41, pp. 16–33.
Khan, R. M. S., Hodge, J. S. and Bassett, H. F. M. (1973) Magnesium in open-heart surgery. *J. Thorac. Cardiovasc. Surg.*, **66**, 185–91.
Kleeman, C. R. and Cutler, R. (1963) The neuro-hypophysis. *Ann. Rev. Physiol.*, **25**, 385–432.
Kleinman, L. H., Yarbrough, J. W., Symmonds, J. B. and Wechsler, A. S. (1978) Pressure-flow characteristics of the coronary collateral circulation during cardiopulmonary bypass. Effects of hemodilution *J. Thorac. Cardiovasc. Surg.*, **75**, 17–26.

Kloner, R. A., Ganote, C. E. and Jennings, R. B. (1974) The 'no-reflow' phenomenon after temporary coronary occlusion in the dog. *J. Clin. Invest.*, **44**, 1496–508.

Kones, R. (1975) Glucose, insulin and potassium therapy for heart disease. *NY State J. Med.*, **1**, 1463–7.

Laks, H., Standeven, J., Blair, O., Hahn, J., Jellinek, M. and Willman, V. L. (1977) The effects of cardiopulmonary bypass with crystalloid and colloid hemodilution on myocardial extravascular water. *J. Thorac. Cardiovasc. Surg.*, 73, 129–38.

Landymore, R. W., Murphy, D. A. and Langley, W. J. (1979) Effect of cardiopulmonary bypass and hypothermia on pancreatic endocrine function and peripheral utilisation of glucose. *Can. J. Surg.*, **22**, 248–50.

Laver, M. B. and Buckley, M. J. (1972) Extreme hemodilution in the surgical patient. In *Hemodilution. Theoretical Basis and Clinical Application* (eds K. Messmer and E. Schmid-Schonbein), S. Karger, Basel, pp. 215–28.

Leaf, A. (1973) Cell swelling: a factor in ischemic tissue injury. *Circulation*, **48**, 455–8.

Lee, W. H., Rubin, J. W. and Huggins, M. P. (1975) Clinical evaluation of priming solutions for pump oxygenator perfusion. *Ann. Thorac. Surg.*, **19**, 529–36.

Leveen, H. H., Schatman, B. and Falk, G. (1959) Cardiac arrest produced by massive transfusions. *Surg. Gynec. Obstet.*, **109**, 502–8.

Lilleaason, P. (1977) Moderate and extreme haemodilution in open-heart surgery. Blood requirements, bleeding and platelet counts. *Scand. J. Thorac. Cardiovasc. Surg.*, **11**, 97–103.

Lilleaasen, P., Frøysaker, T. and Stokke, O. (1978) Cardiac surgery in extreme haemodilution without donor blood, blood products or artificial macromolecules. *Scand. J. Thorac. Cardiovasc. Surg.*, **12**, 249–51.

Litwak, R. S., Gadboys, H. L., Kahn, M. and Wisoff, B. G.(1965) High flow total body perfusion utilizing diluted perfusate in a large prime system. *J. Thorac. Cardiovasc. Surg.*, **49**, 74–90.

Lockey, E., Longmore, D. B., Ross, D. N. and Sturridge, M. F. (1966) Potassium and open-heart surgery. *Lancet*, **1**, 670–5.

Long, D. M., Sanchez, L., Varco, R. L. and Lillehei, C. W. (1961) The use of low molecular weight dextran and serum albumin as plasma expanders in extracorporeal circulation. *Surgery*, **50**, 12–28.

Lowenstein, E., Cooper, J. D., Erdman III, A. J., Geffin, G., Laver, M. B. and Yoshikawa, H. (1975) Lung and heart water accumulation associated with hemodilution. In *Intentional Hemodilution. Bibliotheca Haematologica* (eds K. Messmer and H. Schmid-Schonbein), S. Karger, Basel, Vol. 41, pp. 190–202.

McNamara, J. J., Burran, E. L., Larson, E., Omiya, G., Suchiro, G. and Yamase, H. (1972) Effect of debris in stored blood on pulmonary microvasculature. *Ann. Thorac. Surg.*, **14**, 133–9.

Matheson, N. A. (1966) Renal failure with low-molecular weight dextran. *Br. Med. J.*, **2**, 1198.

Melrose, D. G., Nahas, R., Alvarez, D., Todd, I. A. D. and Dempster, W. J. (1965) Post-operative hypoxia after extracorporeal circulation: a possible graft against host reaction. *Experienta*, **21**, 47–50.

Merikallio, E. (1976) Haemodilution in cardiopulmonary bypass using a gelatine derivative for priming. *Ann. Chir. Gynaecol.*, **65**, 138–44.

Messmer, K. (1977) Acute pre-operative hemodilution: an alternative to transfusion of donor blood. In *Dextran – 30 Years. Acta. Univ. Uppsala* (ed. D. H. Lewis), Almqvist and Wiksell, Stockholm, Vol. 3, pp. 93–110.

Messmer, K., Jesch, F., Schaff, J., Schoñberg, M., Pielsticker, K. and Bouhard, K.

(1978) Oxygen supply by stroma-free hemoglobin. In *Progress in Clinical and Biological Research* (eds G. A. Jamieson and T. J. Greenwalt), A. R. Liss, New York, Vol. 19, pp. 175–90.

Metcalf, W., Papadopoulos, A., Tufaro, R. and Barth, A. (1970) A clinical physiologic study of hydroxyethyl starch. *Surg. Gynecol. Obstet.*, **131**, 255–67.

Mills, N. L., Baudet, R. L., Isom, D. W. and Spencer, F. C (1973) Hyperglycemia during cardiopulmonary bypass. *Ann. Surg.*, **177**, 203–5.

Mischler, J. M. (1984) Synthetic volume expanders – their pharmacology, safety and clinical efficacy in *Clinics in Haematology* vol. 13, pp. 75–92.

Mishler, J. M., Parry, E. S., Sutherland, B. A. and Bushrod, J. R. (1979) A clinical study of low molecular weight hydroxyethyl starch, a new plasma expander. *Br. J. Clin. Pharmacol.*, 7, 619–22.

Moyes, D. G. (1974) Haemodilution with a plasma expander as priming solution in cardiopulmonary bypass. *S-A Mediese Tydskrif*, 1615–16.

Mullerworth, M. H., Currie, T. T., Cockbill, M. T. and Stubbs, A. E. (1973) Repolymerized gelatin as a priming solution for extracorporeal circulation: An experimental study in dogs. *Surgery*, **74**, 666–77.

Murray, J. F., Escobar, E. and Rapaport, E. (1969) Effects of blood viscosity on hemodynamic responses in acute normovolemic anemia. *Am. J. Physiol.*, **216**, 638–42.

Navar, L. G., Guyton, A. C. and Langston, J. B. (1966) Effect of alterations in plasma osmolality on renal blood flow autoregulation. *Am. J. Physiol.*, **211**, 1387–92.

Neville, W. E., Thomason, R. D. and Hirsch, D. M. (1966) Postperfusion hypervolaemia after hemodilution cardiopulmonary bypass. *Arch Surg.*, **93**, 715–23.

Panico, F. G. and Neptune, W. B. (1959) A mechanism to elminate the donor blood prime from the pump oxygenator. *Surg. Forum.*, **10**, 605–9.

Philbin, D. M., Coggins, C. H., Emerson, C. W., Levine, F. H. and Buckley, M. J. (1979) Plasma vasopressin levels and urinary sodium excretion during cardiopulmonary bypass. Comparison of halothane and morphine anesthesia. *J. Thorac. Cardiovasc. Surg.*, 77, 582–5.

Ring, J. and Messmer, K. (1977) Incidence and severity of anaphylactoid reactions to colloid volume substitutes. *Lancet*, **i**, 466–9.

Roe, B. B., Swenson, E. E., Hepps, S. A. and Bruns, D. L. (1964) Total body perfusion in cardiac operations with perfusate of balanced electrolytes and low molecular weight dextran. *Arch. Surg.*, **88**, 128–34.

Rudowski, W. J. (1980) Evaluation of modern plasma expanders and blood substitutes. *Br. J. Hosp. Med.*, **23**, 389–99.

Sade, R. M., Stroud, M. R., Crawford, M. A., Kratz, J. M., Dearing, J. P. and Bartles D. M. (1985) A prospective randomized study of hydroxyethyl starch, albumin and lactated Ringer's solution as priming fluid for cardiopulmonary bypass. *J. Thorac Cardiovasc. Surg.* **89**, 713–22.

Sanchez De Léon, R., Paterson, J. L. and Sykes, M. J. (1982) Changes in colloid osmotic pressure and plasma albumin concentration associated with extracorporeal circulation. *Br. J. Anaesth.*, **54**, 465–73.

Schüpbach, P., Pappova, E., Schilt, W., Kollar, J., Koller, M., Sipos, P. and Vucic, D. (1978) Perfusate oncotic pressure during cardiopulmonary bypass. Optimum level as determined by metabolic acidosis, tissue oedema and renal function. *Vox. Sang.*, **35**, 332–44.

Smith, E. E. and Crowell, J. W. (1967) Role of an increased hematocrit in altitude acclimatization. *Aerosp. Med.*, **38**, 39–43.

Starling, E. H. (1896) On the absorption of fluids from the connective tissue spaces. *J. Physiol. (London)*, **19**, 312–26.

Thomas, D. J. B. and Alberti, K. G. M. M. (1978) Hyperglycaemic effects of Hartmann's solution during surgery in patients with maturity onset diabetes. *Br. J. Anaesth.*, **50**, 185–8.

Thorén, L. (1977) Shock – principles of fluid therapy. In *Dextran – 30 years. Acta. Univ. Ups. Symp. Univ. Uppsala* (ed. D. H. Lewis), Almqvist and Wiksell, Stockholm, Vol. 3, pp. 83–91.

Tobias, M. A. and Fryer, J. M. (1981) Which priming fluids? In *Towards Safer Cardiac Surgery* (ed. D. B. Longmore), MTP Press, Lancaster, pp. 401–26.

Trede, M. (1969) Experimental investigations into the behaviour of coagulation and renal function during high dilution perfusions with glucose, Haemaccel and Rheomacrodex. In *Modified Gelatins as Plasma Substitutes: Bibliotheca Haematologica* (eds P. Lundsgaard-Hansen, A. Hassig and H. Nitschman), S. Karger, Basel, Vol. 33, pp. 553–68.

Utley, J. R., Wachtel, C., Cain, R. B., Spaw, E. A., Collins, J. C. and Stephens, D. B. (1981) Effects of hypothermia, hemodilution and pump oxygenation on organ water content, blood flow and oxygen delivery, and renal function. *Ann. Thorac. Surg.*, **31**, 121–33.

Vasko, K. A., DeWall, R. A. and Riley, A. M. (1973) Hypokalaemia: Physiological abnormalities during cardiopulmonary bypass. *Ann. Thorac. Surg.*, **15**, 347–53.

Vasko, K. A., Riley, A. M. and DeWall, R. A. (1972) Poloxalkol (Pluronic-F68): A priming solution for cardiopulmonary bypass. *Trans. Am. Soc. Artif. Organs*, **18**, 526–31.

Verska, J. J., Ludington, L. G. and Brewer, L. A. (1974) A comparative study of cardiopulmonary bypass with non-blood and blood prime. *Ann. Thorac. Surg.*, **18**, 72–80.

Werner, F. M. (1974) Dextranen of gelatines. *Ned. Tijdschr. Geneeskd.*, **118**, 1121–31.

Westhorpe, R. N., Varghese, Z., Petrie, A., Wills, M. R. and Lumley, J. (1978) Changes in ionized calcium and other plasma constituents associated with cardio-pulmonary bypass. *Br. J. Anaesth.*, **50**, 951–7.

Wickham, N. W. R. and Hardy, R. N. (1982) Artificial blood from fluorocarbons. *Hosp. Update*, **8**, 1432–44.

Willerson, J. T., Curry, G. C., Atkins, J. M., Parkey, R. and Horwitz, L. D. (1975) Influence of hypertonic mannitol on ventricular performance and coronary blood flow in patients. *Circulation*, **51**, 1095–100.

Zubiate, P., Kay, J. H., Mendez, A. M., Krohn, B. G., Hockman, R. and Dunne, E. F. (1974) Coronary artery surgery. A new technique with use of little blood, if any. *J. Thorac. Cardiovasc. Surg.*, **68**, 263–7.

Zuhdi, N., Carey, J. and Greer, A. (1964) Blood, mannitol, dextran, sugar, water and confusion. Presented at the *6th Annual meeting of the South Central Association of Blood Banks*, March 27, Oklahoma City, USA.

Zuhdi, N., McCollough, B., Carey, J. and Greer, A. (1960) The use of citrated banked blood for open heart surgery. *Anesthesiology*, **21**, 496–501.

Zuhdi, N., McCollough, B., Carey, J., Krieger, C. and Greer, A. (1961) Hypothermic perfusion for open-heart surgical procedures: report on the use of a heart–lung machine primed with 5% dextrose in water inducing hemodilution. *J. Int. Coll. Surg.*, **35**, 319–26.

15
Blood cell trauma

GORDON WRIGHT

In the normal cardiovascular system, blood cells are subjected to a variety of physical and biochemical forces. The magnitudes of these forces are variable and, in some cases, they are higher in the normal circulation than they are in cardiopulmonary bypass systems. For example, the lateral pressure experienced by blood cells in the left ventricle exceeds the maximum pressure generated in many cardiopulmonary bypass circuits. Considering the pressure parameter alone, it might seem paradoxical that all cardiopulmonary bypass systems generate more blood cell trauma than the normal human cardiovascular system.

The explanation of this paradox is, of course, that we have considered only one property of the force – its magnitude. We should also consider the nature of the force (sense) and its direction. In mechanical terms, force has the properties of a vector – magnitude, sense and direction of application. Ideally, we should be in a position to describe these force properties for every function of a cardiopulmonary bypass system and relate these to the observed blood cell trauma. The design of circuit components could then include an analysis of relevant force vectors with the object of minimizing blood cell trauma. This is a goal for the future.

For the time being, we have to make the best we can of two incomplete and essentially separate groups of information. On the one hand, we have some important, but somewhat contradictory, data derived from *in vitro* studies of the effects of physical forces upon blood cells; and on the other hand, we have a much larger body of information based upon *in vivo* tests of blood cell trauma in animal experiments and clinical practice.

The plan of the chapter is to examine the effects of physical forces upon blood cells; then to review the effects of cardiopulmonary bypass upon blood cell trauma; and finally to attempt to correlate the two sets of information, and in doing so, make a limited approach to the object of explaining the experimental and clinical results in physical terms. Incidentally, this does not deny the importance of biochemical factors responsible for blood cell trauma, but the present discussion is confined to physical forces, the biochemical factors being included only where they are relevant. Likewise, the discussion will be restricted to trauma to blood cells, the changes in plasma components being included only where they are relevant to this discussion. But first, with an apology to fluid dynamicists, the basic physical concepts must be introduced.

15.1 THE ANALYSIS OF FORCES IN FLUID MOTION

The analysis of forces affecting a fluid at rest requires only one parameter – pressure, or force per unit area. This force is applied normal to the plane of the fluid surface and varies only with density and depth:

$P = \varrho gh$, where P = pressure,
ϱ = fluid density,
g = acceleration due to gravity
and h = height of the column of fluid.

Fluids in motion are subjected to several additional forces. The concept of viscosity, or lack of slipperiness, introduced by Isaac Newton in 1686, is central to an understanding of these forces. No matter what the mean fluid flow through a tube is, the layer of fluid immediately adjacent to the tube wall does not move. The velocity of fluid particles in this narrow region is therefore zero, increasing to maximum at some point in the bulk fluid flow. In some cases, this boundary layer of increasing velocity is narrow. In others, it is wide enough to reach to the central axis of the tube, making the velocity gradient across the tube parabolic in shape (Fig. 15.1). Where there is no lateral movement of fluid, the notion is one of concentric cylinders of fluid of varying velocity and this is known as laminar flow. In the boundary layer, each cylinder of fluid has another cylinder of fluid with a different velocity adjacent to it and a force (shear stress) is applied tangential to the two

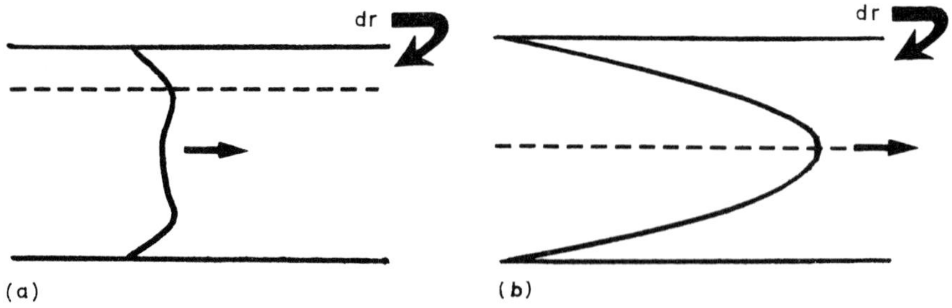

Fig. 15.1 Velocity profiles in laminar flow. (a) Plug flow. (b) Parabolic flow.

surfaces. The magnitude of this force is dependent upon the relative velocities (shear rate = dv/dr) and the absolute viscosity of the fluid (μ). Thus, shear stress (T) is given by the relationship:

$$T = \mu(dv/dr)$$

It should be noted that blood is an unusual fluid in this respect. Whereas most fluids have a constant viscosity that varies only with temperature, the viscosity of whole blood exhibits markedly non-linear properties varying with shear rate, haematocrit and plasma protein concentration (Barras, 1969).

So far, the analysis has been concerned with simple laminar flow. Where there is some lateral movement of fluid as well as axial movement, the concentric cylinders of fluid become disturbed and, when the lateral movement is so great that all fluid particles are moving randomly in all directions, the flow becomes turbulent. In turbulent flow, local velocities are greatly increased, resulting in the generation of much higher shear forces than in equivalent laminar flow. Sudden changes in the diameter of a tube, obtuse bifurcations and an irregular surface configuration increase the tendency of fluid flows to become turbulent. In any case, laminar flow cannot be maintained above a certain critical velocity. In very smooth, straight tubes, it has been found that the transition to turbulent flow occurs when a dimensionless quantity known as Reynold's number (Re) exceeds the value of approximately 2300. Reynold's number is actually a ratio of inertial and viscous forces. The inertial component is represented by fluid momentum (ϱv^2) and this is the force applied when blood cells are projected against a solid surface (wall impact). The viscous component is represented in modified form by shear stress. Thus:

$$Re = \frac{\varrho v^2 \text{ (inertial)}}{\mu v/D \text{ (viscous)}} = \frac{\varrho v D}{\mu}.$$

The increase in energy loss that accompanies a transition from laminar to turbulent flow is revealed as an increase in pressure drop as illustrated in Fig. 15.2.

The value of T (shear stress) in any experimental or clinical situation can be calculated accurately only if the flow conditions are well established. At the entrance to catheters and close to the exit from cannulae, the flow patterns are not established but they are probably never laminar. The distance along the tube for the fully formed flow pattern to become established is known as the inlet length (X) defined as:

$$X = \frac{0.08r(vD)}{\lambda},$$ where r = tube radius,
v = average velocity,
D = tube diameter
and λ = kinematic viscosity.

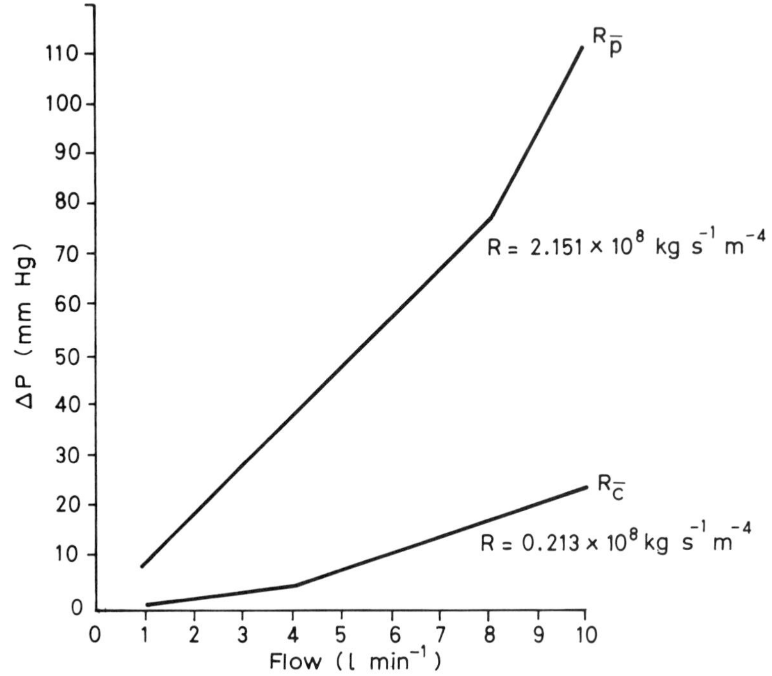

Fig. 15.2 Relationship between flow and pressure drop through two hydraulic resistors. The transition from laminar to turbulant flow is revealed as a change in slope.

The calculated inlet length for laminar flow in a 4 mm diameter tube is 26.7 cm.

Turbulent flows are common in nature. Unfortunately their complexity makes them refractory to fluid dynamic analysis. Possibly the most satisfactory description of shear stress in turblent flow is given by Schlichting (1960) as:

$$T_t = \frac{\varrho e du}{dr} = \frac{0.03 \times 2\Delta P,}{\varrho}$$

where e = eddy current kinematic viscosity
and ΔP = pressure drop

The boundaries of the definition of blood cell trauma are not precise. Here we will include, not only structural damage, but also potentially harmful functional changes, such as increases in the adhesion and aggregation of platelets. This requires a slight widening of the definition of 'physical forces' to include factors involved in surface contact and surface tension. These factors are partly physical and partly chemical. Physical factors that can be important are the surface configuration, electrocharge and surface free energy. Chemical factors determine the wettability of the material and its chemical reaction with the blood cell membrane mucopolysaccharides. Surface tension is present when a liquid is exposed to a gas phase. Molecules in a liquid medium are attracted towards each other by intramolecular forces. These forces are less effective in a gas or vapour because the molecules are further apart, so that the surface layers of a liquid exposed to a gas interface have higher levels of free energy. This extra surface energy is usually described by a statement that there is a surface tension acting parallel to the surface that opposes any attempt to extend the surface. In biological solutions, an important consequence of this energy gradient is that the intramolecular bonds of globular proteins are disrupted and the molecules become elongated and randomly coiled with their polar groups oriented in the interface. One result of this is an increase in the viscosity of liquids containing protein when they are exposed to a gas interface.

We have now considered the most important of the physical forces applied to blood cells in a cardiopulmonary bypass system. These are pressure, shear stress, wall impact and surface phenomena. Although the fluid dynamic analysis given here is somewhat trivial, it covers the essential physical forces applied to blood cells during cardiopulmonary bypass, so it is adequate for our present purpose.

15.2 THE EFFECTS OF PHYSICAL FORCES UPON BLOOD CELLS

In this section, *in vitro* tests on blood samples will be reviewed. The work has been performed under well-controlled conditions in accordance with standard scientific practice, but there are some important differences in results. In this respect, it should be noted that the fragility and reactiveness of blood cells are variable properties which depend to a large extent upon the species of origin, method of collection, anticoagulant, pH, temperature and plasma lipid concentration (Bindslev *et al.*, 1961; Eiseman and Spencer, 1962; Remtsma and Creech, 1962; Rygg, 1973; Wright, 1975; 1976). This, and other factors to be outlined in the appropriate sections below, could well be responsible for the differences in results of tests of blood cell trauma during both *in vitro* and *in vivo* experiments.

15.2.1 Pressure

Blood cells appear to be reasonably tolerant to constant applied pressures, though the effects of high pressures do not appear to have been studied. Experimental work has demonstrated that erythrocytes are capable of withstanding pressures as high as 140 mmHg (18.7 kPa) above atmospheric pressure (Rygg, 1973) and as low as 150 mmHg (20 kPa) absolute pressure

(Wielgorski *et al.*, 1975) with no apparent harmful effects. Similarly, pressure variations up to 300 mmHg (40 kPa) have only insignificant effects upon haemolysis (Blackshear *et al.*, 1967).

15.2.2 Shear stress and wall impact

The importance of shear stress has been recognized in several investigations of blood cell trauma. The usual experimental technique is to shear cells in a viscometer that has stationary and moving parts to which the blood is exposed. Shear rate, and therefore shear stress, is varied by altering the angular velocity of the rotating component. High velocity jets of saline have also been employed to create shear forces.

Nevaril *et al.* (1968) sheared human and rabbit erythrocytes. They observed morphological abnormalities (spherocytes, schistocytes, poikilocytes) and erythrocyte fragments after shearing at 150 Nm^{-2}, but no haemolysis was detected by measuring plasma haemoglobin concentration until the shear stress exceeded 200 Nm^{-2}. Similar values were reported by Leverett *et al.* (1972).

Considerable efforts have been made to reduce the surface effects, air interfaces and turbulence in the design of viscometers, but these factors are thought to be responsible for the disparity in results from experiments on sheared platelets. Thus, Brown *et al.* (1975) measured a significantly reduced platelet content of serotonin after shearing at only 5 Nm^{-2} and acid phosphatase release at 15 Nm^{-2}. These results were criticized by Bernstein *et al.* (1977) who claimed that the apparent low trauma threshold was due to wall impact effects in the viscometer. They generated shear stress in plasma by a high velocity jet of saline and found few structural changes up to 10^4 Nm^{-2}, and only slight to moderate changes in the processes of adhesion and aggregation up to 10^5 Nm^{-2}. However, results similar to those of Brown *et al.* (1975) were subsequently produced by Hung *et al.* (1976), who measured lactic dehydrogenase release at 10–16.5 Nm^{-2}, and by Hardwick *et al.* (1981), who found lactic dehydrogenase and serotonin release at 15 Nm^{-2}. Wall impact forces were also thought to be important by Johnston *et al.* (1975) and the duration of exposure to shear stress was found to be critical by Colantuoni *et al.* (1977).

The effects of shear stress upon leucocytes were investigated by McIntire *et al.* (1978). A shear stress of 7.5 Nm^{-2} significantly inhibited phagocytosis and caused the release of β-glucuronidase in leucocyte suspensions. The authors pointed out that 30 Nm^{-2} is required for inhibition of phagocytosis in whole blood.

Thus, there are two distinct groups of results. In one group, cell damage is reported to occur at shear stress values around 10 Nm^{-2}, while the other group finds no damage up to about 10^4 Nm^{-2}. As an impartial observer, it is difficult to choose between them, but two conclusions appear to be undisputed. These are that blood cells are damaged by high levels of shear stress and that wall impact forces severely damage platelets. Both of these forces are generated in turbulent blood flow.

15.2.3 Surface contact and surface tension

When blood is exposed to a foreign surface, the platelets react by adhering to the surface and to each other. This effect may be mediated by thromboxane A_2 released from the platelets (Gorman, 1979) and it is counteracted in the normal circulation by the secretion of the powerful platelet inhibitor, prostacyclin (PGI_2)(Moncada and Vane, 1978) probably by increasing the plasma concentration of cyclic adenosine monophosphate (cyclic AMP). Whether or not a foreign surface will activate platelet adhesion depends upon both physical and chemical properties of the surface. Physical properties which increase platelet adhesion are roughness, high free energy, a positive electrocharge and poor wettability (Baier, 1977).

Platelet adhesion is not directly affected by the use of anticoagulants, but this may have some effect upon the deposition of protein onto the surface, and this subsequently affects further platelet adhesion to the surface (Salzman *et al.*, 1969; Zucker and Vroman, 1969; Lindon *et al.*, 1978). The previous adsorbance of γ-globulin (Mason *et al.*, 1973) and more especially fibrinogen (Zucker and Vroman, 1969) predisposes platelets to adhesion, while a prior coating of albumin reduces platelet adhesion *in vitro* (Packham *et al.*, 1969; Salzman *et al.*, 1969). Unfortunately, albumin does not appear to have any effect upon platelet loss *in vivo* (Ellison *et al.*, 1980). The interaction between proteins, and therefore platelets, and a physical surface depends largely upon the surface chemical properties. Materials resistant to platelet adhesion include segmented polyurethane, polyether urethane, pyrolytic carbon, polyalkylsulphones, and copolymers of polyether urethane and polydimethyl siloxane (Antifoam A) (Edmunds and Addonizio, 1982).

Surface tension effects were thought to be responsible for the denaturation of globular plasma proteins by Lee *et al.* (1961). The deformation of cell membranes with subsequent disruption was attributed to the attachment of gas bubbles to the cell and a transfer of curvature-related surface energy from the bubbles to the blood cells (Philp *et al.*, 1972). Secondary biochemical and physicochemical sequelae of protein denaturation have been reported by Lee and Hairston (1971) and by Philp *et al.* (1972). Denatured protein may adhere to viable blood cells and result in cellular aggregation, sludging and microthrombosis. The denaturation of erythrocyte membranes results in haemolysis. The release of adenosine diphosphate from these cells induces platelet aggregation (Born *et al.*, 1976) and the aggregated cells release more adenosine diphosphate which promotes further platelet aggregation.

15.3 EXPERIMENTAL RESULTS AND CLINICAL EXPERIENCE

In this section the validity of various indices of blood cell trauma will be examined, followed by a discussion of the results of tests of blood cell trauma performed during experimental and clinical cardiopulmonary bypass. Finally, three particularly controversial aspects of perfusion will be reviewed.

15.3.1 Indices of blood cell trauma

The most obvious damage to blood is indicated by an increase in the plasma haemoglobin concentration. This has been the traditional marker of trauma generated by cardiopulmonary bypass components and procedures. It is obvious from the previous discussion that the three blood cell types react in different ways to similar physical insults. Although haemolysis is a relatively insensitive index, its value as a marker is evident from its almost universal usage. However, the proper interpretation of measurements of plasma haemoglobin concentration requires an appraisal of the physiological mechanisms involved and the measurement techniques employed (Garner, 1973).

Plasma normally contains a protein, haptoglobin which is capable of binding haemoglobin. In the normal circulation, the rate of binding is approximately 1 mg haemoglobin per 1 ml of plasma (Laurel and Nyman, 1957). When the liberation of haemoglobin from damaged erythrocytes does not exceed the capacity of haptoglobin to combine with it, the haptoglobin–haemoglobin complex is removed by the reticuloendothelial system and no free haemoglobin can be detected (Murray *et al.*, 1961). But, if the haptoglobin capacity is exceeded, free haemoglobin circulates in the plasma where it dissociates into its haem and globin moieties. Both moieties combine with plasma albumin to form methaemoglobin and haemopexin respectively (Fleisch, 1959; Heide, 1964). Free haemoglobin can also be excreted by the kidney, but not until the plasma concentration reaches 150 mg per 100 ml plasma.

Nowadays, it is uncommon for such a high level of haemolysis to occur during open-heart operations. The urine is devoid of haemoglobin and free haemoglobin is mainly removed by the reticuloendothelial system at a rate of approximately 5 mg per 100 ml plasma per hour.

It should be noted that the assessment of haemolysis is based upon the measurement of free haemoglobin, but different techniques give different results. As indicated in Fig. 15.3, the benzidine technique of Crosby and Furth (1956) tends to give higher values than the scanning spectrophotometric technique of Blakney and Dinwoodie (1975) and this is probably due to the inclusion of methaemoglobin in results obtained by the benzidine technique.

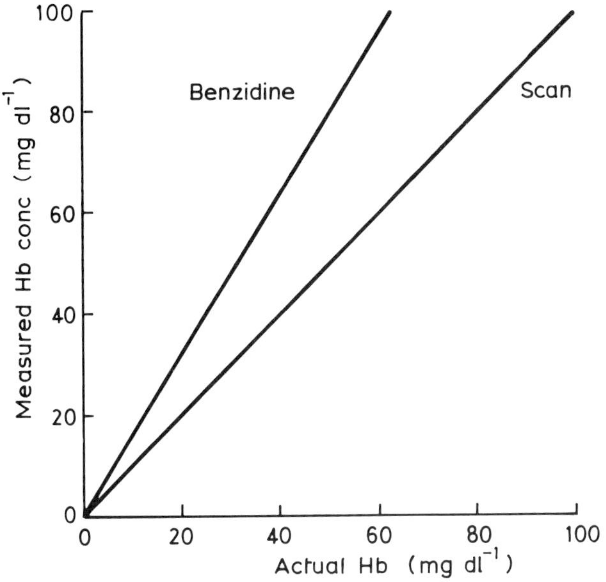

Fig. 15.3 Plasma haemoglobin concentration measured by benzidine and scanning spectrophotometric techniques.

When the benzidine reagent is replaced by orthotolidine, the results tend to be intermediate. A fixed wavelength spectrophotometric technique is often used, but this is less accurate than the scanning technique because of variations in the light absorbance baseline caused by bilirubin and methaemoglobin. In view of this dependence upon the technique used for measuring plasma haemoglobin concentrations, it is regrettable that some papers do not include a reference to the technique employed. The physiological clearance of haemoglobin is not a problem in *in vitro* studies, but even these are not without difficulties. We experienced marked variations in erythrocyte fragility and platelet aggregation in blood samples obtained from the slaughterhouse until we developed a technique for collecting 500 ml of venous blood from live heifers within 30 s.

There are also major problems in assessing platelet and leucocyte trauma. Most commonly, cell counts are used for this purpose, and this is certainly a valuable measurement, but it tells us nothing about the function of surviving cells, or about the fate of damaged cells, i.e. whether they have been destroyed, adsorbed onto physical or biological surfaces, sequestered in organ pools, or incorporated into platelet–leucocyte microthrombi. The dynamic state of platelet and leucocyte populations *in vivo* is a problem for the timing of representative samples for cell counts. The major technical difficulties here are that the results are dependent upon the choice of diluent and counting technique. Thus, we found that platelet counts performed by phase contrast microscopy were approximately 8% higher when cocaine was used in the diluent rather than procaine. The range of error should also be established. In our laboratory, the range of error is ±4%. Finally, it should be remembered that platelet aggregates usually do not enter the counting field.

In vitro tests of cell function are available for both platelets (Hellem, 1960; Born, 1962) and leucocytes (Woltjes *et al.*, 1977), and methods are available for quantifying platelet and leucocyte aggregation (Swank *et al.*, 1964; Solis and Gibbs, 1972). It is apparent that some authors have not understood the differences between platelet adhesiveness (glass bead column), platelet aggregation (Coulter counter or screen filtration pressure) and platelet aggregability (aggregometer).

In studies of cardiopulmonary bypass, further problems arise from changes in the design and manufacture of components and improvements in technique during the history of open-heart surgery, and in the employment of particular devices to represent a group of devices or special procedure. Examples of this are to be found in the literature relating to comparisons of bubble and membrane oxygenators, and pulsatile and non-pulsatile pump systems.

15.3.2 Effects of cardiopulmonary bypass upon blood cell trauma

Many authors have reported their findings of blood cell trauma during cardiopulmonary bypass for both experimental and clinical purposes. The clinical results from 16 open-heart operations during which cardiopulmonary bypass was used for more than 2 hours at the North Staffordshire Royal Infirmary are representative. These are shown in Figs 15.4 and 15.5 for bypasses using a double roller pump set just non-occlusively, a bubble oxygenator and a vacuum suction system. Plasma haemoglobin concentration was measured by the scanning spectrophotometric technique of Blakney and Dinwoodie (1975) and the results were corrected for haemodilution by use of the initial (PCV_1) and subsequent (PCV_2) measurements of packed cell volume:

$$PH_a = \frac{PH_m(1-PCV_2)}{PCV_2(1-PCV_1)/PCV_1}$$

where PH_a = actual plasma Hb; PH_m = measured plasma Hb

Platelet counts were performed by phase-contrast microscopy after the dilution of whole blood in a procaine–saline solution, and the results were corrected using the formula:

$$PC_a = PC_m(PCV_1)/PCV_2$$

where PC = platelet count

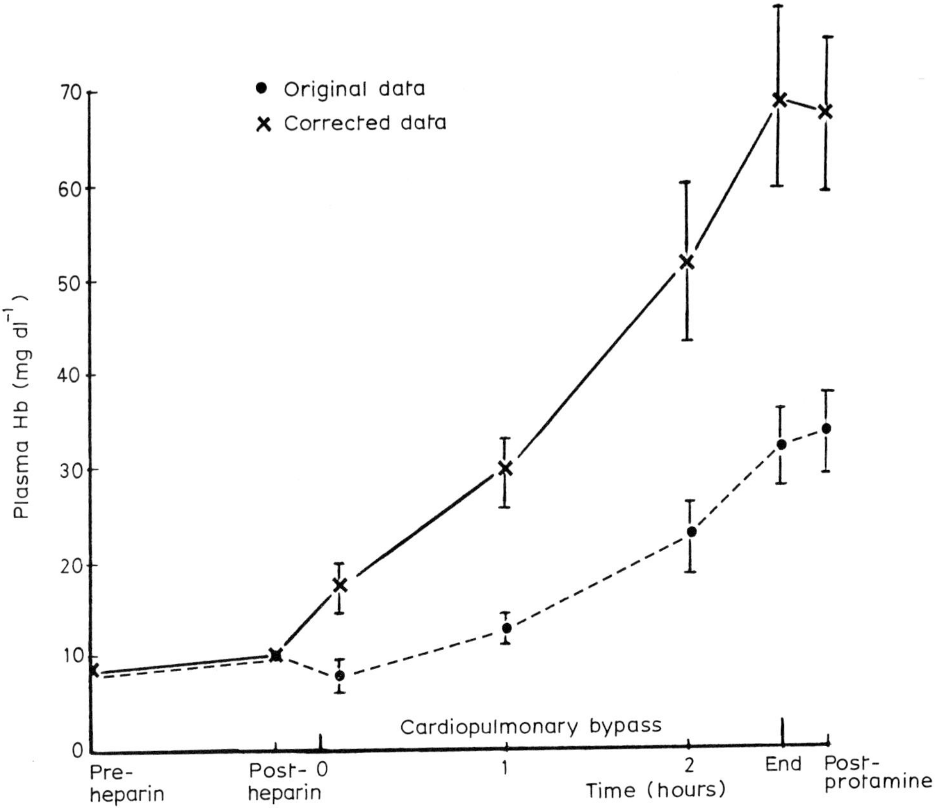

Fig. 15.4 Plasma haemoglobin concentration during open-heart operations. Cardiopulmonary bypass time is indicated in hours.

The pre-operative plasma concentrations of haemoglobin were usually a little higher than the normal range. They increased during the first 5 minutes of cardiopulmonary bypass, while the platelet counts decreased even allowing for haemodilution. Thereafter, there was a steady increase in the rate of plasma haemoglobin accumulation, while the platelet count decreased more slowly.

Haemolysis as an index of erythrocyte trauma is usually expressed as the concentration of haemoglobin in the plasma in mg dl^{-1} or in μM (1 mg dl^{-1} = 620 μM), but for *in vitro* tests the haemolytic index (increase in haemoglobin concentration per 100 litres of blood pumped) or the traumatic index (increase in plasma haemoglobin for each passage of the blood through the circuit) are preferred (Koller and Hawrylenko, 1967). In clinical cases, the results do not vary as much as might be expected considering the possible effects of different components of the extracorporeal circuit, type of operation,

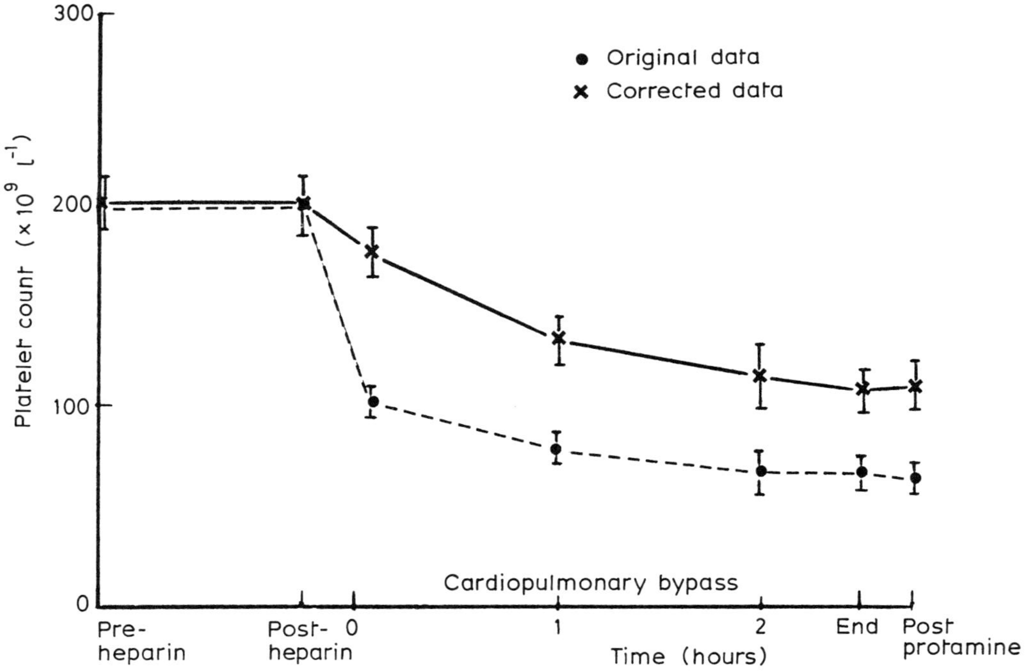

Fig. 15.5 Platelet counts during open-heart operations. Cardiopulmonary bypass time is indicated in hours.

degree of haemodilution and duration of cardiopulmonary bypass. This may be due to some equalization of results as a consequence of patients' clearance mechanisms and suggests that comparative clinical studies should be interpreted with great caution. Typical values for plasma haemoglobin concentration at the conclusion of bypasses of approximately 2 hours duration are in the range 30–40 mg dl^{-1} (Taylor *et al.*, 1978; Wildevuur, 1981; Fig. 15.4). Gas flow rate, haemodilution, type of oxygenator and cardiotomy suction have been thought to be the most important factors.

The only satisfactory way to compare the haemolysis generated by components of the extracorporeal circuit is by *in vitro* tests under standardized conditions. Tests performed in different laboratories are difficult to compare because of differences in protocol. However, this problem did not inhibit Kletschka *et al.* (1975), who were able to conclude that one pump was 'the most atraumatic blood pump in existence' on the basis of a literature survey. Haemolytic indices quoted in their paper ranged from 0.01 to 13 g per 100 litres of blood pumped. Standardized tests were used in the evaluation of four oxygenators by Mortensen (1977). Haemolytic indices ranged from 0.087 to 0.855 g per 100 litres blood pumped compared with a value of 0.016 g per 100 litres blood pumped in controls in which blood was recirculated without an oxygenator in the circuit.

Extracorporeal circulation has a profound effect upon blood platelets. Many workers have reported reductions in platelet counts to 30–50% of the initial value (Schmidt *et al.*, 1961; Kendall and Lowenstein, 1962; Sharp and Eggleton, 1963; Dybkjaer *et al.*, 1964; Gollub, 1964; de Jong *et al.*, 1980). The highest rate of disappearance of platelets from the circulation occurs during the first few minutes of perfusion (Kirby, 1958; de Jong *et al.*, 1980; Wildevuur, 1981; Fig. 15.5). Thereafter, the platelet count decreases more slowly or increases slightly. During the period of partial bypass towards the termination of the perfusion, there is sometimes a slight increase in the platelet count, probably due to the release of platelet pools in the lungs, but a further decrease in the count occurs when protamine sulphate is administered and the platelet count remains below normal for 4–5 days postoperatively (Wildevuur, 1981). By this time, new platelets are produced in the bone marrow and both these and occasional megakaryocytes may be found in peripheral blood smears (Breslow *et al.*, 1968). Subsequently, the platelet count increases, eventually exceeding the pre-operative count by the 7th to 12th postoperative day (Kreel *et al.*, 1960; Breslow *et al.*, 1968; Wildevuur, 1981). Platelet function follows a similar pattern of change, but it appears to recover more rapidly than the platelet count. The subject of platelet function during cardiopulmonary bypass has been recently reviewed by Edmunds and Addonizio (1982). An important feature is that low platelet counts are sometimes, though not always, associated with prolonged bleeding times. Bleeding times return towards normal within 2–4 h of the termination of cardiopulmonary bypass (Harker *et al.*, 1980), but this delay may be of considerable importance because it occurs when the patient's chest is being closed.

Some workers have sought to reduce the levels of platelet destruction, adhesion and aggregation by the use of pharmacological agents including dipyridamole (Mielke *et al.*, 1973), sulphinpyrazone (Birek *et al.*, 1976, prostaglandin E_1 (Addonizio *et al.*, 1977) and prostacyclin (Dewanjee *et al.*, 1981). While providing limited protection of platelets, some of these compounds create additional problems, such as the vasodilating action of prostaglandin E_1. Recently, high hopes have been held for prostacyclin (PGI_2) following successful experimental trials (Longmore *et al.*, 1981), but the short half-life (approximately 2–3 min), high cost and until recently lack of a synthetic analogue have so far prevented its widespread use (see Chapter 16).

Changes in leucocyte counts during extracorporeal circulation have been reported by several authors. The decrease in numbers of leucocytes is just as severe as that of platelets, but Woltjes *et al.*, (1977) and Halie *et al.* (1978) reported that cardiopulmonary bypass had a detrimental effect upon leucocyte phagocytic activity. Differential leucocyte counts show that neutrophil polymorphs are most affected and bone marrow examination reveals myeloid hyperplasia (Brinsfield *et al.*, 1962; Kusserow *et al.*, 1971), possibly resulting from the release of leucopoietic substances from damaged cells or a corticosteroid-induced disturbance in the balance between circulating and marginal pools of leucocytes (Boggs, 1967). Activation of white cells is now the focus of considerable attention. Complement activation, and temporary 'trapping' of white blood cells in the lung may be important aspects. Preoperative leucocyte counts are rapidly restored after concluding the bypass and indeed it is usual for a pronounced leucocytosis to persist for several days postoperatively (Anderson, 1961; Brinsfield *et al.*, 1962).

15.3.3 Oxygenators and blood trauma

The controversy concerning the relative merits of bubble and membrane gas exchange has been a prominent issue among perfusionists since the first clinical perfusion with a membrane oxygenator (Clowes and Neville, 1958). This controversy has been partly concerned with levels of blood trauma in the various devices. Most studies have concluded that membrane oxygenation causes less blood cell trauma than bubble oxygenation (Siderys *et al.*, 1975; Ward and Berry 1975; Heimbecker, 1977; de Jong *et al.*, 1978; Alon *et al.*, 1979; Wildevuur, 1981). However, Tabak *et al.* (1981) were unable to find any difference in erythrocyte survival after recirculation in bubble and membrane oxygenators, and differences in blood cell trauma have been difficult to demonstrate in the clinical situation (Dutton *et al.*, 1974; Liddicoat *et al.*, 1975). As indicated by ten Duis *et al.* (1978) and by

Wildevuur (1981), this is probably due to the overwhelming importance of other factors, especially cardiotomy suction, during open-heart operations compared with experimental cardiopulmonary bypass in animals.

Generally, the lower rate of blood cell trauma in membrane oxygenators is attributed to the absence of a blood–gas interface without further definition of the force vectors involved. The principle of gas exchange (bubble or membrane) has been represented by a single type of device, so that comparisons of bubble and membrane oxygenation are based upon representative forms only. This kind of experimental protocol fails to negate incidental design features such as blood path configuration, type of material, local blood velocities and shear stress which are particular to the design of the device and not to the principle of gas exchange. Also, it has to be remembered that these devices may be operated in a variety of ways. For instance, bubble oxygenators are more traumatic to blood when the gas flow rate is high than when it is low (Rygg, 1973).

15.3.4 Blood pumps

The literature relating to blood cell trauma by blood pumps was reviewed by Kletschka *et al.* (1975). Improvements in the design and machining tolerances of roller pumps have reduced the levels of trauma induced by blood circulation alone. There have been fears that the introduction of pulsatile flow might result in higher levels of blood trauma, but in fact this does not appear to have been the case. Thus, Taylor *et al.* (1978) found no significant difference in haemolysis during clinical perfusions in which the Stockert pump was used in pulsatile and non-pulsatile modes.

Because of the inherent problems of assessing blood cell trauma *in vivo*, we have used a simple *in vitro* method in which two pumps are compared by pumping blood around two similar circuits, each consisting of the pump, two stainless-steel cannulae, a reservoir and a 1 m length of tubing. Each circuit was primed with 400 ml fresh bovine blood anticoagulated with acid citrate dextrose and recirculated with no air interface at $4\,l\,min^{-1}$ for 2 hours. A standard Sarns roller pump was used as a control in each test. Typical results are shown in Table 15.1. These results suggest that the mode of pumping (pulsatile or non-pulsatile) is less important than the design of the pump. Thus, the Oxford–Keele pulsatile pump, which is a ventricle-type pump, induced less blood cell trauma than the Sarns roller pump while the modified roller pulsatile pumps induced more.

High velocities through the arterial cannula are a potential cause of blood cell trauma with pulsatile pumps (Kayser, 1979). Whether or not blood cells will be damaged depends largely upon the dimensions of the input cannula, the shape of the velocity profile, the shear rate, and Reynold's number (Wright and Furness, 1980). A critical point is whether the flow becomes

Table 15.1 Blood trauma induced by pumps *in vitro*. Results of 11 tests with bovine blood

	Standard roller	*Modified roller*	*Compression plate*	*Ventricle*
Δplasma Hb(mg dl^{-1})	59.4	97.7	31.7	17.8
Traumatic index (mg dl^{-1} $stroke^{-1}$)	0.042	0.061	0.021	0.018
Surviving platelets (%)	73.2	101	86.6	19.3
Surviving leucocytes (%)	91.2	118	91.4	63.4
Δ SFP	149	12	−50	−392

turbulent in the cannula. Under the usual conditions of operation, the critical value of Reynold's number will be exceeded during pump ejection. However, the short time available during each pump cycle may not be sufficient for fully formed turbulent flow to become established. Our experience using several pulsatile pumps for experimental cardiopulmonary bypass has been that this is not a source of significant blood cell trauma.

15.3.5 Cardiotomy suction

Those of us who have investigated the various factors responsible for blood cell trauma during cardiopulmonary bypass have little doubt that cardiotomy suction is by far the most important. Representative haematological values for blood samples obtained from the radial artery and cardiotomy reservoir at the end of cardiopulmonary bypass in 35 patients undergoing open-heart operations are shown in Table 15.2. The differences between each pair of data are highly significant by student's *t* and Mann Whitney (Wilcoxon's signed rank sum) tests.

Table 15.2 Haematological indices of blood cell trauma at the end of cardiopulmonary bypass for open-heart surgery. Results for 35 operations.

	Radial artery	*Cardiotomy reservoir*	*P*
Haematocrit	0.24	0.23	0.005
Plasma Hb concn (mgdl^{-1})	28.4	158.5	0.005
Platelet count ($\times 10^9 l^{-1}$)	69.3	50.0	0.005

Statistical significance assessed by student's *t* and Mann Whitney U tests.

Morris *et al.* (1965) claimed that the haemolytic effect of cardiotomy suction was due to contact of the blood with pericardial and epicardial surfaces, but we were unable to detect this effect in dogs (Wright and Sanderson, 1979). However, this factor did appear to be responsible for severe platelet and leucocyte aggregation which could be prevented by washing the pericardium and epicardium with saline before admitting blood to the cardiotomy reservoir.

The critical factor in cardiotomy suction appears to be the simultaneous aspiration of blood and air (Rygg, 1973; ten Duis *et al.*, 1978; Wright, 1978; Wright and Sanderson, 1979; de Jong *et al.*, 1980; Wildevuur 1980). The effect of cardiotomy suction is to cause severe haemolysis, reductions in platelet and leucocyte counts, platelet and leucocyte aggregation, and a depression of platelet function. The use of controlled suction by which air aspiration is avoided greatly reduces these effects (Barthelemy *et al.*, 1978; ten Duis *et al.*, 1978; Wright and Sanderson, 1979; Figs 15.6–15.9). There is also some advantage to be gained by using vacuum rather than roller pump suction (Fig. 15.10) and by the use of cardiotomy reservoirs that incorporate microfilters (Fig.15.11).

15.4 CORRELATION OF PHYSICAL, EXPERIMENTAL AND CLINICAL INFORMATION

In many respects, conclusions are difficult to derive from the published literature on blood cell trauma during cardiopulmonary bypass, because of lack of standardization in test procedures, because the fundamental physical factors have not been identified, and because of technical problems and errors outlined earlier. However, some general conclusions may be acceptable:

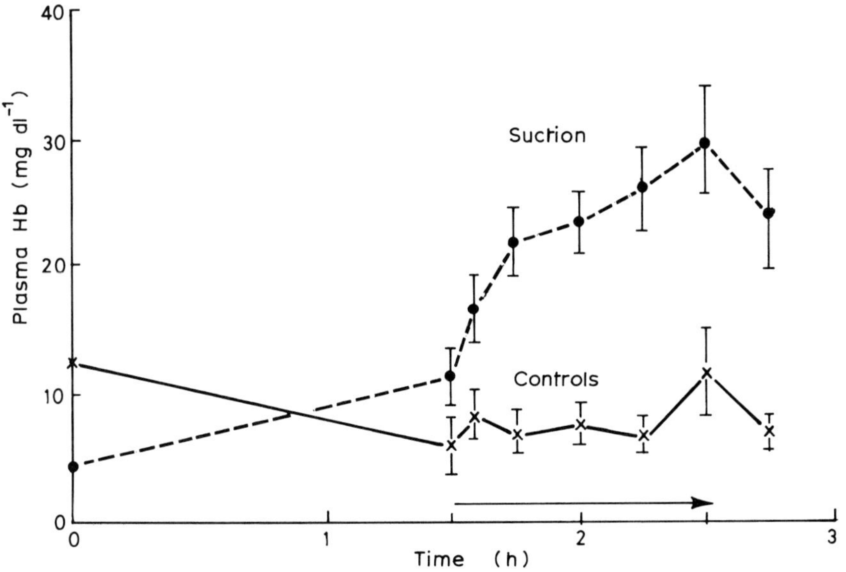

Fig. 15.6 Plasma haemoglobin concentration during *in vivo* cardiotomy suction. Vertical bars indicate standard errors. Arrow indicates duration of suction. (From Wright and Sanderson, 1979.)

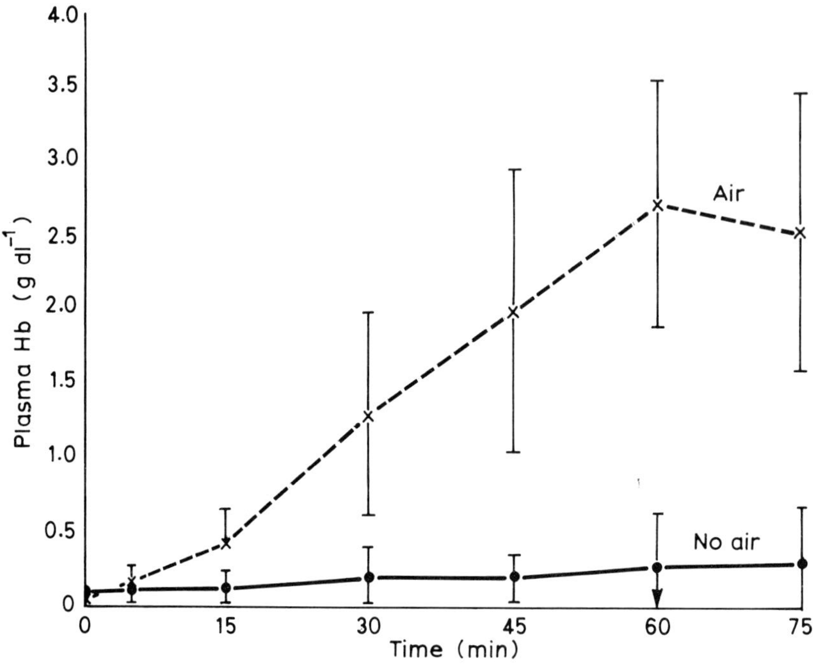

Fig. 15.7 Plasma haemoglobin concentration during *in vitro* suction of blood and air and blood alone. Vertical bars indicate standard errors and arrow indicates end of one-hour suction period. (From Wright and Sanderson, 1979.)

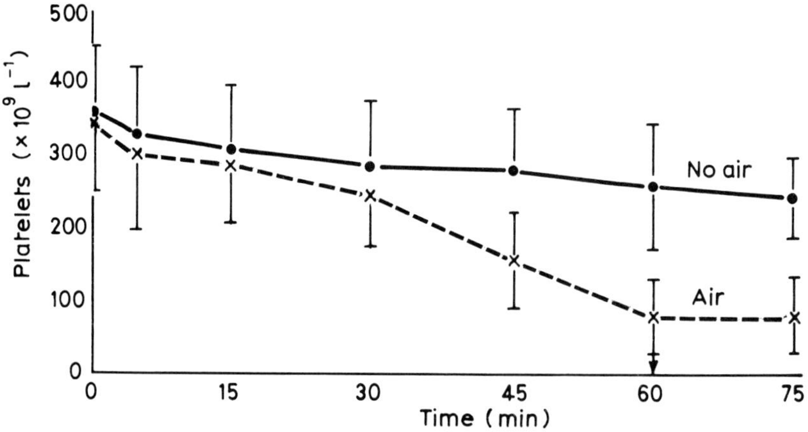

Fig. 15.8 Platelet counts during *in vitro* suction of blood and air and of blood alone. Vertical bars indicate standard errors and arrow indicates end of one-hour suction period. (From Wright and Sanderson, 1979.)

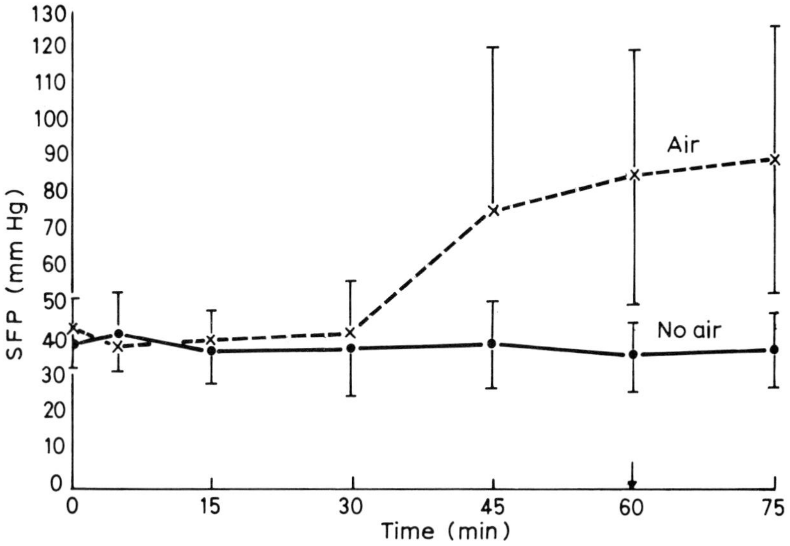

Fig. 15.9 Screen filtration pressure (SFP) during *in vitro* suction of blood and air and of blood alone. Vertical bars indicate standard errors and arrow indicates end of one-hour suction period. (From Wright and Sanderson, 1979.)

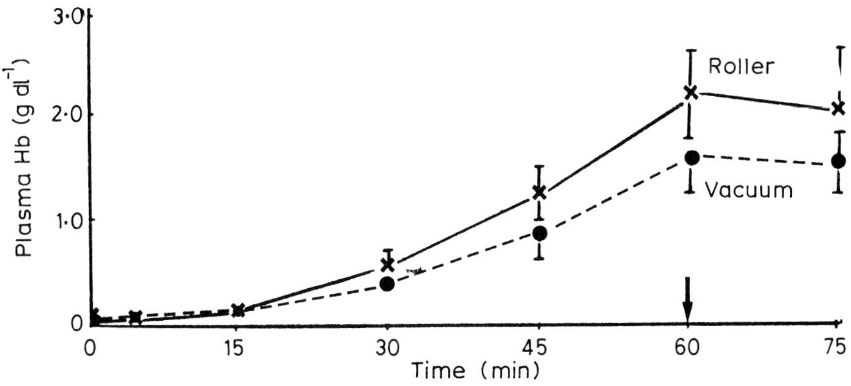

Fig. 15.10 Plasma haemoglobin concentration during *in vitro* suction of blood and air using roller pump and vacuum systems. Vertical bars indicate standard errors and arrow indicates end of one-hour suction period. (From Wright and Sanderson, 1979.)

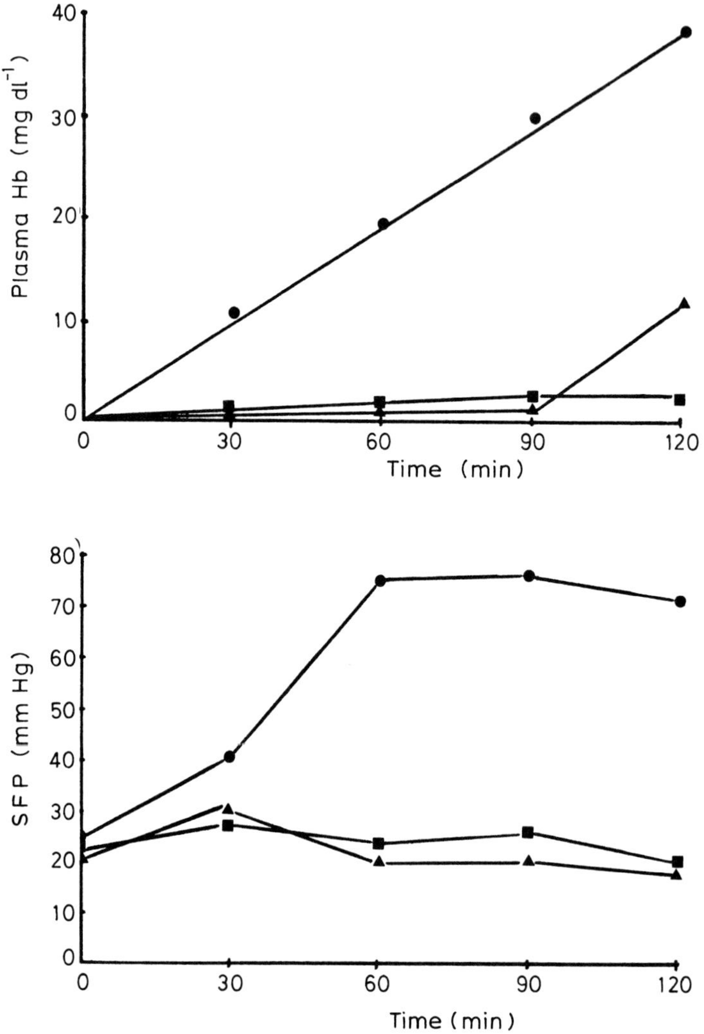

Fig. 15.11 Plasma haemoglobin concentration and screen filtration pressure during *in vitro* suction of blood and air using three cardiotomy reservoirs. Reservoir (■) contained a 20 μm filter. Reservoir (▲) contained a 40 μm filter. Reservoir (●) contained no filter.

(1) The level of blood cell trauma during cardiopulmonary bypass has been reduced by improvements in design, construction and bypass techniques. Nevertheless, it remains as a major problem. Platelet trauma appears to be the most important factor and there has been little improvement in this regard.

(2) Currently available blood pumps cause low levels of blood cell trauma. No adverse effects can be attributed to the introduction of pulsatile pumps.
(3) Membrane oxygenators cause less trauma than bubble oxygenators, but this is not easy to detect in the clinical situation.
(4) Cardiotomy suction is by far the most important cause of blood cell trauma.

A review of the physical factors capable of damaging blood cells reveals that shear stress, wall impact and surface tension are the most important. If blood cell trauma is to be minimized, these forces must be kept as low as possible and this implies that, for any bulk flow rate, the tubes should be as wide and internally smooth as possible, that viscosity of the perfusate should be low and liquid–gas interfaces should be eliminated. Ideally, the critical value of Reynold's number should not be exceeded in order to maintain laminar flow conditions. Unfortunately, physiological requirements override these restrictions during cardiopulmonary bypass and some flow disturbances are inevitable at conventional flow rates used for open-heart surgery. In Fig. 15.12, the diameter of cannula required to keep Reynold's number below

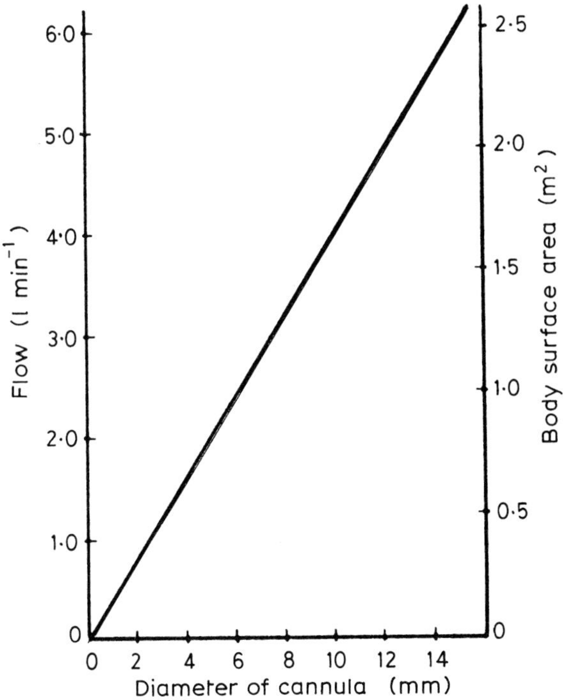

Fig. 15.12 Maximum laminar flow rates that can be achieved through cannulae.

2300 is shown for flow rates up to 6 l min^{-1}. The relationship between body surface area and required cannula diameter is also shown, using the relationship:

$$\text{Flow required (l min}^{-1}) = 2.4 \times \text{body surface area (m}^2).$$

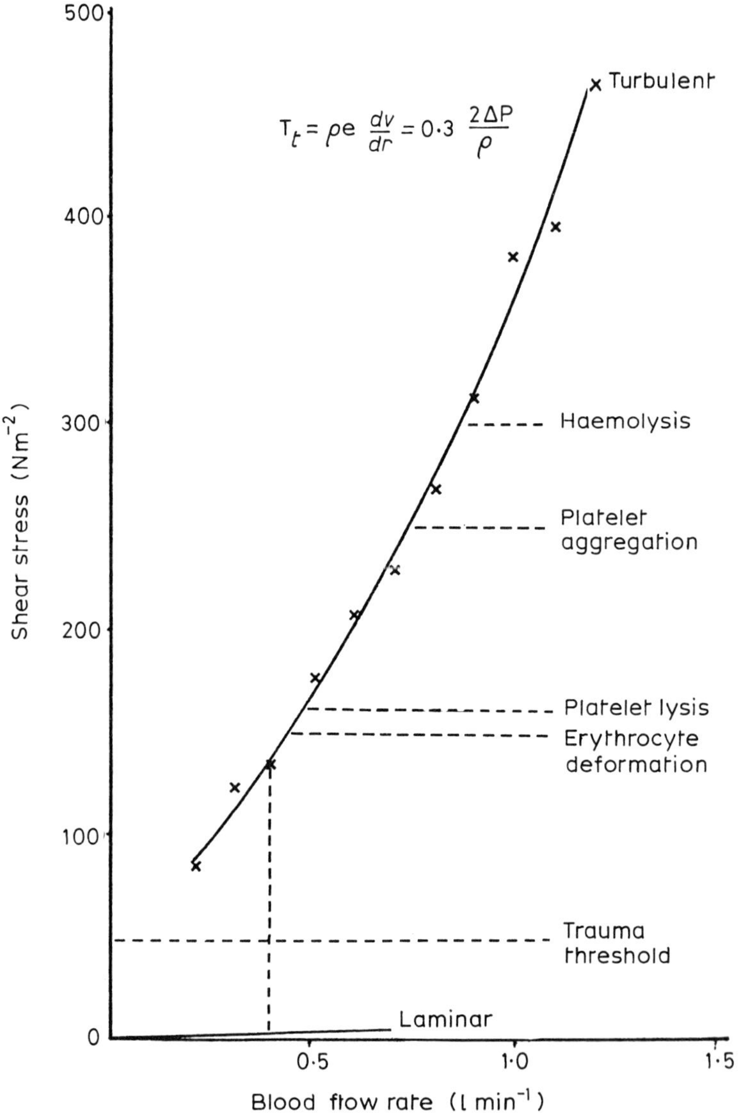

Fig. 15.13 Laminar and turbulent shear stresses for blood and air flowing through tubes of 4 mm internal diameter.

For cardiopulmonary bypass in most adult patients, the tubing and cannulae should be at least 10 mm internal diameter. Even then, flow disturbances will occur at inlet regions and at junctions with cannulae, catheters and connectors. The critical value of Reynold's number may well be lower if the tubing is not perfectly smooth and if the blood reservoir is not stationary. Shear stress, wall impact and surface tension are probably high during cardiotomy suction. The theoretical relationship between blood flow rate through a 4 mm suction catheter and the turbulent shear stress calculated according to Schlichting's (1960) formula and using experimentally derived data, is shown in Fig. 15.13. Some effects of shear stress upon blood cell trauma according to the literature are indicated. Assuming a critical threshold of $50\,\mathrm{Nm}^{-2}$, even the lowest flow rates used during cardiotomy suction are sufficient to cause some blood cell trauma. The results of this model fit well with results of measurements of blood cell trauma during both experimental and clinical cardiotomy suction. High levels of trauma in the suction system are thought to be due to turbulent shear stresses in the inlet catheter when blood and air are aspirated simultaneously (Wright and Sanderson, 1979). The avoidance of air aspiration by the use of a controlled suction system should significantly reduce the levels of blood cell trauma during cardiopulmonary bypass, and only when this has been achieved will it be possible to demonstrate conclusively the effects of improvements in other parts of the system. Further improvements may be made by using vacuum rather than roller pump suction, increasing the diameter of cannulae, tubing and connectors, using membrane rather than bubble oxygenators, and using less thrombogenic materials for the construction of components. The beneficial effects of haemodilution may largely be due to a reduction in plasma viscosity and therefore shear stress associated with velocity gradients through cannulae, connectors and tubing. Low flow techniques and cardioplegia may have contributed by reducing cardiotomy suction requirements.

The general conclusion is that blood cell trauma may be related to physical stresses in the cardiopulmonary bypass system, particularly shear stress, wall impact and surface tension. Attempts to protect the cells from damage by pharmacological methods provide only a second order solution to a problem which is better solved by analysing and then minimizing the relevant physical forces.

REFERENCES

Addonizio, V. P., Macarak, E. M., Niewiarowski, S., Colman, R. W. and Edmunds, L. H. (1977) Preservation of platelets during extracorporeal circulation with prostaglandin E_1. *Trans. Am. Soc. Artif. Int. Organs*, **23**, 439–45.

Alon, L., Turina, M. and Gattiker, R. (1979). Membrane and bubble oxygenator: A clinical comparison in patients undergoing aortocoronary bypass procedures. *Herz*, **4**, 56–62.

Anderson, M. N. (1961) Studies during prolonged extracorporeal circulation. *J. Thorac. Cardiovasc. Surg.*, **41**, 244–51.

Baier, R. E. (1977) The organization of blood components near interfaces. *Ann. NY Acad. Sci.*, **283**, 17–36.

Barras, J.-P. (1969) Blood rheology – general review. In *Modified Gelatins as Plasma Substitutes. Bibliotheca Haematologica.* Karger, Basel, New York, pp. 277–97.

Barthelemy, R., Vives, M., Couzy, H., Morucci, J. P., Puel, P. and Enjalbert, A. (1978). Dispositif de controle automatique des aspirations chirurgicales en chirurgie cardiaque. *Med. Biol. Eng. Comput.*, **16**, 165–8.

Bernstein, E. F., Marzec, U. and Johnston, G. G. (1977) Structural correlates of platelet functional damage by physical forces. *Trans. Am. Soc. Artif. Int. Organs*, **23**, 617–25.

Bindslev, A., Christensen, E. J. and Wandall, H. H. (1961) Hemolysis in dog blood: In vitro experiments. *J. Thorac Cardiovasc. Surg.*, **42**, 55–64.

Birek, A., Duffin, J., Glynn, M. F. X. and Cooper, J. D. (1976) The effect of sulfinpyrazone on platelet and pulmonary responses to onset of membrane oxygenation and perfusion. *Trans. Am. Soc. Artif. Int. Organs.*, **22**, 94–101.

Blackshear, P. L., Dorman, F. D., Bernstein, E. F. and Keller, K. H. (1967) Physical properties of blood that influence the flow and degradation of its constituents in artificial circuits. Digest of the *7th Int. Conf. Med. Biol. Eng.*, Stockholm, p. 24.

Blakney, G. B. and Dinwoodie, A. J. (1975) A spectrophotometric scanning technique for the rapid determination of plasma haemoglobin. *Clin. Biochem.*, **8**, 96–102.

Boggs, D. R. (1967) The kinetics of neutrophil leucocytosis in health and disease. *Semin. Haematol.*, **4**, 359–86.

Born, G. V. R. (1962) Aggregation of blood platelets by adenosine diphosphate and its reversal. *Nature*, **194**, 927–9.

Born, G. V. R., Bergquist, D. and Arfors, K.-E. (1976) Evidence for inhibition of platelet activation in blood by a drug effect on erythrocytes. *Nature*, **259**, 233–5.

Breslow, A., Kaufmann, R. M. and Lawsky, A. R. (1968) The effect of surgery on the concentration of circulating megakaryocytes and platelets. *Blood*, **32**, 393–401.

Brinsfield, D. E., Hoff, M. A., Geering, R. B. and Galletti, P. M. (1962) Haematological changes in long-term perfusion. *J. Appl. Physiol.*, **17**, 531–4.

Brown, C. H., Lemuth, R. F., Hellums, J. D., Leverett, J. B. and Alfrey, C. P. (1975) Response of human platelets to shear stress. *Trans. Am. Soc. Artif. Int. Organs*, **21**, 35–8.

Clowes, G. H. A. and Neville, W. E. (1958) Membrane oxygenator. In *Extracorporeal Circulation* (ed. J. G. Allen), Charles Thomas, Springfield Ill., 81–6.

Colantuoni, G., Hellums, J. D., Moake, J. L. and Alfrey, C. P. (1977) The response of human platelets to shear stress at short time exposures. *Trans. Am. Soc. Artif. Int. Organs*, **23**, 626–31.

Crosby, W. H. and Furth, F. W. (1956) A modification of the benzidine method for measurement of hemoglobin in plasma and urine. *Blood*, **11**, 380–3.

de Jong, J. F., Wildevuur, C. R. H. and Smit Sibinga, C. T. (1978) Cardiopulmonary bypass: analysis of various components of the circuit in canine experiments. *Proc. 3rd Ann. Symp. workshop on blood transfusion.* Groningen-Drenthe, pp. 1–22.

de Jong, J. C. F., ten Duis, H. J., Smit Sibinga, C. T. and Wildevuur, C. R. H. (1980) Hematologic aspects of cardiotomy suction in cardiac operations. *J. Thorac. Cardiovasc. Surg.*, **79**, 227–36.

Dewanjee, M. K., Vogel, S. R., Peterson, K. A., Lim, M. F. and Kaye, M. P. (1981) Quantitation of platelet lysis, platelet consumption on oxygenator, and stabilization of platelet membrane with prostacyclin and ibuprofen during cardiopulmonary bypass surgery in dogs. *Trans. Am. Soc. Artif. Int. Organs*, **27**, 197–202.

Dutton, R. C., Edmunds, L. H., Hutchinson, J. C. and Roe, B. B. (1974) Platelet aggregate emboli produced in patients during cardiopulmonary bypass with membrane and bubble oxygenators and blood filters. *J. Thorac. Cardiovasc. Surg.*, **67**, 258–65.

Dybkjaer, E., Berg, E. and Kissmeyer-Nielsen, I. (1964) Coagulation studies in extracoporeal circulation. *Acta Chir. Scand.*, **128**, 350–61.

Edmunds, L. A. and Addonizio, V. P. (1982) Platelet physiology during cardiopulmonary bypass. In *Pathophysiology and Techniques of Cardiopulmonary Bypass* (ed. J. R. Utley) Williams and Wilkins, Baltimore, Vol. 1, pp. 106–19.

Eiseman, B. and Spencer, F. C. (1962) Effect of hypothermia on the flow characteristics of blood. *Surgery*, **52**, 532–44.

Ellison, N., Addonizio, V. P., Niewarowski, S., MacVaugh, H., Harken, A. H., Colman, R. W. and Edmunds, L. H. (1980) Platelet protection during cardiopulmonary bypass with albumin prime and prostaglandin E_1 infusion. *Anesthesiology*, **53**, S168.

Fleisch, H. (1959) Quantitative determination of methemoglobin and of methemalbumin in the blood. *Helv. Physiol. Pharmacol. Acta*, **17**, 318–28.

Garner, R. (1973) Haematological changes in dogs subjected to extracorporeal circulation of blood or to endotoxin-induced shock. MSc. thesis, University of Keele.

Gollub, S. (1964) Unexplained bleeding after open-heart surgery. *Ann. NY Acad. Sci.*, **115**, 199–224.

Gorman, R. R. (1979) Modulation of human platelet function by prostacyclin and thromboxane A_2. *Fed. Proc.*, **38**, 83–8.

Halie, M. R., Deggeler, K. and Wildevuur, C. R. H. (1978). Extracorporeal circulation, damage to white blood cells and post-operative infection. *Proc. 3rd Ann. Symp. workshop on blood transfusion.* Groningen-Drenthe, pp. 107–18.

Hardwick, R. A., Hellums, J. D., Peterson, D. M., Moake, J. and Olson, J. (1981). Effects of PGI_2 and di-butyryl cyclic-AMP on platelets exposed to shear stress. *Trans. Am. Soc. Artif. Int. Organs*, **27**, 192–6.

Harker, L. A., Malpass, T. W., Branson, H. E., Hessel, E. A. and Slichter, S. J. (1980) Mechanism of abnormal bleeding in patients undergoing cardiopulmonary bypass: Acquired transient platelet dysfunction associated with selective α-granule release. *Blood*, **56**, 824–34.

Heide, K. (1964) On the heme-binding capacity of hemopexin. *Clin. Chim. Acta*, **10**, 460–9.

Heimbecker, R. O. (1977) Progress in extracorporeal circulation. *J. Thorac. Cardiovasc. Surg.*, **74**, 157–8.

Hellem, A. J. (1960) The adhesiveness of human platelets *in vitro*. *Scand. J. Clin. Invest.*, **12**, Suppl. 51, 1–117.

Hung, T. C., Hochmuth, R. M., Joist, J. H. and Sutera, S. P. (1976) Shear-induced aggregation and lysis of platelets. *Trans. Am. Soc. Artif. Int. Organs*, **22**, 285–91.

Johnston, G. G., Marzec, U. and Bernstein, E. F. (1975) Effects of surface injury and shear stress on platelet aggregation and serotonin release. *Trans. Am. Soc. Artif. Int. Organs,* **21**, 413–21.

Kayser, K. L. (1979) Pulsatile perfusion problems. *Ann Thorac. Surg.*, **27**, 284–5.

Kendall, A. G. and Lowenstein, L. (1962) Alterations in blood coagulation and haemostasis during extracorporeal circulation. *Can. Med. Assoc. J.*, **87**, 786–864.

Kirby, C. K. (1958) Discussion of blood changes. In *Extracorporeal Circulation* (ed. J. G. Allen) Charles Thomas, Springfield Ill., p. 264.

Kletschka, H. D., Rafferty, E. H., Olsen, D. A., Clausen, E. W., Hubbard, L. C., Robinson, A. R. and Larson, W. H. (1975) Artificial heart. 3. Development of efficient atraumatic blood pump. A review of the literature concerning *in vitro* testing of blood pumps for hemolysis. *Minn. Med.*, **58**, 756–81.

Koller, T. and Hawrylenko, A. (1967) Contribution to the in vitro testing of pumps for extracorporeal circulation. *J. Thorac. Cardiovasc. Surg.*, **54**, 22–9.

Kreel, I., Zaroff, L. I., Krasna, I. H. and Baronofsky, I. D. (1960) A syndrome following total body perfusion. *Surg. Gyn Obstet.*, **111**, 317–21.

Kusserow, B., Larrow, R. and Nicholls, J. (1971) Perfusion- and surface-induced injury in leucocytes. *Fed. Proc.*, **30**, 1516–20.

Laurel, C. B. and Nyman, M. (1957) Studies on the serum haptoglobin level in haemoglobinaemia and its influence on the renal excretion of haemoglobin. *Blood*, **12**, 493–506.

Lee, W. H., and Hairston, P. (1971) Structural effects on blood proteins at the blood–gas interface. *Fed. Proc.*, **30**, 1615–20.

Lee, W. H., Krumhaar, D., Fonkalsrud, E. W., Schjeide, O. A. and Maloney, J. V. (1961) Denaturation of plasma proteins as a cause of morbidity and death after intracardiac operations. *Surgery*, **50**, 29–39.

Leverett, L. B., Hellums, J. D., Alfrey, C. P. and Lynch, E. C. (1972) Red blood cell damage by shear stress. *Biophys. J.*, **12**, 257–73.

Liddicoat, J. E., Bekassy, S. M., Beall, A. C., Glaeser, D. H. and DeBakey, M. E. (1975) Membrane vs. bubble oxygenator: clinical comparison. *Ann. Surg.*, **181**, 747–53.

Lindon, J., Rosenberg, R., Merrill, E. and Salzman, E. (1978) Interaction of human platelets with heparinized agarose gel. *J. Lab. Clin. Med.*, **91**, 47–59.

Longmore, D. B. (1981) The value of prostacyclins in cardiopulmonary bypass. In *Towards Safer Cardiac Surgery* (ed. D. B. Longmore), MTP, Lancaster, pp. 355–77.

Mason, R. G., Shermer, R. W. and Zucker, W. H. (1973) Effects of certain purified plasma proteins on the compatibility of glass with blood. *Am. J. Pathol.*, **73**, 183–200.

McIntire, L. V., Dewitz, T. S. and Martin, R. R. (1978) Effect of the antiplatelet drug dipyridamole (RAF) on leucocyte reponse to mechanical trauma. *Trans. Am. Soc. Artif. Organs.*, **24**, 310–14.

Mielke, C. H., de Leval M., Hill, J. D., Macur, M. F. and Gerbode, F. (1973) Drug influence on platelet loss during extracorporeal circulation. *J. Thorac. Cardiovasc. Surg.*, **66**, 845–54.

Moncada, S. and Vane, J. R. (1978) Unstable metabolites of arachidonic acid and their role in haemostasis and thrombosis. *Br. Med. Bull.*, **34**, 129–35.

Morris, K. N., Kinross, F. M. and Stirling, G. R. (1965) Hemolysis of blood in the pericardium: The major source of plasma hemoglobin during total body perfusion. *J. Thorac. Cardiovasc. Surg.*, **49**, 250–8.

Mortensen, J. D. (1977) Evaluation of tests for blood damage produced by oxygenators. *Trans. Am. Soc. Artif. Int. Organs.*, **23**, 1–21.

Murray, R. K., Connell, G. E. and Pest, J. M. (1961) The role of haptoglobin in the clearance and distribution of extracorpuscular haemoglobin. *Blood*, **17**, 45–53.

Nevaril, C. G., Lynch, E. C., Alfrey, C. P. and Hellums, J. D. (1968) Erythrocyte damage and destruction induced by shearing stress. *J. Lab. Clin. Med.*, **71**, 784–90.

Packham, M. A., Evans, G., Glynn, M. F. and Mustard, J. F. (1969) The effect of plasma proteins on the interaction of platelets with glass surface. *J. Lab. Clin. Med.*, **73**, 686–97.

Philp, R. B., Inwood, M. J. and Warren, B. A. (1972) Interaction between gas bubbles and components of blood: Implications in decompression sickness. *Aerospace Med.*, **43**, 946–53.

Remtsma, K. and Creech, O. (1962) Viscosity studies of blood, plasma and plasma substitutes. *J. Thorac. Cardiovasc. Surg.*, **44**, 674–80.

Rygg, I. H. (1973) Studies in extracorporeal circulation. The design and development of a heart–lung machine. FADL's Forlag, Copenhagen.

Rygg, I. H. and Valentin, N. (1976) The Rygg–Kyvsgaard pump-oxygenator. In *Current Techniques in Extracorporeal Circulation* (eds M. I. Ionescu and G. H. Wooler) Butterworths, London, pp. 139–69.

Salzman, E. W., Merrill, E. W., Binder, A. and Wolfe, C. F. W. (1969) Protein-platelet interaction on heparinised surfaces. *J. Biomed. Mater. Res.*, **3**, 69–81.

Schlichting, H. (1960) *Boundary Layer Theory*., 4th edn, McGraw Hill, New York.

Schmidt, P. J., Peden, J. C., Brecher, G. and Baranovski, A. (1961) Thrombocytopenia and bleeding tendency after extracorporeal circulation. *New Engl. J. Med.*, **265**, 1181–5.

Sharp, A. A. and Eggleton, M. J. (1963) Haematology and the extracorporeal circulation. *J. Clin. Pathol.*, **16**, 551–7.

Siderys, H., Herod, G. T., Halbrook, H., Pittman, J. N., Rubush, J. L., Kasebaker, V. and Berry, G. R. (1975) A comparison of membrane and bubble oxygenation as used in cardiopulmonary bypass in patients. *J. Thorac. Cardiovasc. Surg.*, **69**, 708–12.

Solis, R. T. and Gibbs, M. B. (1972) Filtration of the microaggregates in stored blood. *Transfusion*, **12**, 245–50.

Swank, R. L., Roth, J. G. and Jansen, J. (1964) Screen filtration pressure method and adhesiveness and aggregation of blood cells. *J. Appl. Physiol.*, **19**, 340–6.

Tabak, C., Eugene, J. and Stemmer, E. A. (1981) Erythrocyte survival following extracorporeal circulation. *J. Thorac. Cardiovasc. Surg.*, **81**, 30–3.

Taylor, K. M., Bain, W. H., Maxted, K. J., Hutton, M. M., McNab, W. Y. and Caves, P. K. (1978) Comparative studies of pulsatile and nonpulsatile flow during cardiopulmonary bypass. 1. Pulsatile system employed and its hematological effects. *J. Thorac. Cardiovasc. Surg.*, **75**, 569–73.

ten Duis, H. J., de Jong, J. C. F., van Asseldonk, A. G. M., Smit Sibinga, C. T. and Wildevuur, C. R. H. (1978) Improved hemocompatibility in open heart surgery. *Trans. Am. Soc. Artif. Int. Organs.*, **24**, 656–61.

Ward, B. D. and Berry, G. L. (1975) Comparative platelet function during prolonged extracorporeal bubble and membrane oxygenation. *AMSECT Proc.*, **7**, 1–14.

Wielgorski, J. W., Cross, D. E. and Nwadike, E. V. O. (1975) The effects of subatmospheric pressure on the hemolysis of blood. *J. Biomech*, **8**, 321–5.

Wildevuur, C. R. H. (1980) Possibilities for improvement of the ECC. *Proc. 3rd Ann. Symp. workshop on blood transfusion*. Groningen-Drenthe, pp. 63–70.

Wildevuur, C. R. H. (1981) Towards safer cardiopulmonary bypass. In *Towards Safer Cardiac Surgery* (ed. D. B. Longmore). MTP, Lancaster, pp. 293–312.

Woltjes, J., ten Duis, H. J., de Jong, J. C. F. and Wildevuur, C. R. H. (1977) Behaviour of leucocytes in extracorporeal circuits (ECC). *Proc. Int. Soc. Artif. Organs.*, August 26–8.

Wright, G. (1975) Pathological effects of intra-arterial blood transfusions in dogs. *Cardiovasc. Res.*, **9**, 685–90.

Wright, G. (1976) L'agrégation cellulaire au cours d'une circulation extra-corporelle. *Les cahiers CECEC*, **6**, 27–37.

Wright, G. (1978) The mechanics of cell trauma in cardiotomy suction systems. *Proc. 3rd Ann. Symp. workshop on blood transfusion.* Groningen-Drenthe, pp. 219–22.

Wright, G. and Furness, A. (1980) To pulse or not to pulse. *Ann. Thorac. Surg.*, **29**, 489.

Wright, G. and Sanderson, J. M. (1979) Cellular aggregation and trauma in cardiotomy suction systems. *Thorax*, **34**, 621–8.

Zucker, M. B. and Vroman, L. (1969) Platelet adhesion induced by fibrinogen adsorbed onto glass. *Proc. Soc. Exp. Biol. Med.*, **131**, 318–20.

16

Heparin, protamine and prostacyclin therapy during cardiopulmonary bypass

K. M. TAYLOR

One area of real progress in cardiopulmonary bypass techniques in recent years has been an increased appreciation of the importance of adequate anticoagulation during the period of extracorporeal circulation. The availability of rapid and relatively accurate tests which can quantitate adequacy or inadequacy of anticoagulation has been a major contribution. It has been appreciated that individual patients respond quantitatively differently to weight-related doses of heparin.

There has also been a marked advance in understanding of the importance of platelet physiology during cardiopulmonary bypass. Platelet activation and aggregation and the release of vasoactive substances from platelet and blood cell microaggregates are developing areas of interest and understanding, where the possible therapeutic advantages of platelet aggregation inhibition with such substances as prostacyclin are being investigated.

16.1 HEPARIN

Heparin is an acid mucopolysaccharide substance with a powerful negative charge. It has widespread effects on the coagulation cascade, mediated through antithrombin III which is also known as heparin co-factor. The effect of antithrombin III thought initially to be an inhibition of the effect of thrombin and fibrinogen is now known to be much wider. Antithrombin III is now thought to inhibit many of the factors in the coagulation cascade, including factors XII, XI, X and IX. The basic effect of heparin in the presence of antithrombin III is to stop the coagulation process. Heparin preparations are commonly obtained from bovine lung or porcine gut. Gut heparin is inferior to bovine lung heparin, being intrinsically more antigenic. However variability in biological activity of different heparin batches has now clearly been demonstrated (McMahon *et al.*, 1975). Batch potency of apparent 100 units to 1 mg formulation may vary by ±30–40%. To batch potency variability must be added individual patient sensitivity to heparin which, as has been shown by many authors including Bull *et al.* (1975a), may be very considerable. Adequacy of heparinization cannot now be assumed on the basis of weight-related dosage without some objective assessment of adequate prolongation of the clotting time.

16.2 PROTAMINE SULPHATE

Protamine sulphate is an organic base opposite in action and charge to the acidic heparin. As expected, it will bind and inactivate heparin at all its activity sites in the coagulation cascade. When bound to heparin, protamine prevents heparin from enhancing the anticoagulant effect of antithrombin III, and therefore allows the normal coagulation cascade to proceed uninterrupted. The potency of protamine is such that it will bind circulating heparin in a 1:1 ratio. However, protamine has a shorter half-life than heparin and although still controversial, the concept of heparin rebound with heparin being released from tissues back into the circulation has led to the adoption of a 1.3:1 protamine to heparin reversal ratio to take account of these two factors. Some have recently challenged the protamine reversal dosage, believing that lower reversal doses can objectively be justified (Dutton *et al.*, 1983).

16.3 COAGULATION FUNCTION TESTS DURING CARDIOPULMONARY BYPASS

16.3.1 Whole blood clotting time (Lee White method)

This standard test of blood coagulation introduced by Lee and White (1913) is the basis for all surface contact tests of coagulation. It depends on the initial activation of factor XII in the cascade by the glass surface of the test tube. It can detect defects involving factors XII, XI, IX and VIII as well as defects of the final common pathway. With the whole blood clotting time (WBCT) test normal coagulation time is around 10 minutes. With adequate heparin anticoagulation the coagulation time will be prolonged to between 40 and 50 minutes. This length of time is clearly inappropriate for the requirements of open-heart surgery and the use of the WBCT has been superseded by the more rapid modification – the activated clotting time (ACT).

16.3.2 Activated clotting time (ACT)

This technique developed by Hattersley (1966) is an accelerated variation of the whole blood coagulation time. Hattersley produced a 10 times acceleration in the clotting process by adding diatomaceous earth. As with the WBCT, a straight-line dose–response curve exists between heparin dose administered and the prolongation of the ACT. This allows the computation of heparin half-life from the ACT dose–response curve which has been incorporated into some microprocessor programmes for calculation and timing of supplemental heparin during the period of cardiopulmonary bypass. It should be noted, however, that the ACT is a devised test of coagulation rather than a true physiological index. The limitations of the test are not fully appreciated. The ACT is less accurate in the context of high heparin dosages, for example where 5 mg kg^{-1} body weight is required for adequate heparinization. It is also inaccurate under conditions of hypothermia. Despite these drawbacks, it has greatly improved the achievement and maintenance of adequate anticoagulation during open-heart surgery. Available systems (for example the Haemochron) are compact and simple to use.

16.3.3 Direct heparin assay systems

More recently newer and more complex systems have been made commercially available which are based upon direct assay of heparin activity and allow accurate choice of the correct initial heparinizing dose for each individual patient. The system will also indicate dosage of supplemental heparin during the operative procedure and will estimate the required protamine reversal dose. This system (Hepcon) does not become inaccurate at high heparin dosage levels or in the presence of hypothermia, since each sample is warmed before the assay is carried out. It is too early to say whether this more complex system will supersede the simpler Haemochron type system, but early results appear encouraging.

16.4 ANTICOAGULATION PROTOCOLS DURING OPEN-HEART SURGERY

Heparin dosage for open-heart surgery has passed through many phases over the years. There has been a steady pendulum-like swing between the advocates of low-dose heparin, 3 mg kg^{-1} or less, and high-dose heparin >3 mg kg^{-1}. Not surprisingly, those groups using low-dose heparin routinely reported an increased incidence of fibrinolysis and depletion of coagulation factors. Those using high-dose heparin reported aggravation of pre-operative coagulation disturbances, and difficulties with reversal. What was clear was the fact that the adequacy of heparinization during open-heart surgery relates directly to the incidence of coagulation disturbances in the postoperative period. The problems associated with inadequate heparinization seemed particularly troublesome when there was a slight, but distinct, tendency towards higher heparin dosage protocols, even in excess of 4 mg kg^{-1} body weight.

As previously indicated, the key to this whole problem was the combined complicating factors of variable heparin potency and individual patient sensitivity to heparin. Studies by Bull *et. al.* (1975a) emphasize that strict adherence to a weight-related heparin dose without measuring adequacy of coagulation time prolongation would mean that a significant number of patients would be either under-heparinized or over-heparinized. Initially a safe range for the activated clotting time was indicated between 300 and 600 s, i.e. 3–6 times normal. This lower limit of 300 s was based upon the coarse evidence of absence of clots in the operative field or in the oxygenator. More refined estimates of the lower limit of the safe range were advanced by Young *et al.* (1978) who used the appearance of abnormal fibrin monomer as the cut-off of the lower limit of the safe range. This increased the safe lower limit to 400 s on the semiautomated ACT. Confirmatory evidence was put forward showing that where the ACT was less than 400 s, considerable fibrin and platelet debris was seen on the oxygenator and surfaces. The process of evolution in safe ACT definition has continued with both Young and Bull suggesting that an ACT between 450 and 500 s at the onset of cardiopulmonary bypass is optimal anticoagulation (Young, 1982, Bull *et. al.*, 1975b). Support for this optimal level of ACT prolongation has come more recently from oxygenator manufacturers, and indeed recent surveys of perfusion practice suggest that the majority of units do use at least 3 mg kg^{-1} body weight as the initial heparinizing dose, with confirmation by ACT that this has achieved prolongation of the ACT to at least 450 s. Repeat estimations of the activated clotting time can be carried out every 45 min during perfusion with incremental heparin given to maintain the ACT in the optimal range. There is still variability in practice with respect to protamine reversal dosage, although a majority appear to use 1.3 mg protamine to 1 mg heparin.

Anticoagulation during paediatric cardiac surgical cases is basically similar. A similar initial heparinizing dosage schedule is employed. Experience in paediatric units has demonstrated that heparin requirements during hypothermic cardiopulmonary bypass are less than those for normothermic perfusion (de Laval, 1984). Some paediatric units employ a higher level of protamine reversal up to twice the heparin dose given in mg protamine sulphate.

16.5 PLATELET AGGREGATION AND PROSTACYCLIN THERAPY DURING CARDIOPULMONARY BYPASS

The importance of platelets and platelet function during cardiopulmonary bypass was, until recently, linked in people's minds, to anticoagulant control and avoidance of coagulation with adequate heparinization. More recently, however, the independent importance of platelet aggregation and disturbances in platelet function have begun to assume real importance in the understanding of the changes produced in blood cell elements during perfusion. Indeed as time passes, it may ultimately be shown that disturbance in platelet function may be the most important haematological consequence of cardiopulmonary bypass.

16.5.1 Platelet structure and function

Platelets are cell fragments derived from megakaryocytes. The internal structure of platelets is a complex tubular and filamentous structure, with diffusely dispersed granules containing a variety of biologically active factors related to coagulation and platelet adhesion, and also a number of potentially pathological vasoactive substances including histamine and serotonin.

Platelets are an inherent part in the blood coagulation cascade. They do, however, have their own separate and discrete haemostatic functions. Platelets adhere both to cell surfaces and to each other, the process known as aggregation. They are increasingly shown to release secretory products into the circulation when activated. Platelets can be stimulated to aggregate by chemical substances including adenosine diphosphate (ADP), serotonin, arachidonic acid and thromboxane A_2. Activated platelets undergo internal structural change with contraction of the tubular and filamentous structure, production of pseudopodia, and also biochemical change with calcium release and the synthesis and ultimate release of thromboxane A_2 and the contents of the platelet secretory granules. These is clearly a potential vicious circle situation, since stimulated aggregating platelets release substances (thromboxane A_2, ADP, serotonin) which will themselves promote further platelet stimulation and aggregation. The release of thromboxane A_2 (Marcus, 1982; Gorman, 1979) is an important feature of platelet activation. Thromboxane A_2 is a powerful platelet activator, but is also an extremely potent local vasoconstrictor. It is clear from this brief review that where platelet activation and aggregation occurs, for example, during cardiopulmonary bypass, the pathological effects may not merely be related to mechanical obstruction of small blood vessels by platelet and blood cell aggregates, but may be related to the pathological effects of the vasoactive substances released from the activated platelets.

As there are many compounds which promote platelet activation, there are similar balancing agents which inhibit platelet activation usually through the central common biochemical pathway of increasing cyclic AMP concentration within the platelet. Platelet inhibitor substances include the prostaglandin substances, prostacyclin (PGI_2), PGE_1, dipyridamole (persantin), and also through a different biochemical mechanism, aspirin and other drugs.

The natural platelet inhibitor substance is prostacyclin, PGI_2. Its effect is seen in the fact that platelets will react with all solid surfaces except those with an endothelial cell lining. Endothelial cells prevent platelet activation by secreting prostacyclin. It must be appreciated that none of the anticoagulants, including full anticoagulation dose heparin, inhibits platelet activation when blood is exposed to synthetic solid surfaces.

The properties of surface materials themselves exert a variable effect on platelets, although at the present time no substance has yet been identified which will prevent platelet activation. Although some relatively thromboresistant materials are known (including polyurethane, polycarbonate, polyesters), the ideal substance for cardiopulmonary bypass circuits exposed to the circulating blood has not yet been identified. Furthermore, the biocompatibility of surfaces does not rest completely upon their tendency to produce platelet activation. Other potentially pathological processes such as protein adsorption and complement activation, must be similarly borne in mind when assessing the total biocompatibility of any surface material.

Pre-coating surfaces with albumin does reduce platelet adhesion (Packham *et al.*, 1969) although this and similar coating techniques have many inherent problems. Blood–gas interfaces are particularly prone to denature plasma proteins and induce massive platelet activation (Vroman *et al.*, 1977; Lee and Hairston, 1971). In this regard, membrane oxygenator systems might be expected to have a lower index of platelet activation than bubble oxygenators. Although studies have demonstrated this phenomenon in *in vitro* circuits, the additional problem of inclusion of cardiotomy suction during clinical open-heart procedures may negate the benefit of the membrane oxygenator as far as platelet activation is concerned.

16.5.2 Platelet physiology during cardiopulmonary bypass

Alterations occur to both the number of circulating platelets and to the function of platelets during conventional cardiopulmonary bypass. Many studies have indicated a rapid initial fall in platelet count at the onset of bypass. Haemodilution accounts for most of the decrease in actual platelet count, although true reductions in platelet counts have been documented in numerous studies. Postoperative platelet counts are diminished for the first few days after open-heart surgery. From around the fifth postoperative day the platelet count rises above pre-operative control values as newly formed platelets enter the circulation. Studies have attempted to demonstrate significant preservation of platelet counts with membrane oxygenation as opposed to bubble oxygenation. Although some studies have shown consistently higher platelet counts in patients perfused with membrane oxygenators, the differences have not been statistically significant.

Platelet function also changes substantially during cardiopulmonary bypass. Studies investigating ADP-induced platelet aggregation as an assessment of platelet function have shown marked impairment of platelet aggregation function from the onset of cardiopulmonary bypass, the function remaining depressed throughout the period of extracorporeal circulation with eventual restoration of function from around 5 days postoperatively (Harker *et al.*, 1980; McKenna *et al.*, 1975).

Evidence of platelet activation during cardiopulmonary bypass is confirmed by studies showing release of platelet factor IV and significant release of thromboxane into the circulation (Davies *et al.*, 1980). Recent studies have also shown significant increases in serotonin and histamine levels during cardiopulmonary bypass. The histamine release profile (Fig. 16.1) suggests considerable release at the onset of bypass which may be related to the *first-pass phenomenon*, and platelet activation as the blood is exposed to the artificial circuit for the first time (Hosking *et al.*, 1984).

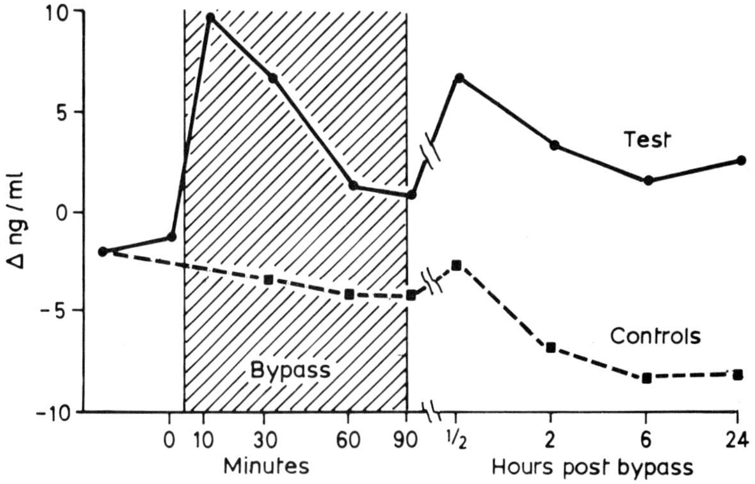

Fig. 16.1 Histamine release during open-heart surgery. The graph shows the rise in plasma histamine levels (ng ml^{-1}) for patients undergoing conventional open-heart surgical procedures (test group) compared with patients undergoing major non-cardiac surgery (control group). The cardiac surgical patients show a marked and highly significant rise in histamine levels persisting into the early postoperative period.

In addition to the release of vasoactive substances from activated platelets, platelet aggregation is known to occur. Platelet aggregates are formed during the period of cardiopulmonary bypass and have been demonstrated in the arterial return line (Dutton *et al.*, 1974), on arterial filter surfaces (Madoc *et. al.*, 1985) and have been demonstrated as peripheral emboli in the brain and other organs.

16.5.3 The use of prostacyclin (PGI_2) and other prostaglandin derivatives

As previously indicated, full heparinization is not the answer to platelet activation during cardiopulmonary bypass. The work of Vane (Moncada *et al.*, 1977) introduced the possibility of using the natural prostaglandin substance, prostacyclin (PGI_2), as an inhibitor of platelet aggregation. A number of experimental and clinical studies have encouraged this approach to preserve platelet numbers and platelet function by temporary inhibition of platelet aggregation (Taylor 1982; Madoc *et al.*, 1985; Longmore, 1981). The prostaglandin substances PGI_2 and PGE_1 have been studied. Prostacyclin with a half-life of about 2–3 min, has been most used and recent work in developing more stable and less vasoactive carbacyclin derivatives (Madoc *et al.*, 1985) is of interest.

Some confusion exists as to the results of the early studies with prostacyclin-based platelet inhibition. Early reports suggested that the demonstrable preservation in platelet numbers during the period of cardiopulmonary bypass was associated with an improvement in platelet function and in particular with a reduction in postoperative bleeding following open-heart surgery. It was suggested that prostacyclin might replace heparin anticoagulation routinely during open-heart surgery. Continuing and more recent studies have clarified this confusion to some extent.

Infusion of prostacyclin or one of its stable carbacyclin derivatives, beginning 30 min before the onset of cardiopulmonary bypass at half dosage ($10\,ng\,kg^{-1}\,min^{-1}$) and assuming full dosage of $20\,ng\,kg^{-1}\,min^{-1}$ by intravenous infusion does produce a significant preservation of platelet numbers during cardiopulmonary bypass. Platelets preserved with prostacyclin also retain significantly better function than control platelets in the postoperative period. The infusion is terminated at the cessation of cardiopulmonary bypass, and with the short half-life of prostacyclin (2–3 min) the expected haemostatic function of normal platelets is rapidly restored. In addition studies have shown that there is a significant reduction in the formation of platelet aggregates during cardiopulmonary bypass with prostacyclin infuion (Table 16.1, Figs 16.2 and 16.3; Madoc *et al.*, 1985; Faichney *et al.*, 1982).

Concern has been expressed regarding the vasodilatory effects of prostacyclin infusion and its ability to produce significant hypotenstion. Some authors have expressed the view that this does present a small but significant problem of haemodynamic management during open-heart surgical procedures. The author's experience has been that a small but insignificant hypotensive effect is seen in patients maintained during cardiopulmonary bypass at normal levels of peripheral vascular resistance. The precipitous falls occasionally reported with prostacyclin's use have in general been in patients who were substantially vasoconstricted prior to the prostacyclin infusion and

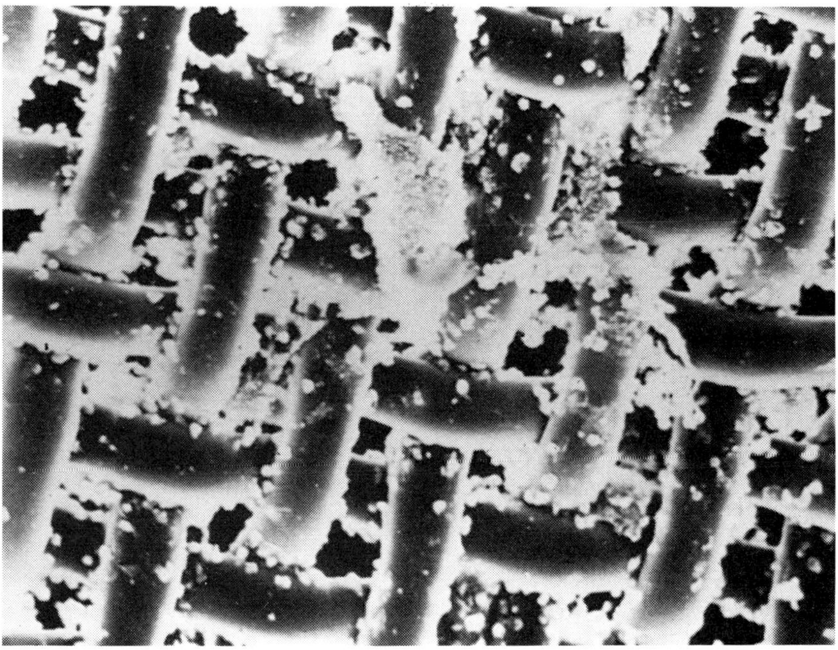

Fig. 16.2 Scanning electron microscopy appearance of microaggregate deposits on the upstream surface of a 40 μm screen filter in the arterial line. The duration of cardiopulmonary bypass was 90 min with adequate heparin therapy maintaining an activated clotting time (ACT)> 400 s throughout perfusion.

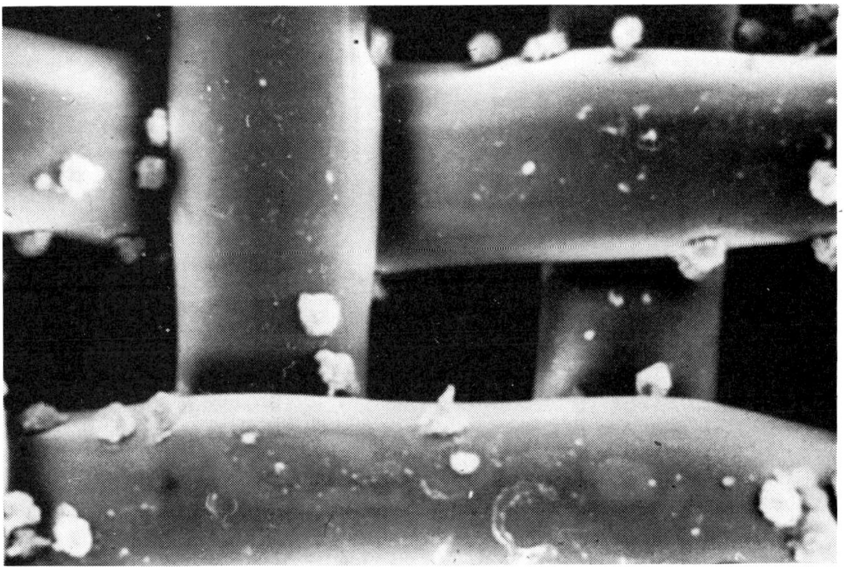

Fig. 16.3 Scanning electron microscopy appearance of the upstream surface of 40 μm screen filter placed in the arterial line. The duration of cardiopulmonary bypass was 90 min. The patient received heparin therapy (ACT> 400 s) plus prostacyclin infusion therapy at a dose during perfusion of 20 ng kg^{-1} min^{-1}.

Table 16.1 Increase in dry weight of 40 μm screen arterial line filters during cardiopulmonary bypass (a) with full heparin therapy and (b) with full heparin therapy plus prostacyclin infusion. The addition of prostacyclin produced a significant reduction in filter weight gain.

	Δ*Filter weight (g)*	
	Heparin	Heparin+ iloprost
Mean	0.05352	0.03751
S.D.	0.00525	0.01207
	Wilcoxon rank sum $p<0.05$	

who were given higher dosages (up to 50 ng kg^{-1} min^{-1}). The carbacyclin derivatives of prostacyclin are said to be less hypotensive in effect. This remains to be tested.

Recent studies have clarified the relative roles of prostacyclin-type therapy, and of heparin anticoagulation. Prostacyclin cannot be used as a replacement for heparin anticoagulation. Recent studies have shown that prostacyclin used alone in the full recommended dosage did not prevent massive coagulation in the extracorporeal circuit in animal experiments (Fig. 16.4). Inhibi-

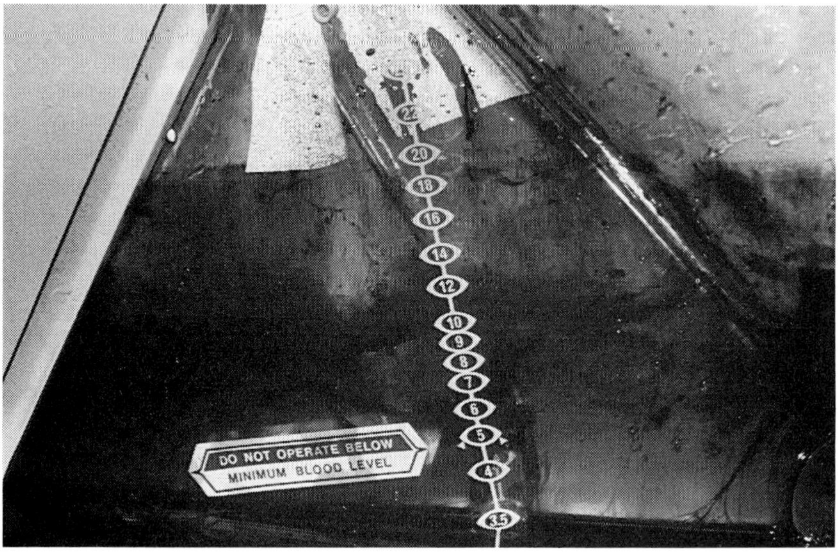

Fig. 16.4 Massive coagulation within oxygenator during experimental *in vivo* perfusion with prostacyclin infusion therapy (20 ng kg^{-1} min^{-1}) but without heparinization.

tion of platelet aggregation is a complementary process to heparin anticoagulation. The potential heparin-sparing effect of additional prostacyclin therapy remains conjectural.

One persistent negative feature of prostacyclin therapy remains its high cost. If continuing studies support the concept that inhibition of platelet aggregation is a useful routine in open-heart surgical practice, widespread use will inevitably be associated with cost reduction. The role of inhibition of platelet aggregation with prostacyclin during open-heart surgery has, to say the least, been controversial. The author believes that enough evidence is now available to indicate that inhibition of platelet aggregation is associated with preservation of platelet numbers and function, and with reduction in platelet aggregation during the period of cardiopulmonary bypass. Whether this significant potential benefit will encourage more widespread clinical use remains to be seen.

REFERENCES

Bull, B. S., Huse, W. M., Braver, F. S. and Korpman, R. A. (1975a) Heparin therapy during extracorporeal circulation. II. The use of a dose–response curve to individualize heparin and protamine dosage. *J. Thorac. Cardiovasc. Surg.*, **69**, 685.

Bull, B. S., Korpman, R. A., Huse, W. M. and Briggs, B. D. (1975b) Heparin therapy during extracorporeal circulation. I. Problems inherent in existing heparin protocols. *J. Thorac. Cardiovasc. Surg.*, **69**, 674.

Davies, G. C., Sobel, M. and Salzman, E. W. (1980) Elevated plasma fibrinopeptide A and thromboxane B_2 levels during cardiopulmonary bypass. *Circulation*, **61**, 808.

De Laval (1984) Personal communication.

Dutton, R. C., Edmunds, L. H. Jr, Hutchinson, J. C. and Roe, B. B. (1974) Platelet aggregate emboli produced in patients during cardiopulmonary bypass with membrane and bubble oxygenators and blood filters. *J. Thorac. Cardiovasc. Surg.*, **67**, 258.

Dutton, D. A., Hothersall, A. P., McLaren, A. D., Taylor, K. M. and Turner, M. A. (1983) Protamine titration after cardiopulmonary bypass. *Anaesthesia*, **38**, 264–8.

Faichney, A., Davidson, K. G., Wheatley, D. J., Davidson, J. F. and Walker, I. D. (1982) Prostacyclin in cardiopulmonary bypass operations. *J. Thorac. Cardiovasc. Surg.*, **84**, 601–8.

Gorman, R. R. (1979) Modulation of human platelet function by prostacyclin and thromboxane A_2. *Fed. Proc.*, **38**, 83.

Harker, L. A., Malpass, T. W., Branson, H. E., Hessel, E. A. II and Slichter, S. J. (1980) Mechanism of abnormal bleeding in patients undergoing cardiopulmonary bypass: Acquired transient platelet dysfunction association with selective granule release. *Blood*, **56**, 824.

Hattersley, P. (1966) Activated coagulation time of whole blood. *J.A.M.A.*, **136**, 436.

Hosking, S., Man, W. and Taylor, K. M. (1984) Histamine release during cardiopulmonary bypass in *Prod. Int. Symp. Frontiers of Histamine Research*, Paris.

Lee, R. I. and White, P. D. (1913) A clinical study of the coagulation time of blood. *Am. J. Med.*, **145**, 495.
Lee, W. H. Jr and Hairston, P. (1971) Structural effects on blood proteins at the gas–blood interface. *Fed. Proc.*, **30**, 1615.
Longmore, D. B. (1981) The value of prostacyclins in cardiopulmonary bypass. In *Towards Safer Cardiac Surgery* (ed. D. B. Longmore), MTP, Lancaster, pp. 355–70.
Madoc, R., Forbes, C. D., Dawson, H., Brannan, J. J. and Taylor, K. M. (1985) Effects of prostacyclin on platelet aggregation during cardiopulmonary bypass. In *30 Years of Extracorporeal Circulation* (eds S. Hagh, F. Sebening) Deutsches Herzentrum, Munchen, p. 363.
Marcus, A. J. (1982) Platelet function and its disorders: Platelet aggregation. In *Textbook of Haemostasis and Thrombosis* (eds R. W. Colman, J. Hirsh, V. Marder and E. W. Salzman). Lippincott Co., Philadelphia, Ch. 23.
McKenna, R., Bachman, F., Whitaker, B., Gilson, J. R. and Weinberg, M. Jr (1975) The hemostatic mechanism after open-heart surgery. *J. Thorac. Cardiovasc. Surg.*, **70**, 298.
McMahon, F. G., Jain, A. K., Ryan, J. R. and Lefton, T. E. (1975) Anticoagulant potency of mucosal and lung heparin. *Clin. Pharmacol. Ther.*, **17**, 79.
Moncada, S., Higgs, E. A. and Vane, J. R. (1977) Human arterial and venous tissues generate prostacyclin (prostaglandin X), a potent inhibitor of platelet aggregation. *Lancet*, **i**, 18.
Packham, M. A., Evans, G., Glynn, M. F., Mustard, J. F. (1969) The effect of plasma proteins on the interaction of platelets with glass surfaces. *J. Lab. Clin. Med.*, **73**, 686.
Taylor, K. M. (1982) Brain damage during open-heart surgery. *Thorax*, **37**, 873–6.
Vroman, L., Adams, A. L., Klings, M., Fischer, G. C., Munoy, P. C. and Solensky, R. P. (1977) Reactions of formed elements of blood with plasma proteins at interfaces. *Ann. NY Acad. Sci.*, **283**, 65.
Young, J. A. (1982) Coagulation abnormalities with cardiopulmonary bypass. In *Pathophysiology and Techniques of Cardiopulmonary Bypass* (ed J. R. Utley), Williams and Wilkins, Baltimore, pp. 88–105.
Young, J. A., Kisker, C. T. and Doty, D. B. (1978) Adequate anticoagulation during cardiopulmonary bypass determined by activated clotting time and the appearance of fibrin monomer. *Ann. Thorac. Surg.*, **26**, 231.

17

Blood conservation during cardiopulmonary bypass – autologous transfusion, cell saving and haemofiltration

D. R. WHEELDON and D. W. BETHUNE

Re-infusion of blood shed during a surgical procedure was first reported 160 years ago (Blundell, 1818). Blood banking and the public awareness of the need for blood for transfusion developed around the time of World War II. Up to 1940 large quantities of blood were not generally available for re-infusion into patients bleeding excessively. Between the wars there were over 1500 reports of autologous transfusion being used in ectopic pregnancy alone (Wilson and Taswell, 1968). Under the impetus of World War II a large network of blood banks was established and homologous transfusion became the conventional method.

The quantity of donor blood and blood products needed for individual open-heart procedures has declined over the years with the introduction of oxygenators requiring reduced priming volumes and the adoption of haemodilution techniques. In the mid 1960s the anticipated donor blood usage for each operation in our Unit was in the region of 15 units whereas now it is 4 units, with further reductions under discussion. Similar requirements are reported in the literature (MacDonald *et al.*, 1982). However, over the same period there has been a steady increase in the number of open-heart operations with even more rapid expansion over the years following the introduction of coronary artery bypass grafting. The result is that the overall demand for blood for open-heart surgery has increased dramatically. This has prompted those involved in cardiac surgery to take a fresh look at autologous transfusion.

Homologous transfusion is associated with a number of potential hazards, (Table 17.1). The total incidence of all reactions is probably less than 5% in

Table 17.1 Complications of homologous transfusion

Haemolytic	Immediate – intravascular Slow – extravascular Delayed – sensitization High antibody titre
Febrile reactions	Leucocyte platelet HLA antibodies Anti IgA, anti Gm antibodies Reaginic IgE and atopic individuals
Bacterial	Heat stable pyrogens *Pseudomonas*
Disease transmission	Viral hepatitis Cytomegalovirus Epstein Barr and mononucleosus Syphilis Herpes Malaria, toxoplasmosis, brucellosis and trypanosomiasis

the UK, and most are mild. However, some reactions may have serious consequences. In addition, the quality of homologous blood declines rapidly with storage (Table 17.2).

Table 17.2 The decline in quality of stored homologous blood

CPD stored bank blood	
Each unit contains 450 ml of blood and 63 ml of citrate-phosphate-dextrose (CPD	
Electrolytes	Serum sodium increases by 20 mmol per litre Serum potassium increases to 20 mmol per litre by 21 days High lactate and ammonia
Erythrocytes	Viability falls to 80% by 21 days 2,3-DPG and ATP levels decline rapidly
Leucocytes	Neutrophils lose all phagocytic activity after 48 hours Some lymphocytes survive 21 days
Platelets	No viable platelets after 24 hours
Coagulation proteins	Factors V and VIII only about 10% after 24 hours Factor XI only about 20% after 24 hours Factors IX and X rapidly decline after 7 days

17.1 AUTOLOGOUS TRANSFUSION

There are three major forms of autologous transfusion:

(1) Pre-donation of blood in the days, weeks and even months preceding elective surgery;

(2) Pre- or peri-operative haemodilution, i.e. the withdrawal of one or two units of whole blood with volume replacements by crystalloid solutions;
(3) The original method of peri-operative salvage and re-infusion of shed blood.

Although the benefits to the patient are similar for all methods, the indications, limitations and risks are different for each.

17.1.1 Pre-operative donation

This method is now rarely used except for patients who may have particularly difficult antibodies for homologous cross matching. The technique may also offer significant advantages when transfusing female patients with child-bearing potential in whom sensitization to homologous transfusion may subsequently be reflected in haemolytic disease of the newborn.

Safe guidelines have been developed for pre-donation programmes. With liquid and frozen storage techniques available donors can deposit one to eight units of blood in the pre-operative period. Weekly phlebotomies performed for as many weeks as required with the last donation no fewer than 72 hours prior to surgery is the usual practice, resulting in five units when stored in CPD (shelf-life 35 days) alone. Other more complicated regimes exist for use in special circumstances. There are numerous clear benefits to pre-depositing blood for autologous transfusion as outlined in Table 17.3. The major drawback to this technique is logistical, particularly for those hospitals serving a large regional population.

Table 17.3 Benefits of autologous transfusion

Elimination of transfusion reactions
Elimination of transfusion transmitted disease
Guaranteed availability of blood
Stimulus to bone marrow*
Less overall use of blood
Less use of homologous blood
Acceptance by some religious groups
Increase in community blood resources

* Pre-deposition only.

17.1.2 Haemodilution

The technique of haemodilution, with or without the withdrawal of one or more units pre-bypass, has become standard for most open-heart units. The degree of haemodilution used (haematocrits 15–30%) and the replacement fluids used vary widely. The lower haematocrit results in a considerable decrease in the number of red cells lost during surgery and also reduces red cell trauma in the cardiopulmonary bypass (CPB) circuit. Animal and clinical studies have demonstrated that the diminished oxygen-carrying capacity of the red cell depleted blood is offset by the increased capillary flow rates achieved as a result of lowered viscosity (Kessler and Messmer, 1975). Large volume additions of crystalloid fluid result in low colloid oncotic pressures which in turn lead to water diffusion into the interstitial space during CPB. This water load may lead to postoperative complications, particularly in children, patients with compromised renal function and those with functional or metabolic pulmonary impairment. Failure to reduce this water load significantly during the first 48 hours post-bypass may be due to the high plasma level of antidiuretic hormone (ADH) commented upon by Philbin *et. al.* (1979) during crystalloid haemodilution and non-pulsatile flow. This massive release of ADH may be caused by the abrupt reduction in blood pressure registered by the aortic and left atrial baroreceptors at the start of bypass.

The low cost and absence of toxicity of balanced electrolyte solutions have proscribed large-scale colloid supplementation. However, there is a mass of theoretical and clinical evidence which indicates some advantages accruing to the partial replacement of crystalloids by cheap colloid substitutes such as Haemaccel, the dextrans or hydroxyethyl starch when available. (Compositions of priming solutions for cardiopulmonary bypass are discussed in detail in Chapter 14.)

17.1.3 Intra-operative autologous transfusion

During the early 1960s when interest in all forms of autologous transfusion resurfaced it was inevitable that intra-operative salvage would attract attention. Despite the technical difficulties with the early techniques which included haemolysis and disseminated intravascular coagulation, in addition to fat and air embolism, the concept of blood salvage and re-infusion is so reasonable that further effort seemed well worthwhile. However, although there have been substantial technical advances over the past 20 years we have yet to develop the ideal autotransfusion system as outlined by Gilcher and Orr (Table 17.4) in 1975.

17.1.4 Autologous transfusion devices

There are at least three types of autologous transfusion devices (ATD) currently available in the UK.

(a) Bentley system

The ATS-200 is a development of the ATS-100 developed by Dr Klebanoff in 1977. The device consists of a roller pump which aspirates blood and air into

Table 17.4 The ideal autologous transfuser

1. Rapid assembly
2. Ease of operation
3. Low cost equipment and software
4. In-line filtration
5. Minimal blood/air interface
6. Simplified and non systemic anticoagulation
7. Red cell concentration facility
8. Removal of cellular and fluid contaminants together with other extraneous debris
9. Rapid return to the patient
10. Safety from air emboli and coagulopathies

a Bentley Q220F hardshell cardiotomy reservoir. The pressure within the reservoir is controlled by adjustment of an air bleed valve. Initially the system was designed to be used with systemic anticoagulation of the patient but it can also be modified to avoid systemic anticoagulation by the addition of local anticoagulant at the suction tip. Filtration and defoaming take place within the reservoir and the salvaged product can be infused by gravity or under pressure. The latter method carries the possibility of air embolism. Added difficulties with this system include the re-infusion of a product of low haematocrit with significant quantities of anticoagulant as well as a range of contaminants both particulate and chemical, some of which have been implicated in the pathogenesis of disseminated intravascular coagulation (Reul, 1974). For this reason the ATS system is not recommended for the infusion of more than five to six units of blood in any individual patient.

(b) Sorenson system

The Sorenson Research Corporation has developed three different autologous transfusion devices. The system marketed in the UK consists of a flexible liner placed within a hard shell vacuum reservoir. A suction tip which mixes CPD anticoagulant with aspirated blood in a ratio of 1:7 delivers the aspirate to the liner via a 170 μm filter. The reservoir is maintained at a negative pressure of 30–60 mmHg (4–8 kPa) by a vacuum regulator. No attempt is made to concentrate or wash the salvaged red blood cells and this system is also somewhat slower than the Bentley system. Modified versions of this system have also been used for postoperative salvage of blood (Schaff, 1978).

(c) Centrifugal cell washers

The concept of collecting specific cellular components from blood for transfusion was pioneered in the mid 1960s by Dr Freireich at the National Cancer Institute in Washington, USA. He recognized the need to collect large numbers of granulocytes from normal donors in order to treat patients with acute leukaemia. Dr Freireich sought the assistance of IBM to produce a suitable machine and from this collaboration the first centrifugal device was developed. The crux of this machine, and all subsequent devices, is the seal designed to permit the transfer of whole blood from the stationary to the rotating portion of the bowl and the transfer of the separated components in the reverse direction. From this development a number of other companies have marketed similar machines as interest in blood component therapy and plasma exchange has increased.

One of the 'family' of such machines is the IBM 2991 Blood Cell Processor which is a portable, automated machine for collecting, packing and washing red cells. This machine became the first device of this sort to be used for peri-operative autologous transfusion.

The Haemonetics Corporation had entered this field at an early stage of development and recognized the potential of a machine designed specifically for peri-operative autologous transfusion. The result was the production of the Cell Saver I and more recently the Cell Saver III. These machines have been used more extensively than any other for autologous transfusion applications. More recently another dedicated autologous transfusion machine has been marketed by Dideco, which is very similar to the Cell Saver systems. Both these machines make use of a hardshell centrifuge bowl in which separation and washing take place. The products are removed serially through a centrally placed channel (Fig. 17.1) starting with the lightest component, the plasma, and ending with the heaviest, the red cells.

The IBM system makes use of a processing bag which is spun in the centrifuge. Red cells are forced to the outside of the bag whilst hydraulic fluid under the flexible membrane is drawn in by centrifugal force and expels the supernatant from the centre of the bag (Fig. 17.2). After washing the bag is removed from the centrifuge and hung up for transfusion to the patient. Table 17.5 provides a comparison of these three machines.

These systems provide a final product of high haematocrit (70%) consisting of washed red cells suspended in saline, free from particulate matter, vasoactive substances and contaminants thus decreasing the chance of coagulation abnormalities. The final product is re-infused by gravity and therefore air embolism is not a concern. Since virtually all contaminants are removed there is no limit to the number of salvaged units which can be re-infused with this system with the proviso that fresh frozen plasma is given to the patient for coagulation support.

17.2 HAEMOFILTRATION

Haemofiltration is a technique which has recently been developed as an alternative to conventional haemodialysis for the treatment of patients in

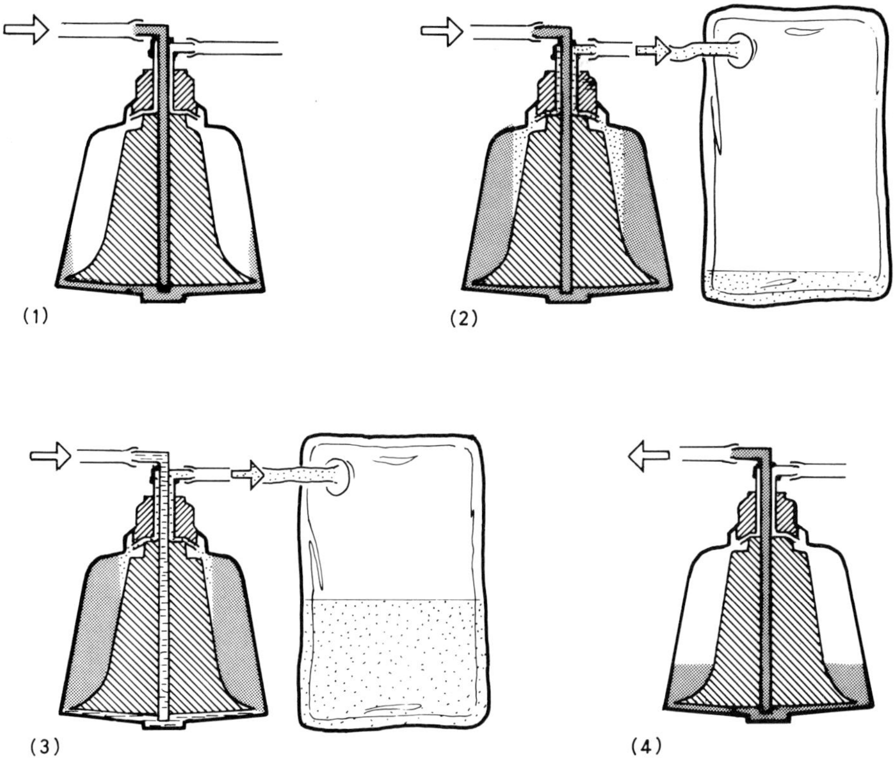

Fig. 17.1 The Haemonetics Cell Saver III. (1) Diluted blood being pumped into spinning centrifuge bowl. (2) Centrifugal force holds red cells in suspension while supernatant is expelled to waste bag. (3) Saline wash being introduced while cell circulation is maintained against the flow of wash solution. (4) Washed cells are returned to perfusion circuit or to transfusion bag.

renal failure (Henderson *et al.*, 1973). Its application in cardiac surgery relates to its principal ability to remove excess fluid from the circulation.

Haemofiltration differs from dialysis in that the membranes used are constructed in a different manner and from different materials. Furthermore, a dialysate fluid is not employed. Solutes of different molecular size and diffusivity are cleared at the same rate as each other by pure convection which is generated by applying a vacuum to the dialysate side of the membrane and a positive pressure to the blood side. High flux dialysers as well as haemofilters can be used for haemofiltration. These membranes have a filtration rate of up to 40% of the blood flow. In order to maintain patient fluid balance a corresponding volume of physiological solution has to be re-infused. The

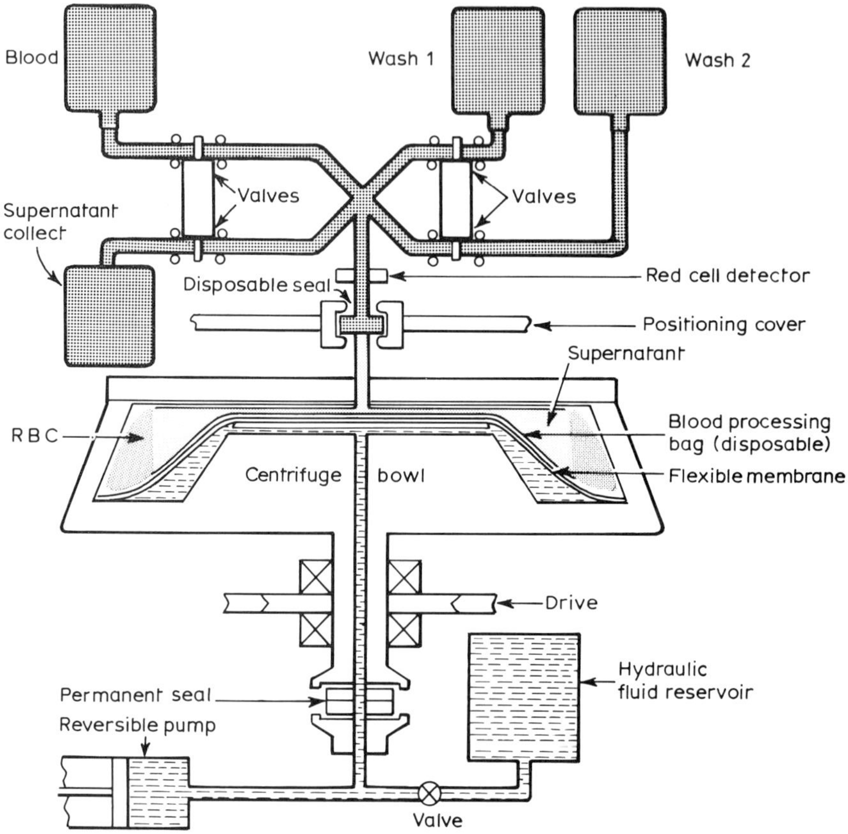

Fig. 17.2 The IBM 2991 Blood Cell Processor.

advantages of haemofiltration over conventional dialysis are that the removal of substances of molecular weight between 2000 daltons and 20 000 daltons is more efficient (Fig. 17.3) and the rate of fluid removal is far greater. This has important implications both with respect to dialysis quality and to the time required to perform adequate dialysis. In addition, haemofiltration patients have been shown to be much more stable haemodynamically (Chaignon *et al.*, 1982).

High flux dialysis and haemofiltration have recently attracted the attention of open-heart teams primarily because both techniques may be used to haemoconcentrate cardiopulmonary bypass (CPB) circuit contents (Hopeck *et al.*, 1981). A few teams, including our own, have also been using dialysis for a number of years as an adjunct to CPB for those patients with known renal insufficiency (Intonti *et al.*, 1981) who undergo open-heart surgery.

Table 17.5 A comparison of three cell washers

Dideco BT 795	*Haemonetics Cell Saver III*	*IBM 2991 Blood Cell Processor*
Designed specifically for autologous transfusion	Designed specifically for autologous transfusion	Originally designed as a laboratory cell processor
Manual operation only	Manual and automatic operation	Semi-automatic serial batch device
Requires dedicated operator	Pre-programmable parameters	Requires dedicated operator
Bi-directional roller pump for fluid handling	Bi-directional roller pump for fluid handling	Gravity feed
Limited safety features	Good safety features	Limited safety features
No air detector	Air detection for safety and trigger for cycle changes	No air detector
Centrifuge a little noisy	Very quiet centrifuge	Fairly quiet centrifuge
Control panel not serviceable	Washable control panel with touch buttons	Control panel not serviceable
Fast	Fast	Fast
Hardware price: £7850	Hardware price: £17 000	Hardware price: £16 000
Disposables: £75	Disposables: £58	Disposables £7

Renal insufficiency in association with cardiac disease can occur in patients with rheumatic fever which causes renal disease as well as cardiac valvular lesions. Dialysis patients frequently develop severe coronary artery disease (Lansing *et al.*, 1968) and are prone to a form of infective endocarditis (Lowrie *et al.*, 1974). Patients with bacterial endocarditis can develop renal failure as a result of circulating antibodies and mycotic emboli. Improvements in perfusion and oxygenation management have encouraged the submission of such patients even with very severe renal dysfunction, to corrective cardiac surgery.

Haemodilution to a haematocrit of 20–30% is now almost universal practice for CPB. This fluid load of 20–40 ml kg^{-1} is poorly tolerated immediately after bypass by patients in renal failure. The use of conventional haemodialysis in the immediate pre- and postoperative period may be limited in these patients due to their reduced cardiac reserve. Intra-operative haemofiltration or high flux dialysis can therefore play a very useful role in the treatment of these patients, both by removing toxic metabolites and by controlling the fluid load. The other major reason for recent interest in haemofiltration is the increasing popularity of multiple dose cardioplegia for

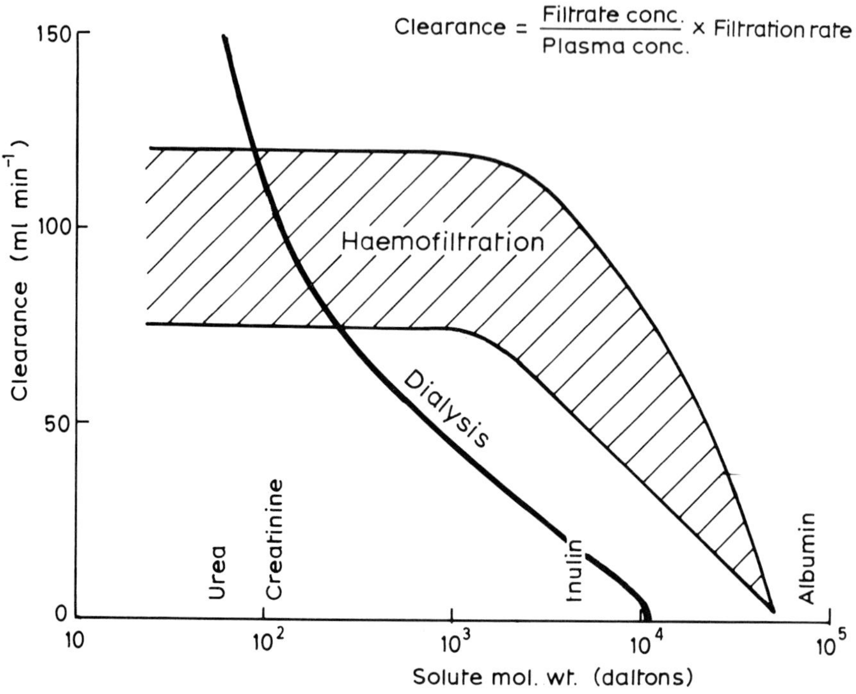

Fig. 17.3 Clearance rates of dialysers and haemofilters for solutes of differing molecular weights.

myocardial preservation (Hearse *et al.*, 1981). This practice frequently leads to further haemodilution, together with an inappropriately high concentration of certain ions, particularly potassium and magnesium.

17.2.1 Haemofilters

There are a number of haemofilters suitable for use during CPB available in the UK at the present time. None was developed specifically for this application. Despite this fact, a number of manufacturers have taken appropriate filters from their dialysis filter range, applied new labelling, added a hard shell reservoir and suitable tubing, and offered them for use during CPB. In fact, several manufacturers of dialysis membranes do have a suitable high flux filter in their range which the perfusionist may include in the circuit.

Table 17.6 lists the specifications of six filters. The first two (Harvey Haemoconcentrator and the Bentley CPB 6000) are sold specifically for CPB application. The examples 3 and 4 have been selected as being suitable alternatives. Only the last two are true haemofilters (Gambro FH-202 and Sartorius SM 400). Fig. 17.4 shows the ultrafiltration rates for these six devices at a blood flow of 300 ml min^{-1} which is about optimum. Higher flows may give rise to haemolysis, and lower flows result in less efficiency.

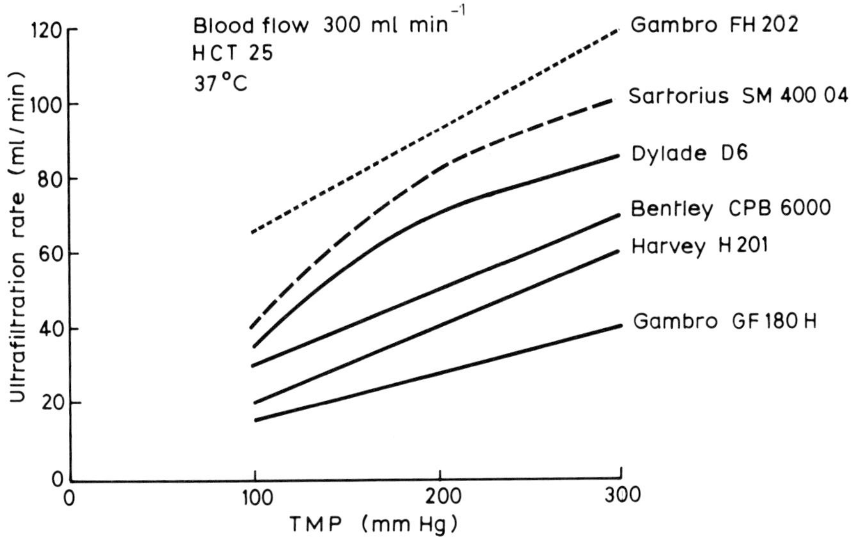

Fig. 17.4 Ultrafiltration rates of dialysers and haemofilters. TMP = transmembrane pressure.

Likewise a transmembrane pressure (TMP) of about 300 mmHg (40 kPa) is well within the sort of value which is easy to maintain using the pipeline theatre wall suction. Assuming an average total circulating blood volume of about 6 litres towards the end of bypass, these devices would allow haemo-concentration from a haematocrit of 20% to one of 25% (removal of 1 litre of fluid within a time frame of 10 minutes (FH-202) to about 20 minutes (Harvey)). These times could be shortened by increasing the TMP. The actual ultrafiltration rate achieved will depend on the blood flow rate through the filter, the nett TMP, haematocrit, protein concentration and temperature (Fig. 17.5).

17.2.2 Membranes

Mass transfer in dialysis depends on the concentration difference on both sides of the membrane, the membrane pore size and the diffusion coefficient within the pore. For the filtration process, mass transfer is dependent on the

Table 17.6 Specifications of some high flux dialysers and haemofilters

	High flux dialysers			*Haemofilters*		
	Harvey H201	*Bentley CPB 6000*	*Dylade D6*	*Gambro GF-180-H*	*Gambro FH-202*	*Sartorius SM 400 04*
Membrane	Cellulose acetate	Cuprophane	Cuprophane	Cuprophane	Polyamide	Cellulose triacetate
Surface area	1.8 m^2	1.36 m^2	2.0 m^2	1.8 m^2	1.2 m^2	0.6 m^2
Priming volume	150 ml	170 ml	96 ml	140 ml	82 ml	28 ml
Max. TMP	600 mmHg (80 kPa)	600 mmHg (80 kPa)	600 mmHg (80 kPa)	600 mmHg (80 kPa)	600 mmHg (80 kPa)	700 mmHg (93.3 kPa)
Blood flow resistance Q_b 300 ml min^{-1}	15 mmHg (2 kPa)	20 mmHg (2.7 kPa)	30 mmHg (4 kPa)	20 mmHg (2.7 kPa)	160 mmHg (21.3 kPa)	280 mmHg (37.3 kPa)
Clearance Q_b 300 ml min^{-1}						
Urea	290	165	270	203	120	145
Creatinine	280	133	250	180	120	120
Price	£74*	not avail.*	£25	£16	£36	£33

*Kit package price.

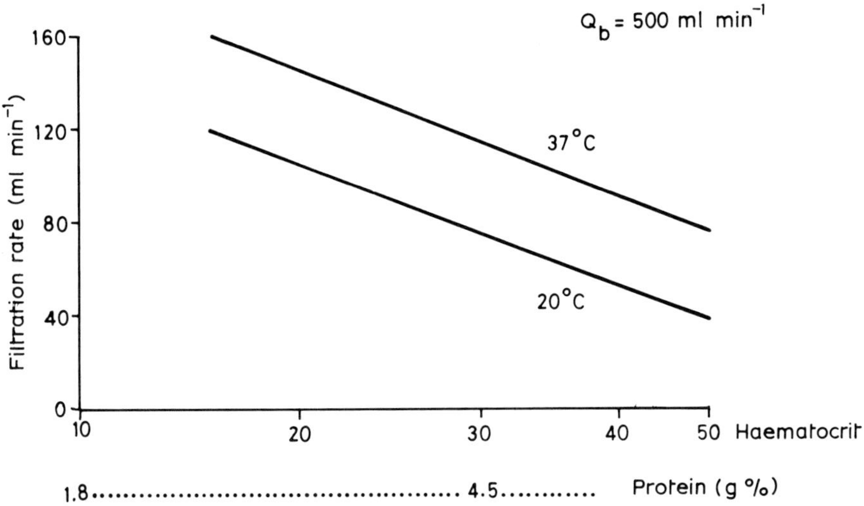

Fig. 17.5 Factors affecting ultrafiltration rate (see text for details).

pore size and the pressure difference between the hydrostatic and the osmotic pressure. Total filtration capacity depends on membrane surface area for both devices.

The structure of the different membranes used for dialysis and haemofiltration augments these differences. Haemofiltration membranes have an asymmetric structure consisting of an ultra thin inner skin (which acts like a micro screen filter) supported on a much thicker macroporous substructure. A dialysis membrane is symmetrical and spongelike in structure containing pores of different sizes distributed throughout the membrane. Features such as high flux capacity depend on the method of manufacture and the chemical properties so induced (particularly with regard to hydration).

When choosing a membrane a number of factors need to be evaluated. For the specific problem of gross fluid overload a pure haemofilter (e.g. the Gambro FH-202) is ideal. For a patient who requires dialysis for the removal of toxic metabolites as well as limited fluid removal, a high flux dialyser with a relatively large effective surface area (e.g. the Dylade D6) is preferable.

However, for general CPB use a filter with a mixture of characteristics will probably provide the best solution and it will be up to each team to decide which membrane best suits their own particular requirements. The haemofilters should probably by reserved for handling gross fluid overload – since they are more expensive and, because of their high resistance, will require a dedicated blood pump for optimum performance. We now use a high flux dialyser (Dylade D6) for both applications. The device is used in the dialysis mode during most of the bypass in patients where metabolite removal is desirable and then converted into the haemofiltration mode towards the end of bypass in order to control the fluid volume (Figs 17.6 and 17.7).

17.2.3 Circuitry

It is possible to place a haemofilter anywhere in the circuit where a convenient shunt can be established. From a safety standpoint, it is preferable to return filtered blood to an area of the circuit which can deal with microbubbles since it is inconvenient and time consuming to debubble this circuit to the same standard as the rest of the CPB circuit when priming.

Introduction of air into the system once primed should be avoided since this will reduce the efficiency of the device. Blood may therefore be drawn off from the circuit: (a) from a port in the venous line, (b) from the arterial reservoir (via the coronary perfusion port if available) or (c) from the arterial line. Filtered blood may be returned to: the venous line, cardiotomy reservoir or to the 'quick prime' port of a hardshell oxygenator. Flow through the circuit may be controlled using a low flow pump or, alternatively, and more simply, by using a controlled resistance applied to a shunt off the arterial line incorporating a rotameter flowmeter of the kind used in dialysis circuits (Fig. 17.8). It is also possible to install the device in a parallel circuit in the arterial line as long as an arterial line filter or bubble trap is employed.

When designing the circuit it is worthwhile bearing in mind that a convenient means of collecting the remaining CPB circuit volume at the end of bypass is desirable. This may involve making a modification to the circuit at the end of bypass – transferring the remaining volume to the cardiotomy reservoir, for example, and forming a small recirculating circuit. The remaining circuit volume may be displaced into this recirculating circuit using a standard electrolyte solution so that bypass can be re-established safely and quickly, if necessary.

17.2.4 Operation

The haemofilter may be set up with the rest of the CPB circuit or added at a later time during the procedure. For instance, a team may elect to use one of these devices only if particular problems of fluid loading occur during the procedure. In this case it will probably be worthwhile to modify the routine circuit in a way which makes this addition safe and simple. On the other hand, other teams may decide to use one of these devices on a routine basis, in which case the device will be set up and primed along with the rest of the circuit. Some of these devices require to be rinsed prior to connection to the patient.

When priming initially with asanguinous fluid, it is helpful to produce a

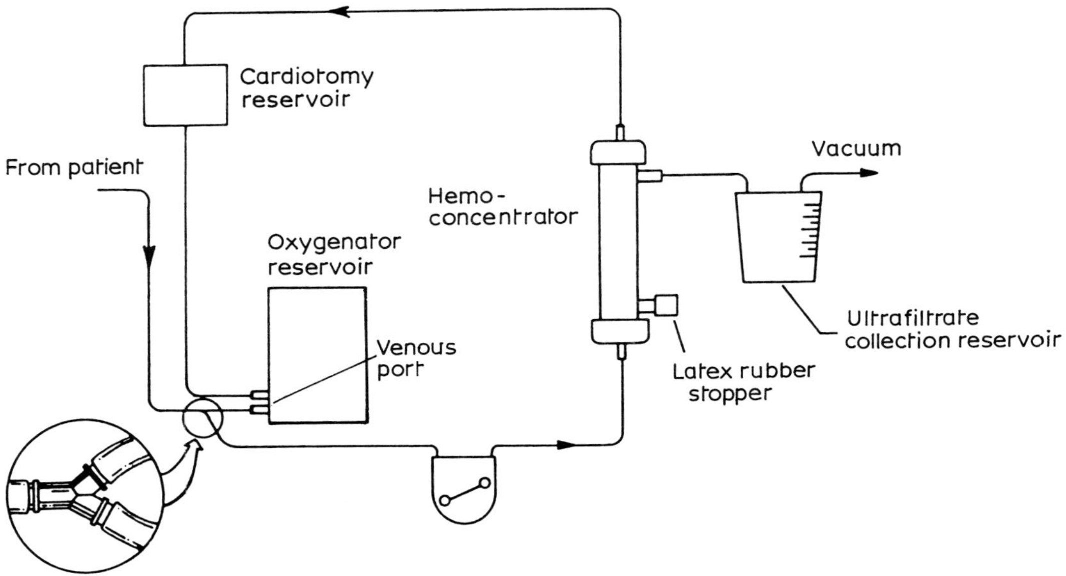

Fig. 17.6 Membrane oxygenator circuit with haemoconcentrator *in situ*. Courtesy of C. R. Bard International.

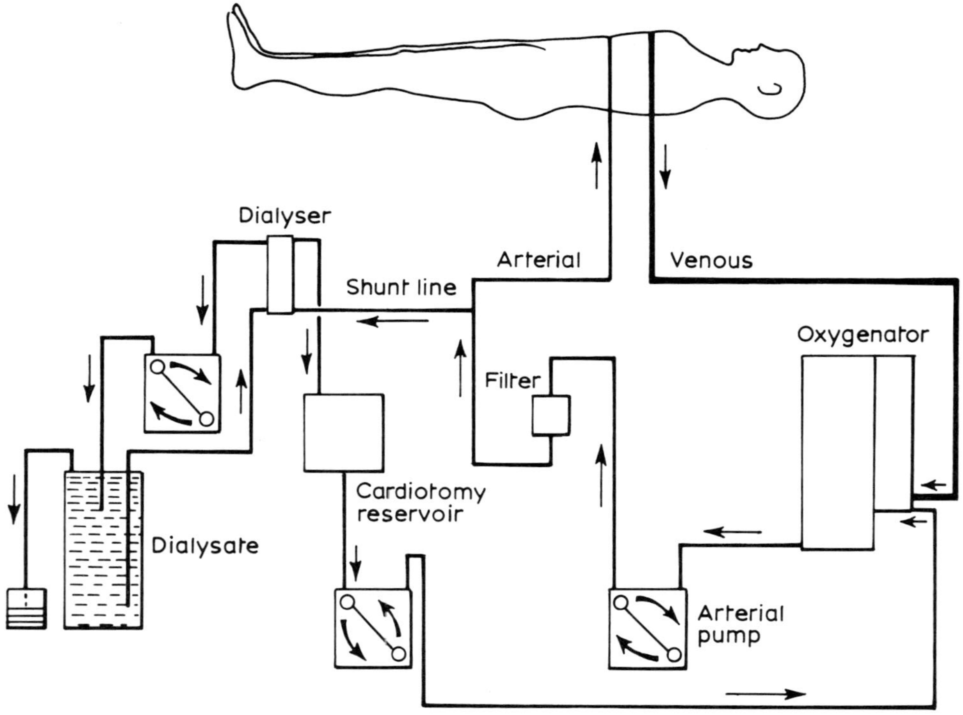

Fig. 17.7 Haemodialysis circuit.

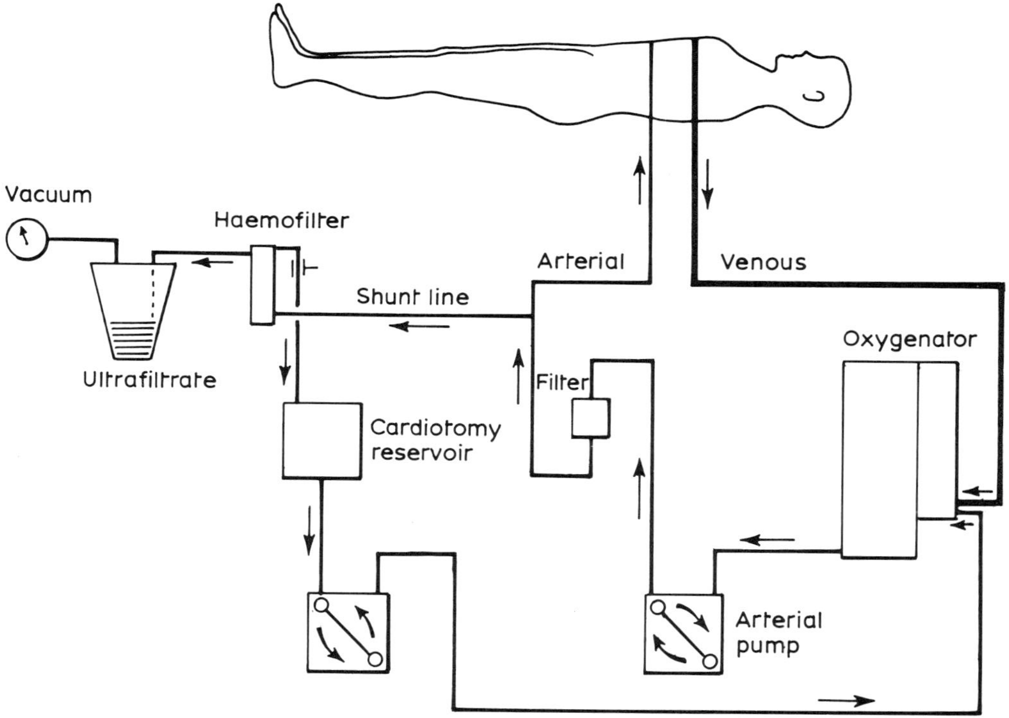

Fig. 17.8 Haemofiltration circuit.

positive pressure (by restricting the outflow) of about 300 mmHg (40 kPa) once the air has been displaced. The vacuum line should be left open to the atmosphere at this stage. This fills the ultrafiltration compartment of the device. If the filter is added at a later stage, perhaps when the bypass has been established for some time or even at the end of the bypass, then the blood pathway should be filled slowly with the vacuum port open to atmosphere. Once most of the air has been removed the blood flow may be increased and vacuum applied according to the desired rate of fluid removal. Once primed with blood it is preferable to maintain a slow flow through the device to avoid sludging.

17.2.5 Fluid control

If the haemofilter is being used purely for the control of fluid load then it will probably be used only towards the final stages of the perfusion. In patients with a pre-operatively expanded blood volume (typically patients with chronic right-sided heart failure) it may be preferable to store the excess volume of blood until the end of the procedure, depending on the haematocrit. Ideally the perfusate should have a haematocrit of around 25% during hypothermia in order to provide optimum viscosity consistent with adequate oxygen carriage. However, if the haemofilter is being used to clear metabolites, ultrafiltration may be carried out during the entire bypass period with volume replacement using one of the standard haemofiltration solutions. Examples of these solutions are given in Table 17.7. As indicated in Fig. 17.3 the clearance of metabolites is related directly to the filtration rate multiplied by the ratio of filtrate concentration to plasma concentration. Since all substances below the cut-off of the membrane are filtered by haemofiltration the filtrate has basically the same concentration in the lower molecular weight range as the filtered medium. Hence clearance by haemofiltration is directly proportional to filtration rate which means that fairly large volumes of ultrafiltration (up to 20 litres) require to be processed in order to remove metabolites from patients in established renal failure.

Table 17.7 Haemofiltration solutions (mmol/l)

	Na	*K*	*Ca*	*Mg*	*Cl*	*Lactate*	*Acetate*	*Glucose*
Gambro HF-1	140	1.0	3.25	1.5	100.1	45	—	2.154
Gambro HF-4	135	3.0	3.75	1.5	109.5	34	—	1.65
Gambro HF-5	140	—	4.0	2.0	111	—	35	—
Boots	143	3.0	1.88	1.0	118	34	—	—
Hartmanns Soln	131	5.0	2.0	—	111	29	—	—

Haemofilters can concentrate down to a haematocrit of 70%, however, it is seldom practical to do this since the ultrafiltration rate falls off in an almost logarithmic fashion with increasing haematocrit and protein concentration – so that a haematocrit of 45% to 55% fulfils most practical requirements.

17.2.6 Heparin removal by ultrafiltration

Heparin is a very heterogenous substance which, depending on its source, may be made up of molecules ranging in molecular weight between 6000 and 22 000 daltons (Goodman and Gillman, 1970). As such, at least a proportion of the heparin in the CPB circuit will be removed by ultrafiltration. When employing haemofiltration during CPB, therefore, heparin monitoring is even more important than usual.

17.3 DISCUSSION

The geometric growth rate of coronary artery bypass procedures as illustrated in our own experience (Fig. 17.9) is beginning to strain blood bank resources. This is becoming increasingly evident in small communities with rapidly expanding cardiac surgical programmes. A number of technical advances in use today can help the perfusionist and surgeon alleviate this problem.

(1) Haemodilution is a widely accepted practice and it has been estimated that this technique has reduced blood bank requirements by as much as 50% (Hallowell *et al.*, 1978). In addition it has also reduced the incidence of serum hepatitis and transfusion reactions (Cosgrove *et al.*, 1979). This has also led to the acceptance of lower postoperative haematocrits in cardiac patients.

(2) The use of appropriate blood component therapy for postoperative bleeding has been shown to be more effective than the use of fresh whole blood (Moran, 1978).

(3) Careful monitoring of activated clotting times (ACT) and lowered protamine to heparin ratios for heparin reversal has also reduced the need for additional blood due to 'heparin rebound' or overdose with protamine (Dutton *et al.*, 1983).

(4) Autologous transfusion has been used intermittently for over 100 years. Techniques such as pre-donation have not gained wide acceptance although immediate pre-operative donation has recently attracted more interest. Pre-donation from the vena cava into heparin has been shown to be the most effective method (Kaplan *et al.*, 1977). The introduction of dedicated cell savers has alleviated many of the problems with autologous transfusion.

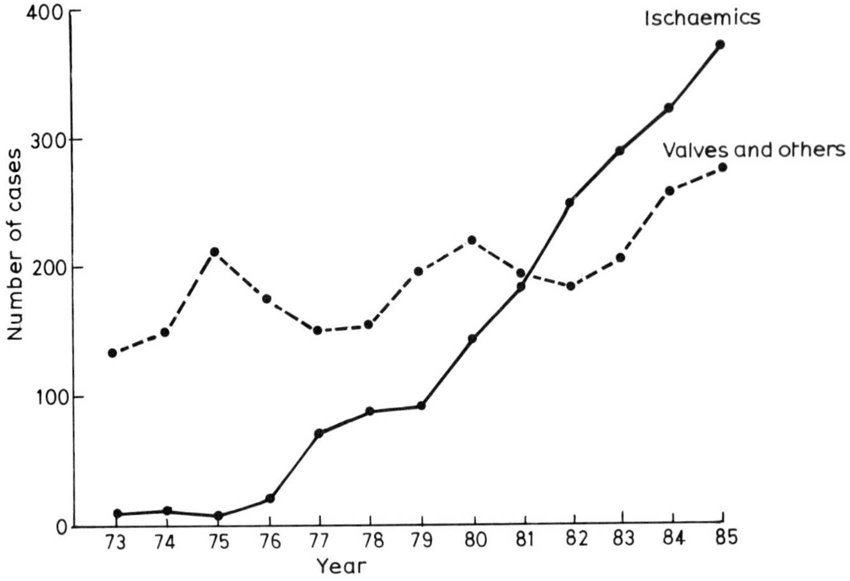

Fig. 17.9 Open heart operations for ischaemic heart disease and congenital heart disease (Papworth Hospital 1973–85).

(5) More recently haemofilters have been used for patient fluid load control with the theoretical advantage over cell savers of conservation of plasma proteins. However, no clinical advantages have been demonstrated when compared with cell savers (Brickley *et al.*, 1982), although both cell savers and haemofilters have been shown to offer clinical advantages in terms of blood usage (Pelley, 1980) and decreased patient fluid load (Brickley *et al.*, 1982; Luckenbach *et al.*, 1980; Sanford *et al.*, 1982) when compared with conventional blood-replacement therapy. The saving of both plasma and formed blood elements by haemoconcentration methods is easily quantifiable but not as easily evaluated qualitatively. However, Orr and Blenko (1978) demonstrated that washed red cells were superior to homologous transfusion with respect to red cell survival and oxygen carriage. Cell washers may also be used for the sequestration of platelet-rich plasma immediately pre-bypass (Cohn *et al.*, 1978).

17.3.1 The future

Haemodilution is well established in CPB practice and it might seem reasonable to expect immediate pre-operative donation to become a routine procedure. This would lower the bypass haematocrit to optimum levels and would also provide a source of active clotting factors immediately post-bypass.

The cell saver is certainly the most versatile machine for autologous transfusion applications and this may become an even more useful device if it can be adapted for continuous processing. Chenoworth *et al.* (1981) have shown that considerable levels of vasoactive substances such as complement (C_3 and C_5) are generated particularly by the cardiotomy suction system. We have confirmed these findings of high complement levels together with high levels of thromboxane and have been able to remove these substances by cell washing. It is also possible that cell washing could reduce the toxic circulating products in patients presenting with active bacterial endocarditis. The major disadvantage of the routine use of cell washers in their present form is the high capital cost (£8000 to £17 000) and the cost of disposables (£7 to £70) per case.

Haemofilters on the other hand are very simple to use and relatively cheap so that it is possible to envisage the routine use of these devices particularly for patient fluid load control. However, haemofilters concentrate all the fluid components of the circuit including any aggregates and cell debris so that a suitable filtration system requires to be established. Finally, there is a further possibility of the use of adsorption columns to remove toxic metabolites in conjunction with haemofiltration to provide a final purified processed product which, physiologically, is as 'normal' as possible.

REFERENCES

Blundell, J. (1818) The transfusion of blood by the syringe. *Med. Chir. Trans.*, **9**, 56.

Brickley, J. M., Kalshoven, J. D., Wilds, S. L. and Dearing, J. P. (1982) A comparison of two methods of post bypass hemoconcentration. *J. Extracorp. Technol.*, **14**, 5.

Chaignon, M., Aubert, M. F., Martin, M., Lucsko, M. and Guedon, J. (1982) Haemodynamic effects of haemodialysis and hemofiltration. *Artif. Organs*, **6**, 27.

Chenoweth, D. E., Cooper, S. W., Hugli, T. E., Stewart, R. W., Blackstone, E. H. and Kirklin, J. W. (1981) Complement activation during cardiopulmonary bypass. Evidence for generation of C3a and C5a anaphylatoxins. *New Engl. J. Med.*, **304**, 9.

Cohn, L. H., Solomon, S., Lee-Son, S., Sandberg, G. and Collins, J. J. (1978) *Sequestration of Platelet-rich Plasma for Patients Undergoing Coronary Bypass Operations*. Haemonetics Blood Conservation Institute, Chicago.

Cosgrove, D. N., Thurer, R. L., Lytle, B. W., Gill, C. G., Peter, M. and Loop, F. D. (1979) Blood conservation during myocardial revascularisation. *Ann. Thorac. Surg.*, **28**, 184.

Dutton, D. A., Hothershall, A. P., McLaren, A. D., Taylor, K. M. and Turner, M. A. (1983) Protamine titration after cardiopulmonary bypass. *Anaesthesia*, **38**, 3.
Gilcher, R. O. and Orr, M. (1975) Intra-operative autotransfusion. *Transfusion*, **15**, 520.
Goodman, L. S. and Gillman, A. (1970) *The Pharmacological Basis of Therapeutics*, 4th edn, Macmillan, London. p. 1447.
Hallowell, P., Bland, J. H., Dalton, B. C., Erdmann, A. J., Lappas, D. G., Lavier, N. B., Philbin, D., Thomas, S. and Lowenstein, E. (1978) The effect of haemodilution with albumin or Ringers lactate on water balance and blood usage in open heart surgery. *Ann. Thorac. Surg.*, **25**, 22.
Hearse, D. J., Braimbridge, M. V. and Jynge, P. (1981) Protection of the ischaemic myocardium. In *Cardioplegia*, Raven Press, New York, Chapter 11, p. 367.
Henderson, L. W., Livoti, L. G., Ford, C. A., Kelly, A. B. and Lysaght, M. J. (1973) Clinical experience with intermittent hemofiltration. *Trans. Am. Soc. Artif. Int. Organs*, **19**, 119.
Hopeck, J. M., Lane, R. S. and Schroeder, J. W. (1981) Oxygenator volume control by parallel ultrafiltration to remove plasma water. *J. Extracorp. Technol.*, **13**, 6.
Intonti, F., Alquati, P., Schiavello, R. and Alessandrini, F. (1981) Ultrafiltration during open heart surgery in chronic renal failure *Scand. J. Thorac. Cardiovasc. Surg.*, **15**, 217–20.
Kaplan, J. A., Cannarella, C., Jones, E. L., Kutner, M. H., Hatcher, C. R. and Dunbar, R. W. (1977) Autologous blood transfusion during cardiac surgery. A re-evaluation of three methods. *J. Thorac. Cardiovasc. Surg.*, **74**, 1.
Kessler, M. and Messmer, K. (1975) Tissue oxygenation during haemodilution. In *Intentional Hemodilution. Bibliotheca Haematologica*, Karger, Basel, Vol. 41, p. 16.
Lansing, A. M., Leb, D. E. and Berman, L. B. (1968) Cardiovascular surgery in end-stage renal failure. *J. Am. Med. Assoc.*, **204**, 682.
Lowrie, E. G., Lazarus, J. M., Hampers, C. L. and Merrill, J. P. (1974) Cardiovascular disease in dialysis patients. *New Engl. J. Med.*, **290**, 697.
Luckenbach, J., Ellison, N., Conaham, T. J. and MacVaugh, H. (1980) External hemoconcentration. A fourth variant of autologous blood transfusion. *J. Extracorp. Technol.*, **12**, 5.
MacDonald, P. M., Hutchinson, J. E., Herring, W., McAfee, T. and Briseno, S. (1982) Utilization of donor blood. *J. Extracorp. Technol.*, **14**, 4.
Moran, J. H. (1978) Immediate centrifugation of oxygenator contents after cardiopulmonary bypass. *J. Thorac. Cardiovasc. Surg.*, **76**, 510–17.
Orr, M. D. and Blenko, J. W. (1978) Autotransfusion of concentrated selected washed red cells from the surgical field: A biochemical and physiological comparison with homologous cell transfusion. Proceedings Blood Conservation Institute.
Pelley, W. B. (1980) Cost-effectiveness of blood conservation. *J. Extracorp. Technol.*, **12**, 6.
Philbin, D. M., Goggins, C. H., Emerson, C. W., Levine, F. H. and Buckley, M. J. (1979) Plasma vasopressin levels and urinary sodium excretion during cardiopulmonary bypass. Comparison of halothane and morphine anaesthesia. *J. Thorac. Cardiovasc. Surg.*, **77**, 582.
Reul, G. J. (1974) Experience with autotransfusion in the surgical management of trauma. *Surgery*, **76**, 546.
Sanford, D. M., Van Sickle, C. and Keen, W. R. (1982) Ultrafiltration/Hemoconcentration. A New Use for the Dialyser. *Proc. Am. Acad. Cardiovasc. Perf.*, **3**.

Schaff, H. (1978) Autotransfusion in cardiac surgical patients after operation. *Surgery*, **84**, 713.

Wilson, J. D. and Taswell, H. F. (1968) Autotransfusion: Historical review and preliminary report on a new method. *Mayo Clin. Proc.*, **43**, 26–35.

18
Microemboli: gaseous and particulate

D. T. PEARSON

The functional replacement of the heart and lungs by a pump oxygenator during open-heart surgery is known to be associated with multi-organ damage predominantly affecting the brain (Aberg, 1974; Editorial, 1982; Taylor, 1982; Tufo *et al.*, 1970), kidneys (Abel *et al.*, 1976; Hiberman *et al.*, 1979) and liver (Collins *et al.*, 1983). The brain appears to be particularly susceptible to damage in this context though the precise mechanisms involved in the wide variety of cerebral damage syndromes which may be evident in the postoperative period are not clearly understood but are the subject of research and evaluation in many cardiac surgical centres throughout the world.

Despite overall improvements in cardiopulmonary bypass technology over recent years, a wide variety of disturbances in cerebral function ranging from mild psychosis to overt focal and diffuse neurological damage continue to be seen following cardiac surgery (Bojar *et al.*, 1983). It is of major concern that subclinical cerebral injury leading to transient or permanent intellectual impairment, which can only be detected by expert psychometric testing, is reported to be a common sequelae of open heart surgery (Aberg, 1974; Aberg *et al.*, 1982, 1983).

Systemic arterial microembolism has been suggested as an important cause of brain damage (Brennan *et al.*, 1971; Slogoff *et al.*, 1982) though abnormalities in cerebral blood flow have also been implicated (Hendriksen *et al.*, 1983; Matsumoto *et al.*, 1981; Sanderson *et al.*, 1972). Coronary artery disease is often part of a generalized systemic arteriopathy involving cerebral as well as other blood vessels. Patients having coronary artery surgery may as a result be more susceptible to damage from microemboli and alterations in cerebral blood flow due to hypotension and abnormal arterial blood gases. The maintenance of adequate cerebral perfusion is essential in all patients who are supported by a pump oxygenator. Reduced cerebral perfusion, resulting from systemic arterial hypotension, may precipitate cerebral damage

(Stockard *et al.*, 1974) as may failure of autoregulation of the cerebral blood flow when arterial PO_2 (PaO_2) and arterial PCO_2 ($PaCO_2$) levels are abnormal (DeWall, 1975) though the optimal level of $PaCO_2$ during hypothermic cardiopulmonary bypass is yet to be established (Hendriksen *et al.*, 1983). The use of more objective, sensitive and quantitative indices of brain damage may contribute to the understanding of a complication which can nullify the benefits of cardiac surgery involving the use of cardiopulmonary bypass (Aberg *et al.*, 1982; Taylor *et al.*, 1980).

The more important aetiological factors involved in cerebral dysfunction following open heart surgery are shown in Table 18.1. Some of these will be considered in this chapter, in particular gaseous microemboli (GME). Factors involved in the production of these microemboli and methods of reducing the quantity entering the systemic arterial circulation will be described.

Table 18.1 Cerebral dysfunction during open-heart surgery: aetiological factors

Haemodynamic
Age of patient
Duration of bypass
Systemic arterial blood pressure on bypass
Cerebral blood flow on bypass
Non-pulsatile flow on bypass
Embolic
Gaseous microemboli from
(a) heart and pulmonary veins
(b) pump oxygenator
Foreign material from
(a) oxygenator, cardiotomy reservoir and tubing circuit (cotton fibres, silicone, plastic chips)
(b) pump tubing (spallation)
(c) operative equipment (talc, thread, dust, cloth particles)
Red blood cell, platelet and leucocyte aggregates
Fibrin
Denatured protein
Calcium and arterio-sclerotic debris
Fat globules
Toxic
Freon
Plasticizers
Ethylene oxide residues

18.1 GASEOUS MICROEMBOLI

18.1.1 Gaseous microemboli from the pump oxygenator system

Gaseous microemboli may originate from

(1) The oxygenator (Pearson *et al.*, 1981)
(2) The heat exchanger (Clark *et al.*, 1975)
(3) The cardiotomy reservoir (Loop *et al.*, 1976; Pearson *et al.*, 1974)
(4) Roller pumps (Bass and Longmore, 1969)

(a) Bubble oxygenators

The fundamental requirement of any oxygenator, used for clinical perfusion, is the provision of adequate gas exchange without damage to formed blood elements and without the introduction into the systemic arterial circulation of gaseous and particulate microemboli. It has been described in the literature that oxygenators (a) release GME (Austen and Howdry, 1965; Gallagher and Pearson, 1973; Pearson *et al.*, 1981; Selman *et al.*, 1967) (b) damage formed blood elements (Van den Dungen *et al.*, 1982; Wright and Sanderson, 1976) and (c) do not enable the perfusionist to maintain physiological levels of PaO_2 and $PaCO_2$ during cardiopulmonary bypass (DeWall, 1975; Newland *et al.*, 1982; Pearson *et al.*, 1985).

During recent years the design trend in bubble oxygenators has been towards an increase in oxygen transfer at lower gas to blood flow ratios (Pearson *et al.*, 1983). This 'apparent' improvement in performance is achieved by a reduction in the bubble size in the oxygenating column thus increasing gas to blood surface area contact, and may be expected to result in inadequate CO_2 clearance and increased GME in the arterial blood (Galletti and Brecher, 1962).

Nine commercially available bubble oxygenators were evaluated during clinical perfusion in adult patients (body weight 60–65 kg) to assess the relationship between gas to blood ratio, GME production and arterial blood gases. All patients were maintained at a pulsatile flow rate of $4\,l\,min^{-1}$ from the oxygenator using a Cobe Stockert pump (Cobe Laboratories Inc., Lakewood, CO) and data were collected when the patient temperature had fallen from 37 to 28°C. During this period there was no addition of fluid from the cardiotomy reservoir and GME originating in the priming fluid or heat exchanger could not interfere with the results. Gas flow rates to the oxygenator (100% oxygen) were delivered from back pressure compensated anaesthetic rotameters. Arterial blood samples were analysed for PaO_2 and $PaCO_2$ using a Corning 175 blood gas analyser (Corning Medical Ltd, Halstead,

Essex, UK) and the results were corrected for the difference between the blood temperature and that of the analyser's electrodes.

The transducer of the TM8 Microbubble Activity Monitor (Technique Laboratories, Hartley Witney, Hants, UK) was fixed over the arterial line approximately 1 metre from the oxygenator outlet. A transducer of this device propagates a continuous narrow beam of ultrasound into the blood passing from the oxygenator. When GME pass this beam, the receiving transducer picks up modifications to the signal which are then processed by the electronic unit to provide a digital display in the size range selected on the sensitivity control. It is recognized that the use of ultrasound to detect GME in blood vessels and extracorporeal circuits has limitations (Furness and Wright, 1979; Moulinier and Mausurel, 1979; Nishi, 1972; Pearson *et al.*, 1981) and may give rise to errors of measurement of bubble size and GME numbers. Any errors associated with transducer coupling can be avoided by careful attachment of the transducer. The ultrasonic device used in this work does detect a representative sample of the GME passing the transducer head and enables different oxygenators to be compared. It has important advantages compared with other devices described in the literature (Sakauye *et al.*, 1982; Daniels *et al.*, 1979; Grulke *et al.*, 1973) of being non-invasive and easy to apply in the clinical environment.

(i) Oxygenator reservoir level

An inverse relationship between oxygenator arterial reservoir blood level and GME production was demonstrated for all the nine oxygenators evaluated, four of which are shown in Fig. 18.1. The gas to blood flow ratio was maintained constant for each oxygenator during this assessment. The most dramatic changes occurred with the Shiley 100A HED oxygenator (Shiley Laboratories Inc., Irvine, CA) and little effect was noted in the Bentley Q-200A oxygenator (Bentley Laboratories Inc., Irvine, CA) even though the gas to blood ratio was greater. Alteration in oxygenator arterial reservoir blood level also influenced gas transfer. The inverse relationship is depicted for two oxygenators in Fig. 18.2 (values for other oxygenators lie between these values). As the volume of blood in the arterial reservoir increases, the dynamic hold up time of the oxygenator is prolonged, allowing more time for defoaming to occur and as a result, reducing the GME in the arterial blood. It is recognized that gas transfer in most bubble oxygenators occurs within the oxygenating column and on the large surface area of the defoamer. As increases in arterial reservoir level encroach upon the defoamer, oxygen transfer and PaO_2 fall.

(ii) Gas to blood flow ratio

In each oxygenator, correlation of numbers of GME in the arterial blood with temperature corrected values for PaO_2 and $PaCO_2$ were made. The blood

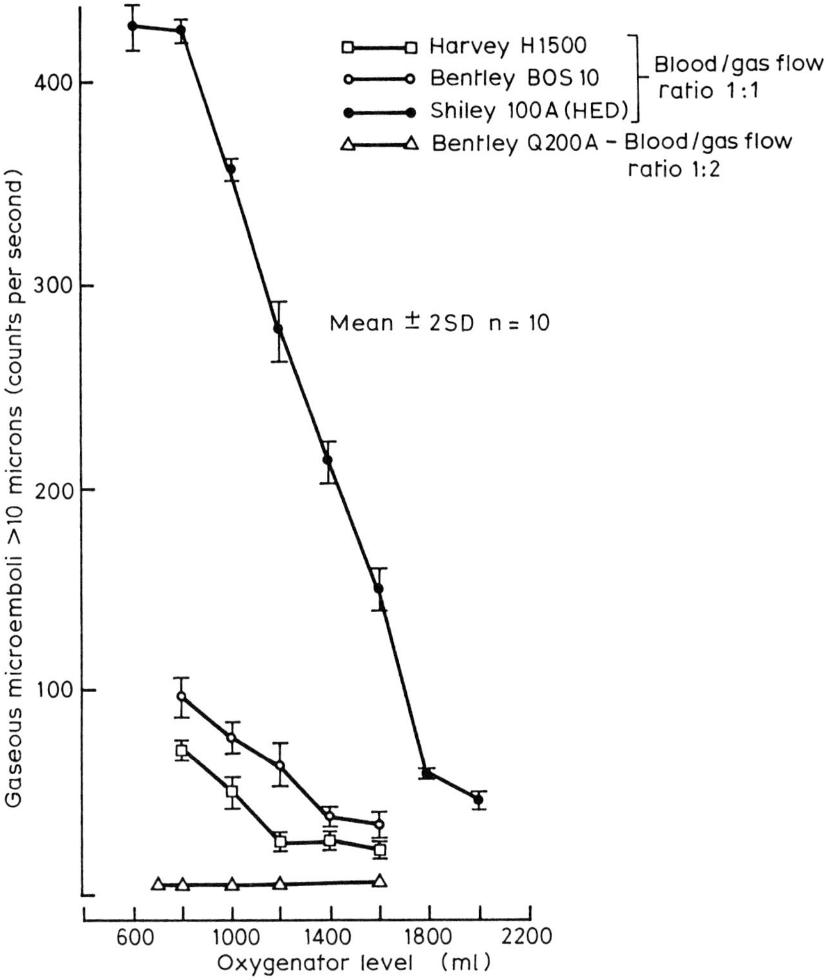

Fig. 18.1 Numbers of gaseous microemboli detected in the arterial line of four bubble oxygenators with respect to arterial reservoir blood level. (Reproduced with permission from Pearson *et al.*, 1983.)

flow rate was maintained constant at $4\,l\,min^{-1}$ and the gas flow rate (100% oxygen) increased in $1.0\,l\,min^{-1}$ increments from 1.0 to $4.0\,l\,min^{-1}$. The results are shown in Fig. 18.3 and indicate that as the gas to blood flow is increased for each oxygenator there is a concomitant rise in both PaO_2 and number of GME detected in the arterial line together with a fall in $PaCO_2$.

Marked differences are demonstrated between the oxygenators in their ability to produce physiological blood gases and in their defoaming capabilities at a given gas to blood flow ratio. High gas to blood flow ratios are not

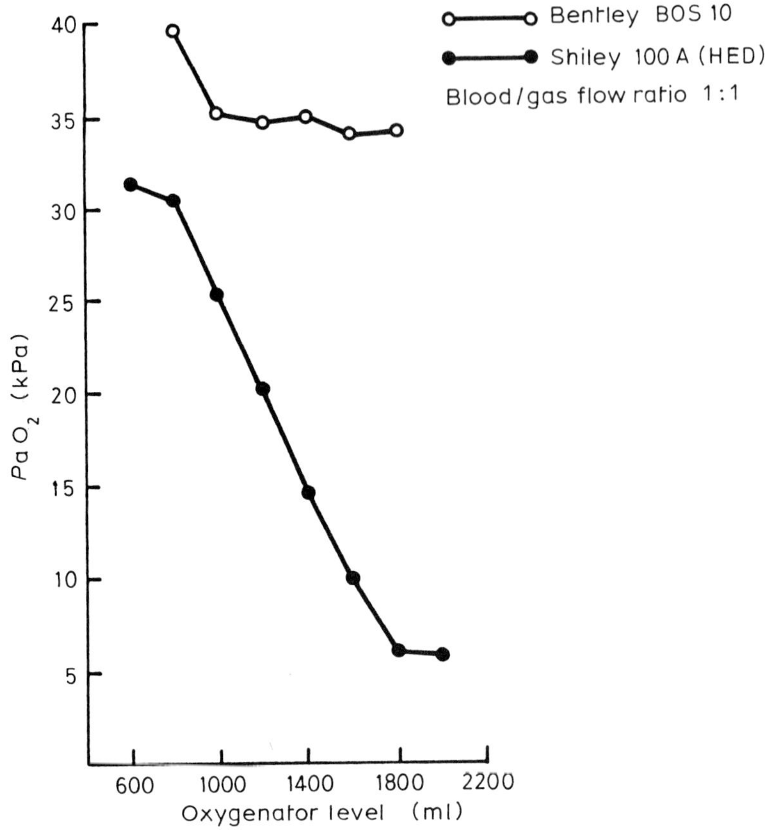

Fig. 18.2 Changes in arterial PO_2 with respect to arterial reservoir blood level in two bubble oxygenators. (Reproduced with permission from Pearson *et al.*, 1983.)

always associated with high levels of GME in the arterial blood from the oxygenator. The Harvey H-1000 (Bard Cardiopulmonary, Santa Ana, CA) and the Bentley Q-200A are able to produce acceptable levels of PaO_2 and $PaCO_2$ with the generation of less GME at higher gas to blood flow ratios than other oxygenators tested. These two oxygenators have been superseded by more 'efficient' products.

During clinical perfusion for open-heart surgery in randomly selected adult patients, the total number of GME detected by the TM8 device were measured during the total bypass period and the values expressed as the mean number of microemboli per litre of arterial blood. The results of 89 perfusions are shown in Table 18.2 and demonstrate no significant difference in GME count when either of the two bubble oxygenators (Harvey H-1500 and Bentley BOS 10) was used. A statistically significant reduction in GME was achieved by the introduction of a Pall arterial line filter (Pall Biomedical Ltd,

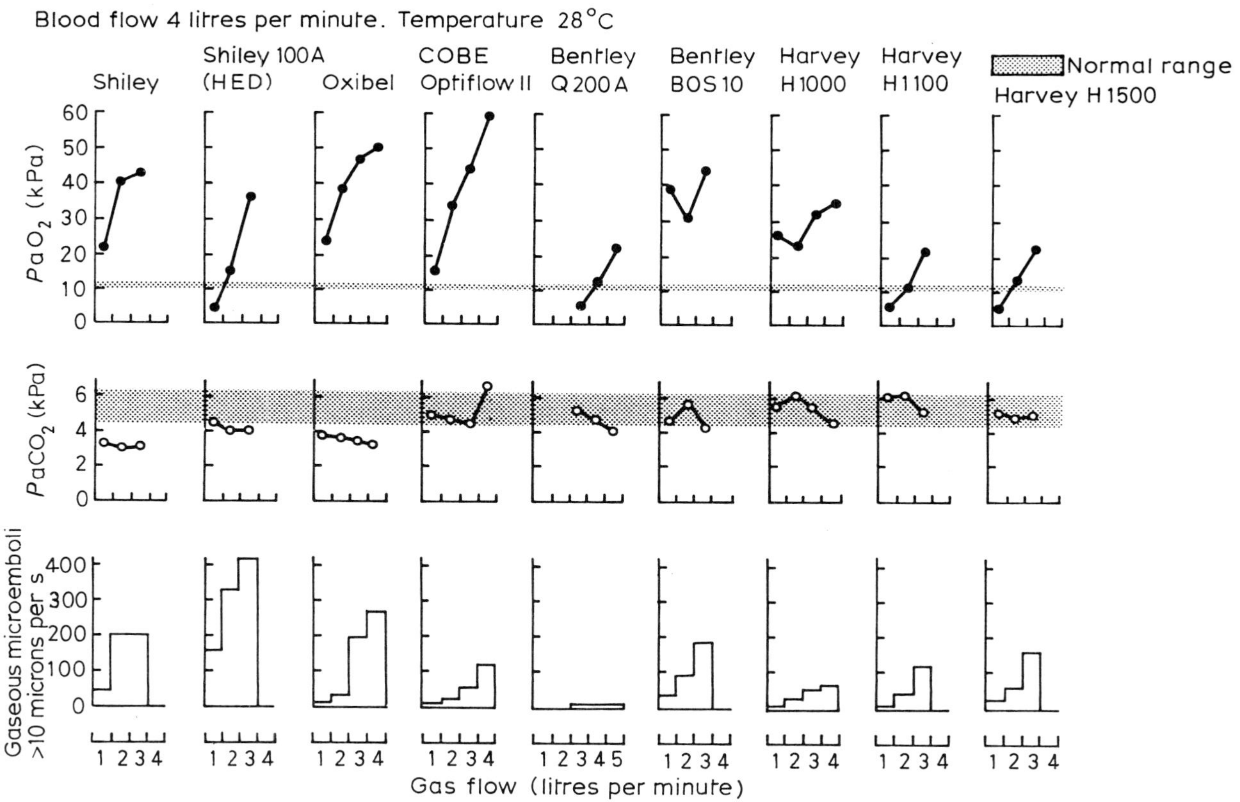

Fig. 18.3 Relationship between numbers of gaseous microemboli detected in arterial line of nine bubble oxygenators and arterial blood gases. Effect of alterations in gas:blood flow ratio. (Reproduced with permission from Pearson *et al.*, 1983.)

Table 18.2 Oxygenators and gaseous microemboli. Clinical perfusion for open heart surgery in adults. Gaseous microemboli >10 $\mu m\, l^{-1}$ arterial blood (mean±SEM)

Bentley BOS 10	n=25	1447±547	
Harvey H-1500	n=22	1383±204	n.s.
Harvey H-1500 with Pall filter	n=6	488±124	$p<0.05$
Travenol TMO	n=36	51±12	$p<0.001$

Portsmouth, UK) into the circuit. The lowest number of GME were found when a Travenol TMO membrane oxygenator (Travenol Laboratories, Deerfield, IL) was used (vide infra). A scattergram of the data presented in Table 18.2 is displayed in Fig. 18.4 to demonstrate a degree of overlap between the values for numbers of GME in the arterial line of bubble and membrane oxygenators and confirm that the results for many individual bubble oxygenators were below the median value for the Harvey H-1500 with an arterial line filter. The results of the evaluation suggest that the use of a membrane oxygenator or the addition to the circuit of an arterial line filter is not the most comprehensive solution to effecting a dramatic reduction in GME load to the patient and other factors must be involved.

A more detailed analysis during clinical perfusion in adult patients of 21 Harvey H-1500 oxygenators is shown in Fig. 18.4 with respect to the mean PaO_2 and GME production. Arterial PO_2 was measured continuously using an in-line polarographic electrode (Orange Medical Instruments, High Wycombe, UK) (Claremont *et al.*, 1984; Parker *et al.*, 1983). To facilitate comparison of GME activity and PaO_2, the relatively high frequency GME signal was electronically processed using a simple peak detector and a low pass filter. This circuit has a time constant of approximately 2 min, similar to the response time of the in-line PO_2 electrode. Figure 18.5 shows a comparison of the unfiltered and filtered GME activity together with counts taken every two minutes directly from the digital display of the TM8 Microbubble Activity Monitor. Those patients in whom the mean PaO_2 was below 20 kPa during the period of cardiopulmonary bypass received a significantly lower number of GME than a similar group of patients in whom the PaO_2 was above 20 kPa (Table 18.3).

The results of continuous monitoring of PaO_2 and GME in the arterial line of a Harvey H-1500 oxygenator are shown for two adult patients during cardiopulmonary bypass in Fig. 18.6. In the upper trace, by altering the gas flow rate to the oxygenator (100% oxygen), the perfusionist attempted to keep the PaO_2 to within the normal range. In the lower trace, the perfusionist was unaware of the values obtained from the in-line PO_2 electrode and adjusted the gas flow rate (100% oxygen) according to his experience and values obtained by intermittent arterial blood sampling and analysis for PO_2.

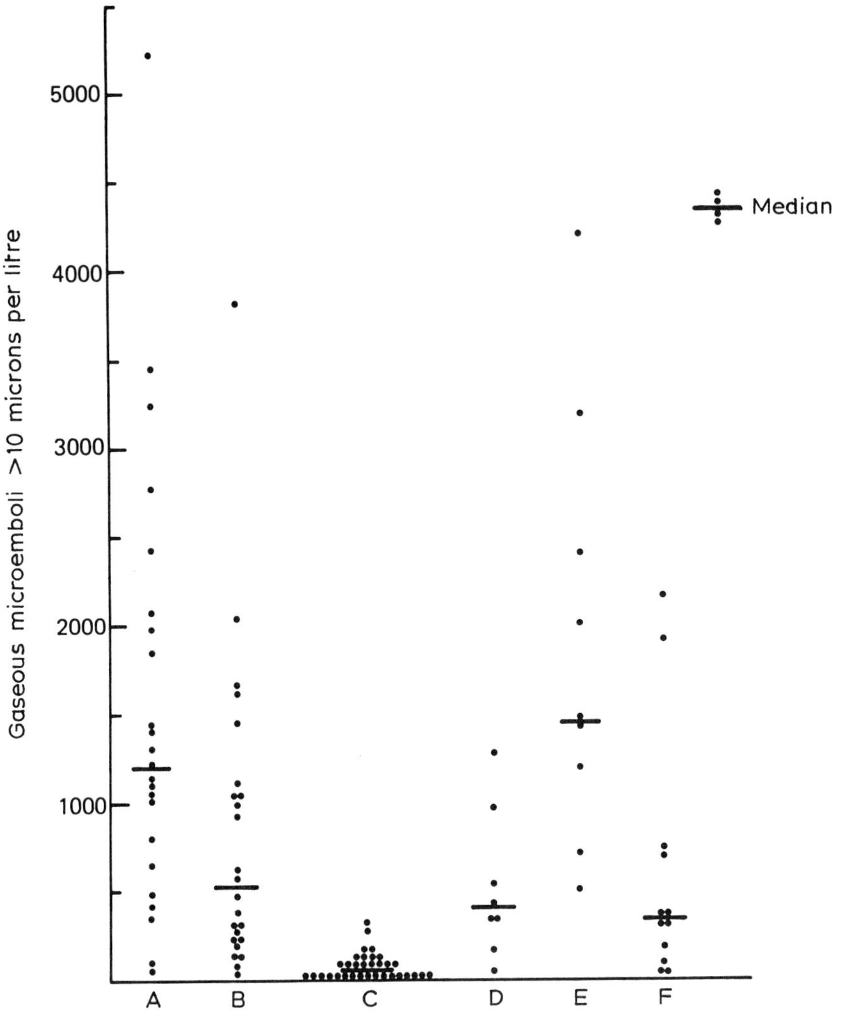

Fig. 18.4 Scattergram of gaseous microemboli (mean number per litre of arterial blood) detected in arterial line during clinical cardiopulmonary bypass. A, Harvey H-1500; B, Bentley BOS 10; C, Travenol TMO; D, Harvey H-1500+Pall arterial line filter; E, Harvey H-1500 (mean PaO_2>20 kPa); F, Harvey H-1500 (mean PaO_2 <20 kPa).

The traces establish the close direct relationship between PaO_2 and GME detected in the arterial line and confirm that the GME load to the patient can be dramatically reduced by maintaining the PaO_2 at physiological levels. In both patients, the $PaCO_2$ was monitored by intermittent arterial blood

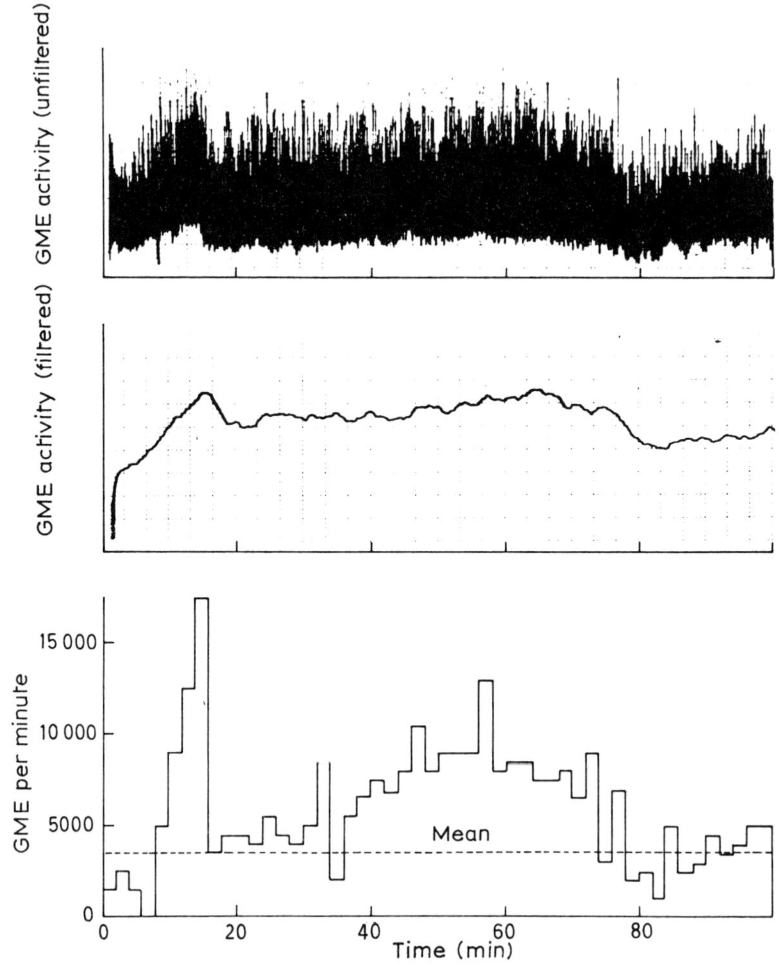

Fig. 18.5 Comparison of unfiltered and filtered GME activity with counts taken at 2 minute intervals directly from the digital display of the TM8 Microbubble Activity Monitor.

Table 18.3 Harvey oxygenator (H-1500): Effect of arterial PO_2

Clinical perfusion for open-heart surgery in adults.
Gaseous microemboli >10 μm l^{-1} arterial blood (mean±SEM)

PaO_2> 20 kPa	1902±378	n = 9	$p<0.01$
PaO_2 <20 kPa	634±194	n = 12	

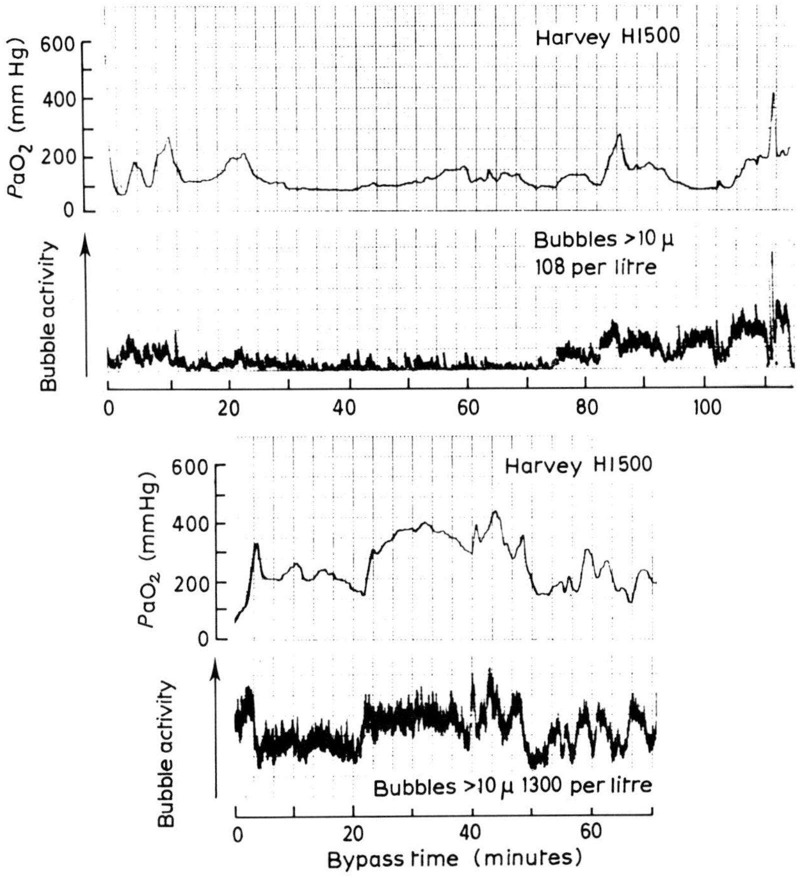

Fig. 18.6 Continuous monitoring of PaO_2 and arterial line GME in two patients during cardiac surgery using the Harvey H-1500 bubble oxygenator. (Reproduced with permission from Pearson *et al.*, 1983.)

sampling and adjusted to within the normal range by the addition of varying amounts of CO_2 to the gas flow to the oxygenator.

The above evaluations suggest that in bubble oxygenators whilst there are many factors involved in the ability of the perfusionist to control the PaO_2 and $PaCO_2$ at physiological levels, such control has an important influence upon the GME load to the patient during cardiopulmonary bypass. The performance characteristics of 33 bubble oxygenators (23 Harvey H-1500 and 10 Bentley BOS 10) have been evaluated during clinical perfusion of adult patients undergoing cardiopulmonary bypass surgery for acquired or ischaemic heart disease (Pearson *et al.*, 1985). For each oxygenator, patients were randomly allocated to one of two groups. Patients in both groups had continuous monitoring of PaO_2 using an in-line polarographic electrode and intermittent measurement of PaO_2 and $PaCO_2$ at 15 minutes intervals. However, in group C (continuous PaO_2 data), all these data were available to the perfusionist, whereas in group I (intermittent PaO_2 data), the PaO_2 data from the in-line electrode were deliberately withheld to simulate current clinical practice. Using the data available, the perfusionist manually adjusted the flow rates of oxygen and carbon dioxide in an attempt to maintain physiological blood gas levels.

There was no statistically significant difference between the four patient groups with respect to patient weight, height, body surface area, age, hypothermic temperature during bypass and total bypass time. Tables 18.4 and 18.5 contain the mean values for various measured parameters in each patient group of the two oxygenator series. The results of a statistical comparison between patient groups I and C (Student's *t* test) and between oxygenators is shown in Tables 18.4, 18.5 and 18.6. There was no significant

Table 18.4 Control of arterial PO_2: Harvey H-1500 oxygenator

Patient Group	*Group I (mean±SD)*	*Group C (mean±SD)*	
Number of patients	11	12	
GME per litre	1768±1046	601±678	$p<0.01$
Arterial PO_2 (kPa)	31±5	13±2	$p<0.001$
O_2 flow ($l\,min^{-1}$)	2.1±0.4	1.9±0.3	NS
Blood flow ($l\,min^{-1}$)	4.1±0.5	4.1±0.4	NS
Gas/blood flow ratio	0.6±0.1	0.5±0.1	
Arterial reservoir level (ml)	1300±200	1200±200	NS
Arterial PCO_2 (kPa) during rewarming	5.8±0.7	6.3±0.7	$p<0.01$

NS, not significant

Table 18.5 Control of arterial PO_2: Bentley BOS 10 oxygenator

Patient group	*Group I (mean±SD)*	*Group C (mean±SD)*	
Number of patients	5	5	
GME per litre	1458±693	536±311	$p<0.05$
Arterial PO_2 (kPa)	36±8	19±6	$p<0.01$
O_2 flow ($l\,min^{-1}$)	1.5±0.5	0.7±0.3	$p<0.02$
Blood flow ($l\,min^{-1}$)	3.7±0.2	3.9±0.2	
Gas/blood flow ratio	0.42±0.10	0.18±0.06	
Arterial reservoir level (ml)	1100±100	1100±200	NS
Arterial PCO_2 (kPa) during rewarming	5.5±0.6	7.6±0.8	$p<0.01$

NS, not significant

Table 18.6 Statistical comparison of Harvey H-1500 and Bentley BOS 10 oxygenators

Patient group	*Group I*	*Group C*
Oxygenator	H-1500/BOS 10	H-1500/BOS 10
GME per litre	NS	NS
Arterial PO_2	NS	$p<0.01$
Arterial PCO_2 during rewarming	NS	$p<0.01$
Oxygen flow	$p<0.05$	$p<0.001$
Blood flow	NS	NS

NS, not significant.

difference between the arterial reservoir level and blood flow rate in the four patient groups.

In both oxygenators, there were statistically higher levels of PaO_2 and GME in group I when compared to group C. When the Harvey H-1500 was compared to the Bentley BOS 10 oxygenator, there was no difference in the mean PaO_2 values in group I, but in group C the range of PaO_2 values was narrower and the mean value significantly lower in the Harvey H-1500 oxygenator. Gas : blood flow ratios in the Bentley BOS 10 were lower than in the Harvey H-1500. In the Harvey H-1500 series, there was no significant difference in gas : blood flow ratio between groups I and C even though the mean PaO_2 and mean GME counts were highly significantly lower in group C. In the Bentley BOS 10 oxygenator series, a significant difference in gas : blood flow ratio was demonstrated between groups I and C.

It was anticipated that since the PaO_2 was adjusted by regulation of oxygen flow to the oxygenator, the significantly lower PaO_2 in group C compared with group I would be accompanied in both oxygenators by a significant reduction in oxygen flow. Specific levels of PaO_2 do not result from specific oxygen flow rates and are a function of many factors. Blood flow, temperature, pH, venous blood oxygen content and arterial reservoir level can affect the PaO_2 as may the addition of blood and electrolyte solution to the circuit. The gas flow rate needed to maintain a particular level of PO_2 will vary from patient to patient as well as throughout bypass. In the Bentley BOS 10 oxygenator, the lower PaO_2 in group C, as compared with group I, was associated with a lowered gas flow rate to the oxygenator. This was not found with the Harvey H-1500.

Currently available bubble oxygenators have been demonstrated to have adequate oxygenation capabilities at total gas flow rates lower than the devices which they supersede (Pearson *et al.*, 1983). This greater 'efficiency' can result only from an increased gas–blood surface area which it is believed is due to a reduction in the size of the bubbles in the oxygenating column (Ferguson *et al.*, 1967), though other factors such as increased turbulence in the oxygenating column and the amount of gas transfer occurring in the defoamer may be relevant. The defoamer, however, is not as efficient at defoaming the smaller bubbles which remain after gas transfer as it is at removing larger bubbles and this may explain why the lower oxygen flow rates in the Bentley BOS 10 when compared with the Harvey H-1500 did not result in lower GME counts (Table 18.6).

At low gas : blood flow ratios, CO_2 removal by the oxygenator may be impaired. Statistically higher values for $PaCO_2$ were found during the rewarming period in group C as compared with group I for both oxygenators (Tables 18.4 and 18.5), the Bentley BOS 10 having greater difficulty in clearing CO_2 than the Harvey H-1500 in patient group C. Problems with CO_2 clearance using the Bentley oxygenator have been described by other investigators (Kemna and Docherty, 1978; Walton *et al.*, 1982).

It has been demonstrated, assuming complete equilibration between the blood and gas in the oxygenating column of a bubble oxygenator, that the minimum gas : blood flow ratio for acceptable CO_2 clearance at normothermia is approximately 1:1 (Galletti and Brecher, 1962). During the rewarming phase of cardiopulmonary bypass, there is a need to increase CO_2 clearance as CO_2 production increases and decreased solubility of CO_2 occurs as the temperature rises. The low gas : blood flow ratios used in the two oxygenators evaluated during clinical perfusion were associated with impaired CO_2 clearance especially when the gas flow rate was reduced in an attempt to reduce the PaO_2 to within the physiological range. The relationship between GME activity and PaO_2 throughout cardiopulmonary bypass is shown for two typical patients using a Bentley BOS 10 oxygenator. In Fig. 18.7 (group I) and Fig. 18.8 (group C) the direct relationship between PaO_2 and GME is confirmed. Control of the PaO_2 to nearer physiological levels may present the perfusionist with the dilemma of accepting an abnormally high $PaCO_2$ or increasing the gas : blood flow ratio with a consequent rise in GME counts and in PaO_2 to above physiological levels as shown in Fig. 18.8.

The overall pattern of gas transfer demonstrated in clinical evaluation of the two bubble oxygenators described is one of excess oxygenation if CO_2 clearance is adequate and inadequate CO_2 clearance when physiological levels of PaO_2 are present. This was confirmed during the evaluation of the 23 Harvey H-1500 oxygenators. Arterial blood gas samples were evaluated at 15 minute intervals through each bypass. Temperature corrected values for PaO_2 and $PaCO_2$ are shown as a scattergram superimposed upon the normal ranges in Fig. 18.9. When intermittent control of PaO_2 is used, normal $PaCO_2$ values are associated with excessively high PaO_2 values, previously demonstrated to correlate with high levels of GME activity. Control of PaO_2 to within the physiological range (values will vary with temperature and be lower than the range indicated during hypothermia (Severinghaus, 1966), arterial haemoglobin oxygen saturation being maintained above 95%) is associated with more values for $PaCO_2$ above the normal range.

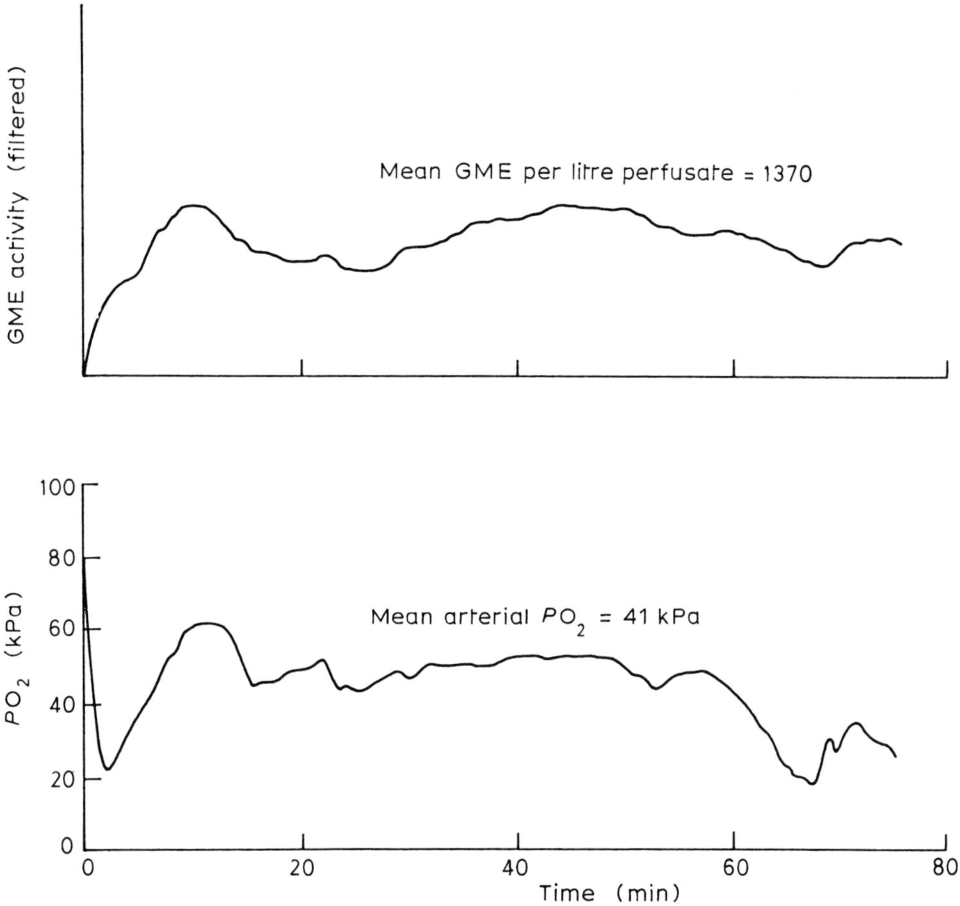

Fig. 18.7 Filtered GME activity in arterial line and PaO_2 during clinical perfusion using a Bentley BOS 10 bubble oxygenator. Group I (intermittent).

Hypothermia is used extensively during cardiac surgery and arterial blood gas measurements are corrected for body temperature. Evidence is accumulating which suggests that maintenance of $PaCO_2$ at 5.33 kPa and pH 7.4 is detrimental to myocardial performance and cerebral blood flow (Becker *et al.*, 1981; Matthews *et al.*, 1984). Temperature correction of $PaCO_2$ and pH should not be used (Ream *et al.*, 1984) and the flow of carbon dioxide to the oxygenator to be adjusted to maintain $PaCO_2$ at 1.33 kPa and pH 7.75 at 22°C (Matthews *et al.*, 1984). It may be impossible to achieve this degree of respiratory alkalosis within the confines of normal PaO_2 values and a low GME count using currently available bubble oxygenators, particularly

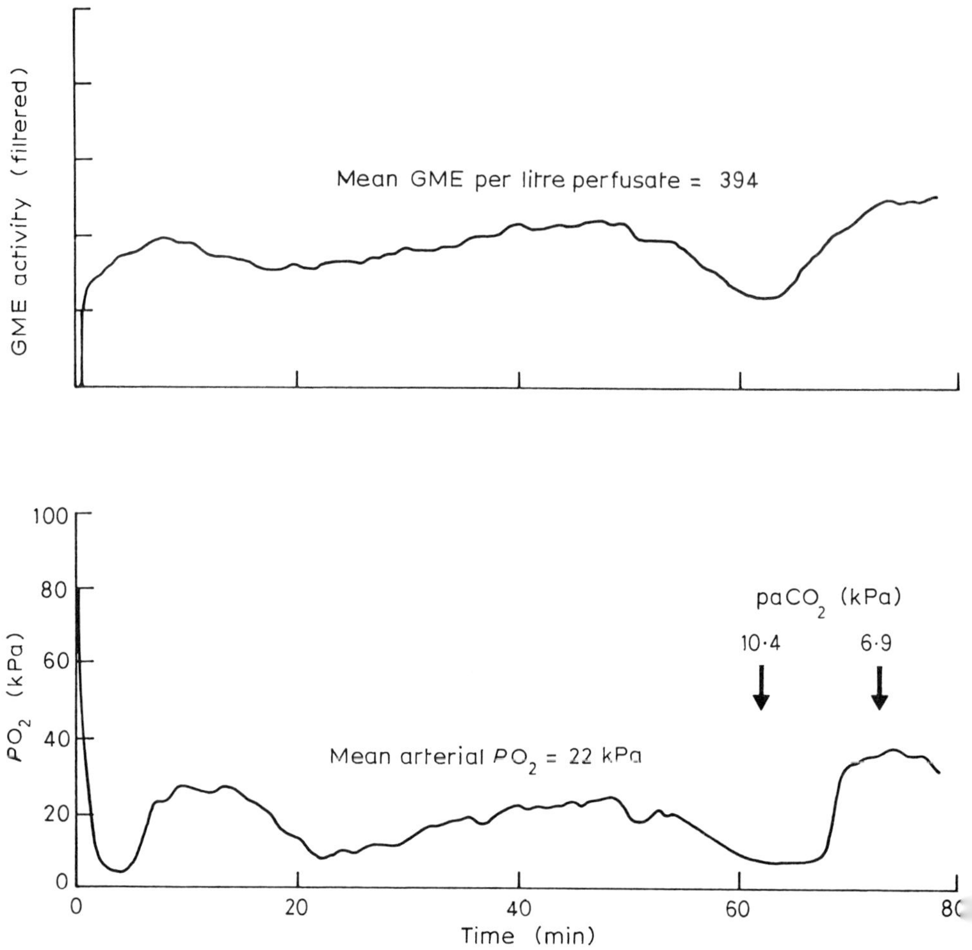

Fig. 18.8 Filtered GME activity in arterial line and PaO_2 during clinical perfusion using a Bentley BOS 10 bubble oxygenator demonstrating inadequate clearance of CO_2 (see text). Group C (continuous).

during hypothermia. A balance between improved cerebral blood flow with a low $PaCO_2$ and microvascular blockade by microemboli with a high PaO_2 is a perfusion dilemma during cardiopulmonary bypass.

The use of an in-line PO_2 electrode in conjunction with a detailed knowledge of the bubble oxygenator clinical performance characteristics significantly improves the management of blood gas levels during cardiopulmonary bypass and can dramatically reduce the number of GME in the

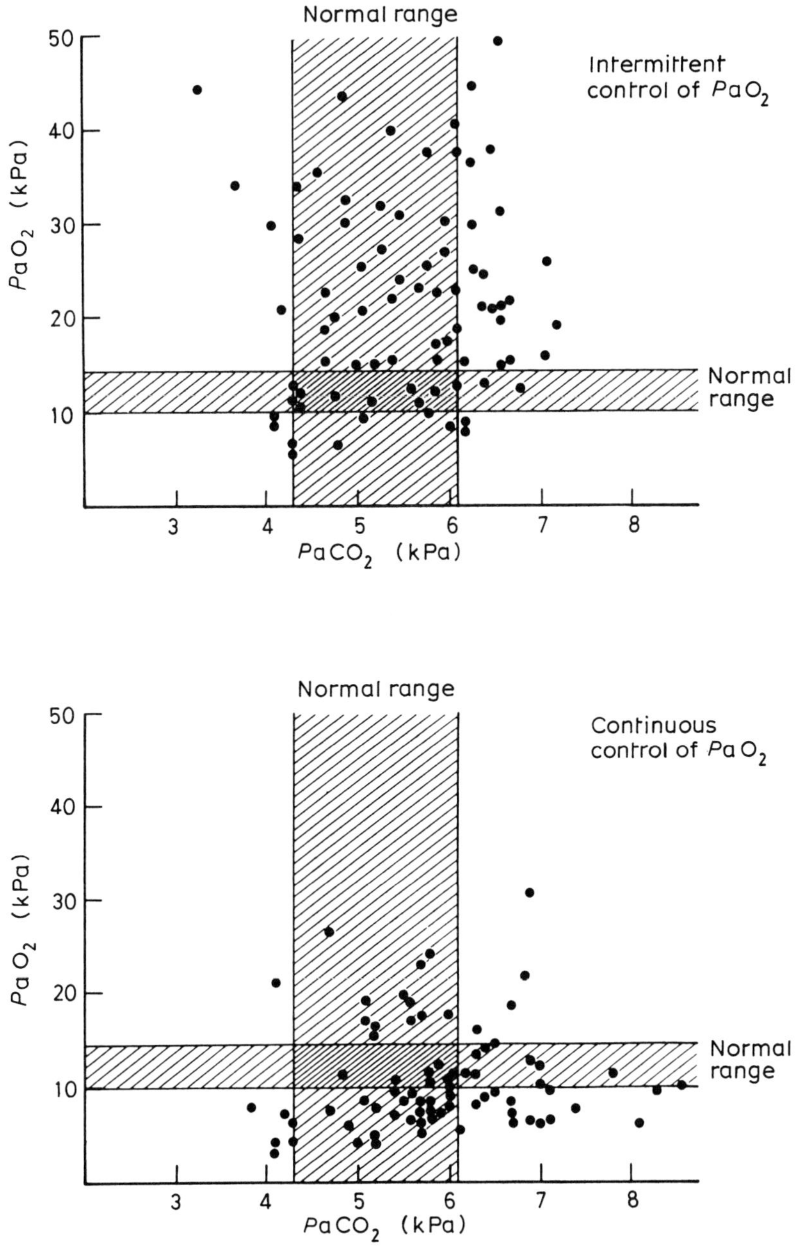

Fig. 18.9 Scattergram of temperature-corrected values of PaO_2 and $PaCO_2$ in Harvey H-1500 oxygenator series in patient groups I (intermittent control of PaO_2) and C (continuous control of PaO_2). Shaded areas indicate normal range of values for PaO_2 and $PaCO_2$.

arterial blood. The electrode introduces a foreign surface of negligible area into the cardiopulmonary bypass circuit. Arterial line filtration (vide supra) has also been shown to reduce the number of GME (Loop *et al.*, 1976; Patterson and Twitchell, 1971) but only at the expense of the introduction of a large foreign surface into the circuit with the potential for aggregation of formed blood elements, particularly when inadequate control of heparin anticoagulation may occur. Careful filter priming is essential if the introduction of more GME is to be avoided (Wellons and Nolan, 1973).

The time constants associated with changes in PaO_2 during cardiopulmonary bypass do not permit intermittent sampling to determine adequately, and hence allow control of, the PaO_2. This can only be achieved by the use of the in-line PO_2 electrode together with manual or automated regulation of gas flow. Since a PO_2 electrode does not take into account alterations in P_{50} due to shifts in the oxygen haemoglobin dissociation curve during hypothermia, further benefit may be derived from the addition of an arterial saturation electrode (Bentley oxy-stat) to the circuit, allowing further reduction in PaO_2 within the confines of full saturation of the haemoglobin with oxygen.

The maintenance of physiological levels of PaO_2 may facilitate reduction in the life span of the gaseous microemboli in the arterial line and systemic arterial circulation. A low PaO_2 will increase the gradient between the bubbles (100% oxygen) and the blood favouring more rapid dissolution than would occur if the PaO_2 was higher than necessary. Whilst it has been recommended that the use of an inert sweep gas (nitrogen) in a bubble oxygenator may be used to control the PaO_2 during hypothermia (Berger, 1979) and independent control of $PaCO_2$ can be achieved using helium (Groom *et al.*, 1982), the safety of these manoeuvres is yet to be established.

(b) Membrane oxygenators

It has not been possible to detect GME originating from membrane oxygenators. The use of a TM8 Microbubble Activity Monitor on the arterial line leading from a series of Travenol TMO membrane oxygenators used for clinical perfusion showed a substantial and significant reduction in GME when compared with the two bubble oxygenators even when an arterial line filter was used (Fig. 18.4 and Table 18.2). A comparison of continuous measurement of PaO_2 and unfiltered GME for a Harvey H-1500 bubble oxygenator and Cobe CML membrane oxygenator is shown in Fig. 18.10. The familiar high level of GME activity and positive relationship to PaO_2 are demonstrated with the Harvey H-1500. The abrupt rise in both PaO_2 and GME towards the end of bypass is due to a rise in oxygen flow to correct inadequate CO_2 clearance. By comparison, the GME activity in the Cobe CML is small and occurs in discrete bursts, unrelated to the PaO_2. The effect

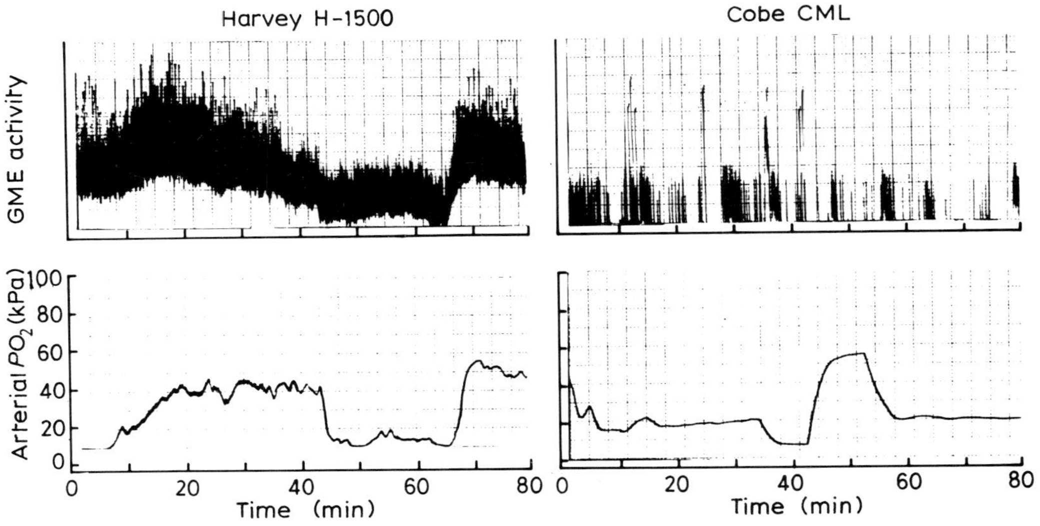

Fig. 18.10 Recordings during clinical cardiopulmonary bypass, using a Harvey H-1500 bubble oxygenator and Cobe CML membrane oxygenator, of unfiltered GME activity in the arterial line and PaO_2.

of a rise in the oxygen concentration of the gas flowing to the oxygenator is demonstrated to cause a rise in PaO_2 but no change in GME.

Gaseous microemboli detected in the arterial line of membrane oxygenators have been shown to originate from

(1) Cardiotomy suction
(2) GME present in priming fluid
(3) Admission of drugs, cold fluid and blood to the oxygenator
(4) Heat exchanger during rewarming
(5) Entrainment of air at venous cannulation sites
(6) Tapping of the oxygenator

Whilst these causes of increased GME activity apply to both bubble and membrane oxygenators, they are particularly relevant in membrane oxygenators which do not contain inherent defoaming material and arterial reservoirs which could reduce the number of GME entering the arterial line and systemic arterial circulation (Pearson *et al.*, 1981). The GME detected in the Cobe CML membrane oxygenator were due to injection of drugs into the venous line and the intermittent admission of cardiotomy suction.

(c) Heat exchanger

It has been demonstrated *in vitro* and inferred during clinical perfusion that a temperature gradient between the water inflow to the heat exchanger and the blood of greater than 10°C on rewarming causes a significant increase in GME in the arterial blood (Clark *et al.*, 1975). It is important to maintain as low a gradient as possible commensurate with an acceptable rate of rise in patient temperature. The decrease in solubility of gases in the blood with rise in temperature is liable to generate GME especially if the temperature gradient is high. Most currently available bubble oxygenators have heat exchangers incorporated into the oxygenating column so that GME generated during rewarming are presented to the defoamer and may not be released from the oxygenator. The theoretical benefits of this heat exchanger position have not been confirmed.

(d) Cardiotomy reservoir

Most oxygenators in common use alter the blood in a manner that is detrimental to the tissues being perfused and these effects are exaggerated after blood has been aspirated from the heart with resultant red cell destruction and the formation of gas and particulate emboli. Several authors have identified cardiotomy suction as a potent source of both particulate (Page *et al.*, 1974; Solis *et al.*, 1974) and gaseous microemboli (Pearson *et al.*, 1978; Loop *et al.*, 1976). The high levels of cellular aggregation and trauma caused by cardiotomy suction can be considerably reduced by the avoidance of air aspiration (Wright and Sanderson, 1979).

Cardiotomy reservoirs do not completely remove all the bubbles from the blood passing through them so that when the blood is returned to the oxygenator, the GME passing along the arterial line increases (Gallagher and Pearson, 1973; Loop *et al.*, 1976). Phasic peaks in ultrasonic echoes attributable to GME were detected on the arterial line of a bubble oxygenator following intermittent admission of cardiotomy suction blood from a cardiotomy reservoir during clinical perfusion (Fig. 18.11). The bubbles generated by cardiotomy suction are qualitatively different from those originating in the oxygenator, consisting of mainly nitrogen, a relatively insoluble gas. The persistence of these emboli after passage through both the defoamer of the cardiotomy reservoir and oxygenator indicates their relative stability.

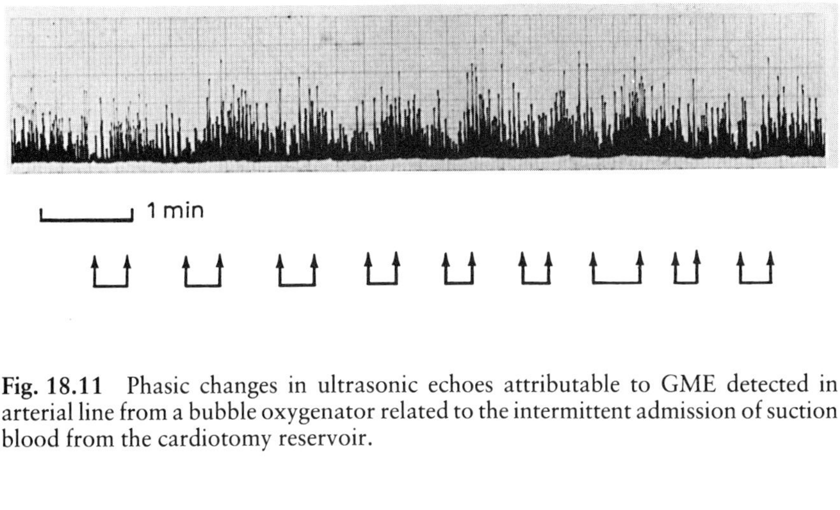

Fig. 18.11 Phasic changes in ultrasonic echoes attributable to GME detected in arterial line from a bubble oxygenator related to the intermittent admission of suction blood from the cardiotomy reservoir.

The ability of commercially available cardiotomy reservoirs to remove bubbles from aspirated blood has been investigated *in vitro* using a simulated cardiopulmonary bypass circuit and TM8 Microbubble Activity Monitor (Pearson *et al.*, 1978, 1981). An analysis of the design features of the reservoirs assessed by correlation of their *in vitro* performance with the overall configuration of the reservoir, type of defoamer and pore size of the incorporated filter material suggested that optimal efficiency could be achieved by

(1) Direct injection of blood into defoamer so as to avoid blood turbulence at reservoir inlet
(2) Ensuring that the flow pattern of blood through the reservoir allows all blood to pass through the defoamer

(3) Incorporation of integral micropore filtration
(4) Not allowing defoamed and filtered blood to fall freely into the storage part of the reservoir with resultant splashing and generation of GME

Most of the commercial cardiotomy reservoirs currently available fulfil these ideal design criteria though blood turbulence at the reservoir inlet ports continues to be an unfavourable feature of some devices causing unnecessary further admixture of gas with the blood and increasing the GME load to the reservoir (Pearson *et al.*, 1981). Experiments *in vitro* have demonstrated that GME are detectable at the reservoir outlet following admission of bubble-free blood to the device. The incorporation of micropore filtration material into the reservoir is an extremely efficient means of removing GME from aspirated blood but adds a large foreign surface to the total oxygenator circuit with the potential of inducing aggregation of formed blood elements and the increase in dynamic hold up at high blood flows may occasionally present problems for the perfusionist.

Alterations in perfusion technique will influence the defoaming performance of cardiotomy reservoirs (Pearson *et al.*, 1978). If blood is stored in the reservoir for as long as possible within the confines of an adequate level in the oxygenators, not only will maintenance of a higher level reduce splashing of the defoamed blood but GME will have more time to settle out. The greater proportion of air to blood in the aspirate from the open heart and pericardium, the more difficult it is for the cardiotomy reservoir to remove the GME. The speed of the suction pumps should be monitored continuously so as to allow as low an admixture of air with blood as is commensurate with the surgical technique. Whilst vacuum suction has been found to cause slightly less cellular aggregation and blood trauma than roller pump suction (Wright and Sanderson, 1979), the avoidance of air aspiration is the most important factor in reducing the blood damage and GME production of cardiotomy suction.

(e) Roller pumps

It has been reported (Bass and Longmore, 1969) that negative pressures which are generated behind each pump roller are potentially capable of causing GME formation by cavitation. During *in vitro* experiments at different blood PO_2 levels with variation in roller occlusion settings and pulsatile–non-pulsatile flow using a Cobe Stockert pump, these findings have not been confirmed.

(f) Other sources of gaseous microemboli from the pump oxygenator

Following priming of Harvey H-1500 oxygenators, the priming solution

(Plasmalyte 148: Travenol Laboratories) was circulated through an arterio-venous connection at 4.6 l min^{-1} with a gas flow rate of 2.0 l min^{-1} simulating the flow rates of clinical perfusion. The temperature of the priming solution was maintained at 37°C and arterial reservoir at the 1000 ml level. A carefully primed Pall arterial line filter together with a bypass line was incorporated into the circuit. GME could be detected in the recirculated priming solution, the number being significantly reduced when the filter was in circuit (Table 18.7). The large number of GME entering the systemic

Table 18.7 Harvey oxygenator (H-1500) with Pall arterial line filter

Recirculation of non-cellular priming solution.
Fluid flow rate 4.6 l min^{-1}
Gas flow rate (100% oxygen) 2.0 l min^{-1}
Gaseous microemboli >10 $\mu m\ s^{-1}$ in arterial line (mean±SEM, n = 6).

With filter	188±28	$p<0.001$
Without filter	416±36	

arterial circulation at the start of bypass have a long life span (Bethune, 1980) and may be responsible for the documented reduction in renal (Moghissi *et al.*, 1969) and cerebral (Braithwaite, 1973; 1974) blood flow which can occur at this time. It has been recommended (Bethune, 1976) that the oxygenator should be flushed with CO_2 and primed with warm fluids which are circulated without a gas supply to the oxygenating column. By this technique the number of GME which are introduced into the patient at the start of bypass can be reduced. When the priming fluid is incorporated within the patient at the start of bypass, the pressure difference between free and dissolved gases in the circulating blood will favour growth of any GME originating from the prime. Nitrous oxide, being a highly soluble gas, will tend to come out of solution causing enlargement of the GME of air and oxygen introduced in the priming solution. When used as an anaesthetic agent, nitrous oxide should be discontinued some ten minutes prior to the start of cardiopulmonary bypass to allow its elimination via the lungs. It is also advisable that any cold fluids should be warmed prior to their addition to the cardiotomy reservoir and oxygenator during bypass, thus preventing gas from being liberated from solution.

18.1.2 Gaseous microemboli originating in the heart and pulmonary veins (surgical air)

Gaseous microemboli may enter the systemic arterial circulation in association with (Gallagher and Pearson, 1973):

(1) cannulation of the heart and aorta

(2) following removal of the aortic clamp
(3) entrainment of air at venous cannulation sites
(4) following restoration of effective cardiac action

(a) Cannulation of the heart and aorta

Cannulation of the aorta, insertion of caval or right artial cannulae through the right atrial wall in the presence of an atrial septal defect and placement of left atrial or apical left ventricular vent cannulae may admit GME into the systemic arterial circulation.

(b) Following removal of aortic clamp

If the left heart is opened air may collect between the aortic clamp and aortic valve. Even when the root of the aorta is vented through the suture line or wide bore needle, GME are released into the systemic arterial circulation when the aortic clamp is removed.

(c) Entrainment of air at venous cannulation sites

Air may be entrained into the venous line to the oxygenator due to inadequate snaring of the site of insertion of the right atrial cannulae and during right atrial venting of cardioplegic solution. A large proportion of this air, which is not always visible to the naked eye, will pass through both bubble and membrane oxygenators to enter the arterial line. Whilst the use of a partial clamp on the venous line to raise venous pressure may reduce the entrainment of air, it must be recognized as a major source of GME during cardiopulmonary bypass.

(d) Following restoration of effective cardiac action

Following cardiotomy for a septal defect, or during exposure of left-sided heart valves, cardiac ejection is prevented until the heart is filled with blood, air pockets are displaced and bubbles trapped in muscular trabeculae are finally removed. Many techniques have been described to avoid the hazards of systemic air embolism and include the insertion of a drain in the left ventricle attached to suction (Miller *et al.*, 1963). This may be combined with induced ventricular fibrillation (Nicks, 1969; Senning, 1952), flooding of the operative field with CO_2 (Burbank *et al.*, 1965; Nichols *et al.*, 1958) and aspiration of the pulmonary veins and cardiac chambers with a needle (Taber *et al.*, 1970). Vents may be placed into the left side of the heart via the right superior pulmonary vein and air removed from the aorta using a wide bore needle either freely draining into the pericardium or attached to controlled suction. Other techniques include closure of the left atrium under blood, ventilation of the lungs to evacuate pulmonary venous air and positioning the patient in a head down position. Many of these techniques are relatively ineffective (Pearson *et al.*, 1983) and none have completely eliminated the incidence of air embolism (Gallagher and Pearson, 1973).

Using an *in vivo* technique in which GME were detected in the carotid artery and tubing of the left heart vent, the efficiency of documented methods of removal of GME from the left heart have been assessed. It has been established that the most effective method of removing GME from the left heart following cardiotomy is to allow a free flow of blood from the pulmonary veins and left atrium to pass through an actively beating left ventricle (Pearson *et al.*, 1983). If a high mean aortic pressure is maintained during the venting period, blood will be preferentially discharged into the low resistance left heart vent and the potential danger of ejection of GME into the systemic circulation via the aortic valve will be reduced. The inverse relationship between mean aortic pressure during left heart venting and the bubble activity detected in the carotid artery following termination of bypass in 19 patients having left-sided prosthetic valve replacement surgery is shown in Fig. 18.12 and confirms the value of this method.

The large number of techniques and their relative complexity which have been described to remove air from the left heart prior to termination of cardiopulmonary bypass is probably evidence of their inefficiency. Recent work by Slogoff *et al.* (1982) has shown an incidence of postoperative cerebral dysfunction more than twice as high in patients undergoing intracardiac than in patients having extracardiac operations. The data suggest that air or particulate microemboli originating in the heart and aorta are the major causes of cerebral damage. It is interesting to note that patients evaluated in this series were perfused using a variety of bubble oxygenators without arterial line micropore filtration. Following the original description of use of an ultrasonic detector over the carotid artery to detect GME during open heart surgery (Gallagher and Pearson, 1973), the technique has been supplemented by 2-D echocardiography using a phased array ultrasonic probe placed behind the aortic root through the oesophagus (Krebber *et al.*, 1982). It was confirmed that whilst bubbles could originate in the oxygenator and the bubble activity could be reduced by arterial line filtration, the largest quantity of bubbles was seen when the heart started ejecting following cardiotomy, even after comprehensive de-airing procedures. It was further demonstrated in animals, using a technique described by Taylor *et al.* (1980) to assess cerebral damage, that cardiopulmonary bypass with cardiotomy produced a greater rise in cerebrospinal fluid enzymes, indicative of brain damage, than when cardiotomy was not performed.

Whilst specific extracorporeal components have been evaluated with respect to their GME production, the general principles and deductions are

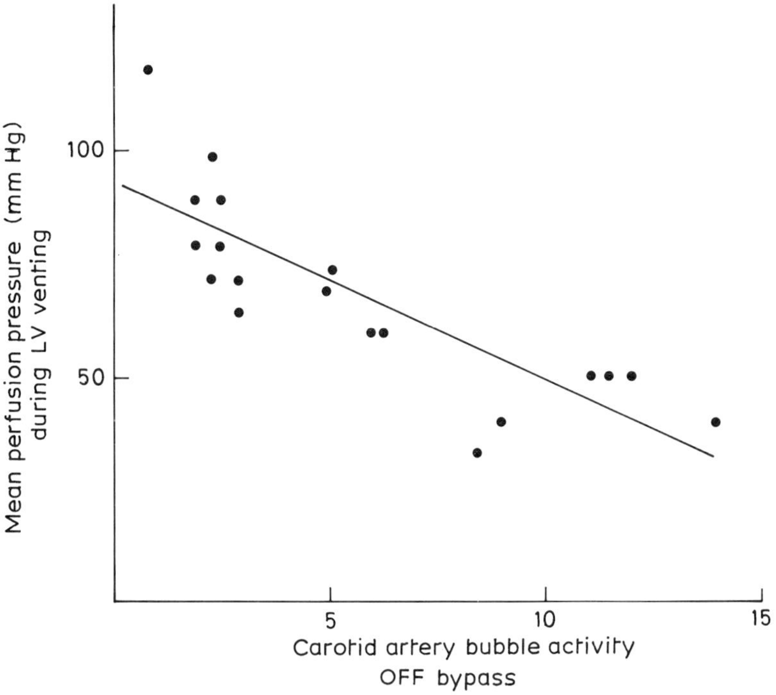

Fig. 18.12 Relationship between mean perfusion pressure (systemic arterial pressure) during left ventricular venting and bubble activity measured ultrasonically in the carotid artery after termination of bypass in 19 patients having left-sided prosthetic valve replacement surgery.

relevant to oxygenators and cardiotomy reservoirs from other manufacturers. It is important to recognize that the gas transfer characteristics of an oxygenator (or more correctly, a gas transfer device) can only be evaluated using in-line sensors for PaO_2 and $PaCO_2$ since the time constants associated with changes in these parameters do not allow for intermittent sampling to reflect adequately oxygenator performance. Further, if performance comparisons are to be made between devices from different manufacturers it is essential that the assessment be carried out during clinical perfusion and the ability of the perfusionist to control the blood gases at physiological levels form an important part of the evaluation. In currently available bubble oxygenators, conflict between desired CO_2 clearance and control of PaO_2 and GME using manual or automatic adjustment of gas flow rate must be appreciated during clinical perfusion as must the influence of arterial reservoir blood level upon PaO_2 and GME. The independent control of PaO_2 and $PaCO_2$ in membrane oxygenators which may be achieved by adjustment of gas flow rate and oxygen and carbon dioxide concentrations in the gas is not influenced by reservoir levels and unrelated to GME production. However, GME in the priming fluid, uncontrolled admission of cardiotomy suction and unrecognized entrainment of air at venous cannulation sites may produce higher levels of GME in the arterial line of a membrane oxygenator than can occur in a well-supervised perfusion using a bubble oxygenator. The use of an arterial line filter has been advocated and demonstrated to reduce GME in the arterial line (Semb *et al.*, 1982). It is at best only a partial solution to a problem best solved by attention to factors involved in the production of the emboli and may add to the embolic load if incorrectly primed (Wellons and Nolan, 1973).

All patients having cardiac surgery using cardiopulmonary bypass receive a variable amount of GME from extracorporeal components and surgical sources (Fig. 18.13). The quantity and quality of GME entering the systemic arterial circulation has been demonstrated to be as dependent upon inter-related surgical, anaesthetic and perfusion techniques as the equipment used.

18.2 PARTICULATE MICROEMBOLI

18.2.1 Foreign material emboli

Foreign particles may be present on blood contact surfaces of commercially available extracorporeal components of the cardiopulmonary bypass system.

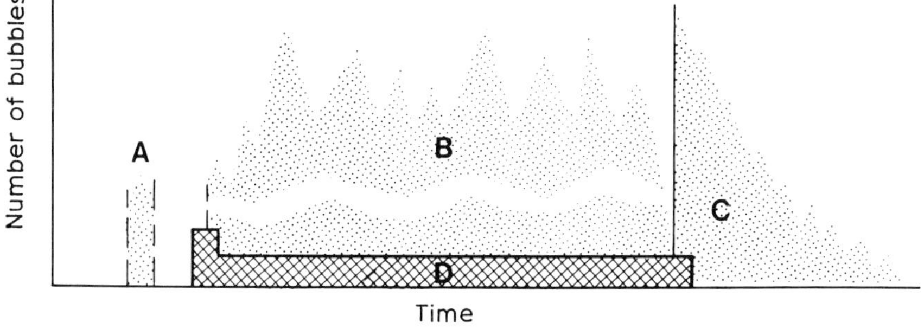

Fig. 18.13 Schematic diagram indicating source and type of GME entering the systemic arterial circulation during open-heart surgery using cardiopulmonary bypass. (Reproduced with permission from Pearson, 1981.)

Reed *et al.* (1974) have evaluated the degree of particulate contamination in seven commercially available bubble oxygenators. Recirculation of the priming solution through a filter with a pore size of 5 µm resulted in the removal of large quantities of particulate matter consisting of cotton fibres, plastic chips and unidentifiable material. The use of a washing and micropore filtration technique during the preparation of the pump oxygenator prior to priming was reported to result in a significant reduction in the incidence of neurological complications. The retention of amorphous debris on a 0.8 µm pore size pre-bypass filter following flushing of a Travenol TMO membrane oxygenator is shown in Figs 18.14 and 18.15.

An additional source of particulate emboli has been identified in relation to spallation of plastic tubing particles into the lumen of the conduits of the pump oxygenator by the erosive and fatiguing action of the roller in the pump head (Kurusz *et al.*, 1980). The numbers and size of the particles, up to 300 µm in diameter, which may be generated is dependent upon the type and batch of tubing used in the roller pump, the degree of occlusion setting and speed of rotation. Spallation is more likely to occur with silicone rubber than with polyvinyl or polyurethane tubing.

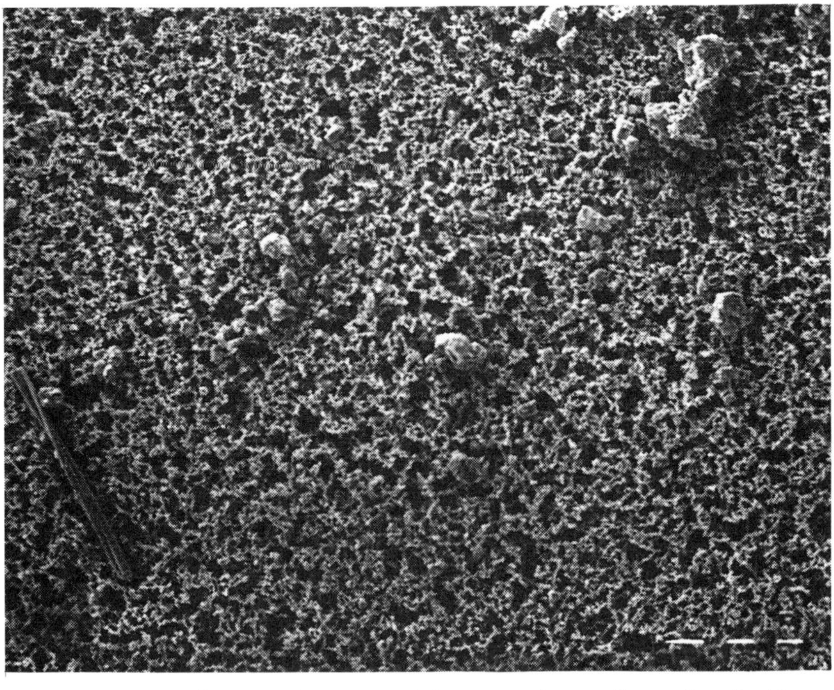

Fig. 18.14 SEM of contaminants on 0.8 µm membrane filter after flushing a Travenol TMO membrane oxygenator. (Scale bar = 1 µm.) (Reproduced with help and permission from Pall Bioimedical Ltd, Portsmouth, UK.)

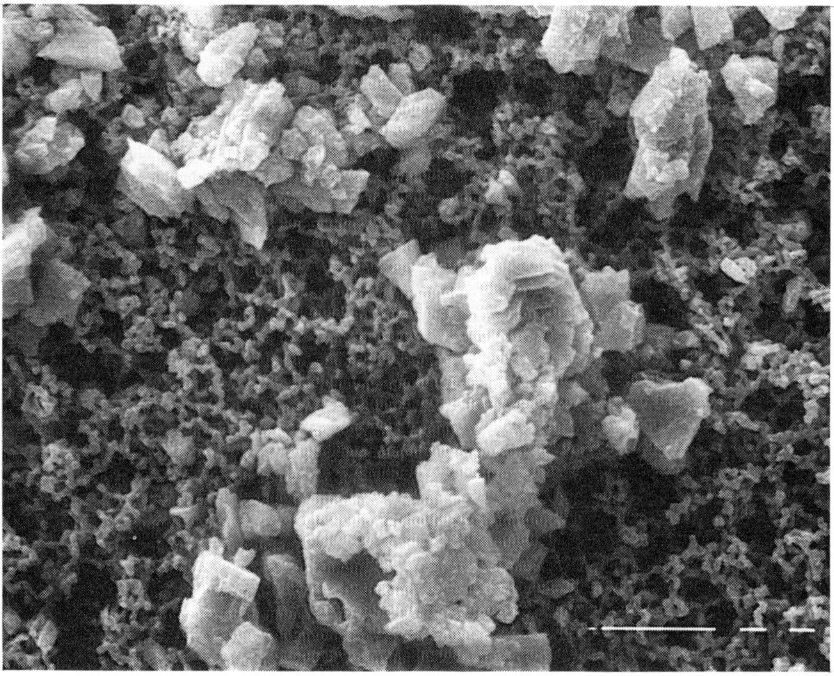

Fig. 18.15 Magnification of top right particles shown in Figure 18.14. (Scale bar = 1 μm) (Reproduced with help and permission from Pall Biomedical Ltd, Portsmouth, UK.)

A silicone, dimethyl polysiloxane, is used as a defoaming agent in bubble oxygenators and cardiotomy reservoirs (Lindberg *et al.*, 1961). Valentin and Vilhelmsen (1976), confirming the extensive literature concerning the release of silicone into the blood from the oxygenator, have described the presence of silicone in the brain and kidneys of patients who did not survive the operative procedure.

Several authors have identified the cardiotomy suction as a potent source of particulate emboli (Caguin and Carter, 1963; Clarke *et al.*, 1976; Solis *et al.*, 1975). These emboli include fibrin, fat, platelet aggregates, calcium, arterio-sclerotic debris and foreign material introduced by the operative equipment (talc, thread, dust, cloth particles and even hair). Denatured proteins produced as the result of the gas–blood interface may result in the formation of fat emboli and red cell aggregates (Lee *et al.*, 1961). Histological studies (Hill *et al.*, 1969) and the results of psychometric testing (Aberg and Kihlgren, 1977) indicate that it is essential to include micropore filtration in the cardiotomy system to remove these emboli.

18.2.2 Blood derived emboli

It is well established that donor blood contains particulate emboli (Solis *et al.*, 1974; Wright and Sanderson, 1976). Debris accumulates in the blood at an amount and rate dependent upon the duration of storage and type of anticoagulant used (Swank, 1961). The debris consists of intact and fragmented red cells, leucocyte and platelet aggregates, fibrin and denatured proteins. These emboli are not removed by the standard filter supplied with blood administration sets and are known to cause blockage of the pulmonary capillary bed as described during massive intravenous transfusion of blood to patients in haemorrhagic shock (McNamara *et al.*, 1970; Moseley and Doty, 1970; Jenevein and Weiss, 1964). Donor blood added to the priming fluid or transfused intravenously during cardiopulmonary bypass is not filtered in the lungs but enters the arterial circulation directly. Micropore filtration can remove these emboli (McNamara *et al.*, 1972; Patterson and Twichell, 1971; Solis and Gibbs, 1972) and should be used during cardiopulmonary bypass since there is evidence that microembolic cerebrovascular blockade resulting from infusion of donor blood may effect postoperative cerebral function (Patterson *et al.*, 1974).

Fibrin may form within extracorporeally circulated blood in areas of stagnant flow, turbulence and cavitation and on rough surfaces. Cardiopulmonary bypass circuits contain large areas of foreign surface with a multitude of intraluminal projections and sites of non-streamlined blood flow where fibrin deposits are prone to develop. The exposure of blood to a foreign surface results in rapid protein absorption dominated by fibrinogen (Baier and Dutton, 1969) with consequent adhesion of platelets and leucocytes (Baier, 1977). Fibrin deposition in the extracorporeal circuit is more likely to occur if the coagulation cascade is not adequately inhibited by heparin. Measurement of whole blood activated clotting time (ACT) during extracorporeal circulation (Bull *et al.*, 1975a,b) is essential during cardiopulmonary bypass since neither heparin dosage nor plasma heparin levels can predict the magnitude of clinical heparin effect and the degree of anticoagulation (Esposito *et al.*, 1983). Abts *et al.* (1978) have demonstrated increased numbers of microemboli downstream of arterial filters when the ACT was deliberately reduced. The appearance of a fibrin monomer in the plasma during cardiopulmonary bypass if the ACT is allowed to fall below 400 s has established this value as the safe lower limit to provide coagulation-free perfusion (Young *et al.*, 1978). Figures. 18.16 and 18.17 show photomicrographs of the upstream surfaces of arterial line filters with different degrees of anticoagulation during cardiopulmonary bypass and emphasize the importance of measurement of ACT during cardiopulmonary bypass. The potential for thrombosis and cellular adhesion is considerable with these devices and may result in systemic arterial embolization (Kursz, 1981). In a study of prostacyclin and heparin anticoagulation during cardiopulmonary bypass, the fluctuating pressure differentials during perfusion were suggestive of the accumulation and release of material from the arterial line filters (Longmore *et al.*, 1979).

Thrombocytopenia associated with cardiopulmonary bypass has been attributed to the adhesion of platelets to the foreign surfaces of the bypass components, consumption of platelets in disseminated intravascular coagulation, platelet aggregation induced by heparin and protamine, mechanical

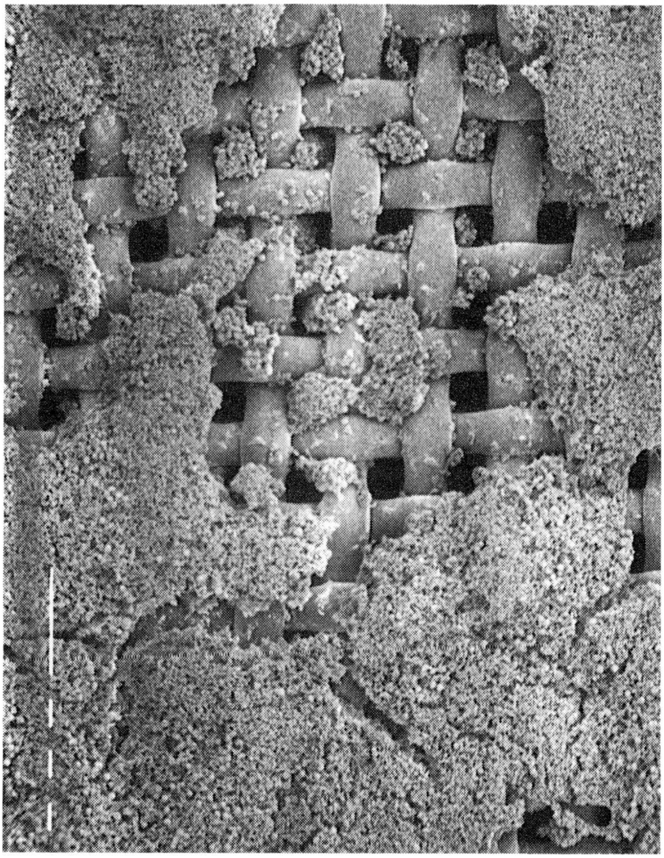

Fig. 18.16 SEM of upstream surface of Pall EC3840 40 μm screen filter. (Large left hand scale bar = 100 μm). Surface covered by aggregated platelets as a result of inadequate heparinization. ACT <300 s after one hour of bypass. Operation: mitral valve replacement; bypass time: 97 min; blood flow rate: 3.6 l min^{-1}; haematocrit: 40%. (Reproduced with help and permission from Pall Biomedical Ltd, Portsmouth, UK.)

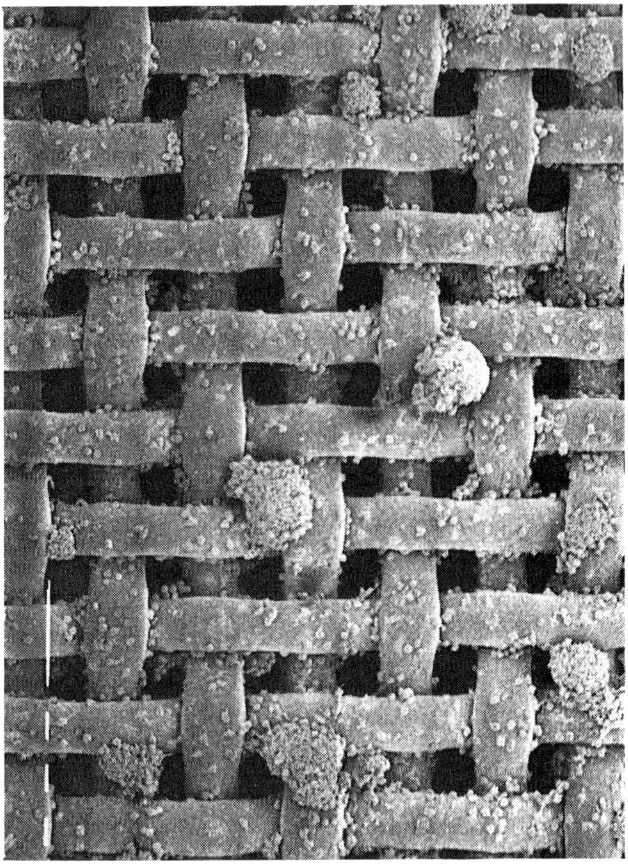

Fig. 18.17 SEM of upstream surface of Pall EC3840 40 μm screen filter. (Large left hand scale bar = 100 μm). Normal heparinization with ACT >400 s throughout procedure. Surface of filter shows captured platelet (degenerated) aggregates. Operation: triple coronary bypass grafts; bypass time: 133 min; blood flow rate: 4.3 l min^{-1}; haematocrit: 34%. (Reproduced with help and permission from Pall Biomedical Ltd, Portsmouth, UK.)

damage to platelets and haemodilution by pump priming solutions (McKenna *et al.*, 1975). Cardiopulmonary bypass is associated with a 30–50% fall in the pre-operative platelet count (Woods *et al.*, 1967) and alteration in platelet function (Bicks *et al.*, 1976; Tamari *et al.*, 1975). The platelet aggregation is induced by contact with foreign surface and thrombin generated during the operation (Baier and Dutton, 1969; Beurling-Hardbury and Galvan, 1978). The normal pattern of alteration in platelet count during cardiopulmonary bypass is for a rapid fall to occur in the first five minutes of perfusion followed by a period of stabilization. A further decrease follows the administration of protamine sulphate (Hope *et al.*, 1981). The initial decrease is consistent with the finding that platelet adhesion to biomaterials is favoured by the formation of blood–gas interfaces on the surface of the biomaterial (Ward *et al.*, 1974) and gaseous microemboli (Butler and Hills, 1983; Butler, 1983). The use of techniques to eliminate GME during priming of oxygenators (Bethune, 1976) and arterial line filters (Wellons and Nolan, 1973) may limit the degree of platelet aggregation and embolization at the start of perfusion.

Thrombocytosis and circulating platelet aggregates may be associated with postoperative neurological dysfunction (Preston *et al.*, 1979) and it is assumed that increased postoperative bleeding results from reduced platelet numbers and defects in their function. The attractive concept of pharmacological inhibition of platelet activation during cardiopulmonary bypass by prostacyclin has been demonstrated not only to preserve platelet numbers and reduce platelet aggregation (Longmore *et al.*, 1979; Radegran *et al.*, 1982) but also to reduce the weight increase and microaggregate deposition of platelets, fibrin and leucocytes on screen filters placed in the arterial line (Faichney *et al.*, 1982; Walker *et al.*, 1981). Aren *et al.* (1983) have confirmed preservation of platelet numbers and reduced aggregation when prostacyclin is used during clinical cardiopulmonary bypass as well as demonstrating reduced postoperative chest drainage and the need for blood transfusion. Heparin is known to increase the sensitivity of platelets to aggregating stimuli (Ellison *et al.*, 1978). The reduced requirements for heparin when prostacyclin is used during extracorporeal circulation may further reduce the incidence of platelet aggregation. It is thus possible that the use of prostacyclin may have many important therapeutic advantages including a valuable role in the reduction of microembolic visceral injury during cardiopulmonary bypass.

Biogenic amines, such as serotonin, are released when platelets aggregate. Serotonin in the presence of ADP promotes platelet adhesiveness and aggregation thus contributing to the microembolization by further aggregating platelets and contributing to the mechanical occlusion by inducing arteriolar vasoconstriction. Histamine is also released from platelets and mast cell containing aggregates and can result in the escape of plasma proteins from the blood into the surrounding tissues. During shock and hypothermia the release of a heparin-like substance contributes to the platelet aggregation induced by biological amines such as adrenaline and noradrenaline (Swank, 1982).

Activation of complement by certain materials and conditions during cardiopulmonary bypass has been shown to result in an increase in the adhesiveness and aggregability of neutrophils. The nylon tricot defoamer used in some bubble oxygenators is a potent complement activator and this material should be avoided in extracorporeal devices (Chenoweth *et al.*, 1981). More leucocytes have been observed adherent to Bentley nylon filter medium than Pall polyester medium (Kursz, 1981). Complement-mediated neutrophil aggregation in the pulmonary capillaries is an important factor in the genesis of pulmonary endothelial injury and increased capillary permeability of the post-perfusion lung syndrome (Hammerschmidt *et al.*, 1981). The clinical significance of the sequestration of aggregated leucocytes which have been discovered in tissue biopsies following cardiopulmonary bypass (Ts'ao *et al.*, 1973) is not due to the resultant mechanical blockage but the release of the lysosomal granules into the circulation and surrounding tissues (Goldstein and Perez, 1980). The proteolytic enzymes will destroy structural proteins and the highly toxic oxygen-free superoxide radicals cause injury to enzyme systems and attack cell membranes (Newman, 1983). Studies *in vitro* have demonstrated the capacity of corticosteroids to stabilize lysosomal membranes, prevent complement-induced aggregation and superoxide damage to endothelial cells. A study of corticosteroid pretreatment has indicated a potential beneficial effect in reducing brain damage as assessed by a biochemical marker technique (Taylor *et al.*, 1983). Although the use of steroids has been advocated in the treatment of pulmonary cellular damage (Wilson, 1972), substantial evidence of clinical efficiency is lacking (Bihari and Tinker, 1982).

Most authorities would agree that the principal aetiological factors associated with the diffuse cerebral damage syndromes which can follow the use of cardiopulmonary bypass are related to diffuse microembolism and altered perfusion blood flow. It is increasingly evident that the brain would appear to be more resistant to imperfect perfusion than was previously recognized (Taylor, 1983) though the definition of safe thresholds for flow, pressure and pulsatility at the different temperatures of open-heart surgery are yet to be defined. Age and prolonged extracorporeal circulation increase the risk of brain damage but whether perfusion pressure is a determinant of postoperative neurological dysfunction has been questioned (Kolkka and Hilberman, 1980; Slogoff *et al.*, 1982).

Measurement of cerebral blood flow during cardiac operations has demonstrated an uncoupling of flow and metabolism during hypothermia, the raised cerebral blood flow being suggestive of microvascular blockade by emboli (Hendriksen *et al.*, 1983). Many emboli enter the systemic arterial circulation during cardiac surgery, the quantity and quality being dependent upon the equipment used and the surgical and perfusion techniques. Whilst the use of arterial line filters is advocated to reduce the embolic load to the patient, careful attention to priming and patient anticoagulation status are essential prerequisites of their use. The use of micropore filtration in the cardiotomy suction system is mandatory. Recognition that 'surgical air' is an important cause of postoperative neurological dysfunction is of concern since the recommended techniques for de-airing the heart are proven to be relatively ineffective and warrant further evaluation.

Pharmacological intervention during cardiopulmonary bypass in the form of platelet aggregation inhibition and modification of inflammatory cell behaviour are of great potential importance too not only as a means of reducing the numbers of emboli but also of preventing the subsequent release of vasoactive substances.

The number of microemboli, both gaseous and particulate, which enter the systemic circulation during open-heart surgery are mainly dependent on interrelated surgical, anaesthetic and perfusion techniques rather than the equipment used. Knowledge of the factors involved in the production of the emboli and methods of reducing the quantity entering the systemic arterial circulation can improve the quality of patient care during open-heart surgery.

> The success of a perfusion depends not as much on the perfusion system as how it is applied. De Wall (1975)

REFERENCES

Abel, R. M., Buckley, M. J., Austen, W. G., Barnett, G. O., Beck, C. H. and Fischer, J. E. (1976) Acute postoperative renal failure in cardiac surgical patients. *J. Surg. Res.*, **20**, 341–8.

Aberg, T. (1974) Effect of open heart surgery on intellectual function. *Scand. J. Thorac. Cadiovasc. Surg.* (Suppl. 15).

Aberg, T., Ahlund, P. and Kihlgren, M. (1983) Intellectual function after open heart surgery. *An. Thorac. Surg.*, **36**, 680–3.

Aberg, T. and Kihlgren, M. (1977) Cerebral protection during open heart surgery. *Thorax*, **32**, 525–33.

Aberg, T., Ronquist, G., Tyden, H., Ahlund, P. and Bergstrom, K. (1982). Release of adenylate kinase into cerebrospinal fluid during open heart surgery and its relationship to postoperative intellectual function. *Lancet*, **i**, 1139–42.

Abts, L. R., Beyer, R. T., Galletti, P. M. *et al.* (1978) Computerized discrimination of microemboli in extracorporeal circuits. *Am. J. Surg.*, **135**, 535–8.

Aren, C. A., Feddersen, K. and Radegran, K. (1983) Effects of prostacyclin infusion on platelet activation and post-operative blood loss in coronary bypass. *Ann. Thorac. Surg.*, **36**, 49–54.

Austen, W. G. and Howdry, D. H. (1965) Ultrasound as a method to detect bubbles and particulate matter in the arterial line during cardiopulmonary bypass. *J. Surg. Res.*, **5**, 283–4.

Baier, R. E. (1977) The organisation of blood components near interfaces. *Ann. NY Acad. Sci.*, **283**, 17–36.

Baier, R. E. and Dutton, R. C. (1969) Initial events in interactions of blood with a foreign surface. *J. Biomed. Mater. Res.*, **3**, 191–206.

Bass, R. M. and Longmore, D. B. (1969) Cerebral damage during open heart surgery. *Nature*, **222**, 30.

Becker, H., Vinten-Johansen, J. *et al.* (1981) Myocardial damage caused by keeping pH 7.40 during systemic deep hypothermia. *J. Thorac. Cardiovasc. Surg.*, **82**, 810–20.

Berger, E. C. (1979) *The Physiology of Adequate Perfusion.* CV Mosby, St Louis, p. 34.

Bethune, D. W. (1976) Organ damage after open heart surgery. *Lancet*, **ii**, 1410–11.

Bethune, D. W. (1980) Life span of gaseous emboli and organ damage. In *Psychic and Neurological Dysfunctions after Open Heart Surgery* (eds H. Speidel and G. Rodewald) Georg Thieme Verlag, Stuttgart and New York, pp. 92–9.

Beurling-Hardbury, G. and Galvan, C. A. (1978) Acquired decrease in platelet secretory ADP associated with an increased postoperative bleeding in post-cardiopulmonary bypass patients and in patients with severe valvular heart disease. *Blood*, **52**, 13–23.

Bicks, R. L., Schmalhorst, W. R. and Arbegast, N. R. (1976) Alterations in haemostasis associated with cardiopulmonary bypass. *Thromb. Res.*, **8**, 285–302.

Bihari, D. J. and Tinker, J. (1982) Steroids in intensive care. *Br. J. Hosp. Med.*, **28**, 323–30.

Bojar, R. M., Najafi, H., de Laria, G. A., Serry, C., Goldin, M. D. (1983) Neurological complications of coronary revascularisation. *Ann. Thorac. Surg.*, **36**, 427–32.

Braithwaite, M. A. (1973) Detection of neurological damage during open heart surgery. *Thorax*, **28**, 464–72.

Braithwaite, M. A. (1974) Cerebral blood flow and metabolism during open heart surgery. *Thorax*, **29**, 633–8.

Brennan, R. W., Patterson, R. H. and Kessler, J. (1971) Cerebral blood flow and metabolism during cardiopulmonary bypass: evidence of microembolic encephalopathy. *Neurology*, **21**, 665–6.

Bull, B. S., Huse, W. M., Brauer, F. S. and Korpman, R. A. (1975b) Heparin therapy during extracorporeal circulation II. The use of a dose–response curve to individualize heparin and protamine dosage. *J. Thorac. Cardiovasc. Surg.*, **69**, 685–9.

Bull, B. S., Korpman, R. A., Huse, N. M., Briggs, B. D. (1975a) Heparin therapy during extracorporeal circulation I. *J. Thorac. Cardiovasc. Surg.*, **69**, 674–84.

Burbank, A., Ferguson, T. B. and Burford, T. H. (1965) Carbon dioxide flooding of the chest in open heart surgery. *J. Thorac. Cardiovasc. Surg.*, **50**, 691.

Butler, B. D. (1983) Gaseous microemboli: Concepts and considerations. *J. Extracorp. Technol.*, **15**, 148–55.

Butler, B. D. and Hills, B. A. (1983) Role of lung surfactant in cerebral decompression sickness. *Aviat. Space Environ. Med.*, **54**, 11–15.

Caguin, F. and Carter, M. G. (1963) Fat embolism with cardiotomy with the use of cardiopulmonary bypass. *J. Thorac. Cardiovasc. Surg.*, **46**, 665–72.

Chenoweth, D. E., Cooper, S. W., Hugli, P. E., Stewart, R. W., Blackstone, E. H. and Kirklin, J. W. (1981) Complement activation during cardiopulmonary bypass: Evidence for generation of C3a and C5a anaphylatoxins. *New Engl. J. Med.*, **304**, 497–503.

Claremont, D. J., Padgin, T. M. and Walton, N. (1984) Continuous monitoring of blood PO_2 in extracorporeal systems. An *in vitro* evaluation of a re-usable oxygen electrode. *Anaesthesia*, **39**, 362–9.

Clark, R. E., Dietz, D. R. and Miller, J. G. (1975) Continuous detection of microemboli during cardiopulmonary bypass in animals and man. *Circulation*, **54**, 74–8.

Collins, J. D., Bassendine, M. F., Ferner, R. *et al.* (1983) The incidence and prognostic importance of jaundice following cardiopulmonary bypass surgery. *Lancet*, **i**, 1119–24.

Daniels, S., Paton, W. D. M. and Smith, E. B. (1979) Ultrasonic imaging system for the study of decompression induced gas bubbles. *Undersea Biomed. Res.*, **6**, 197–207.
DeWall, R. (1975) What constitutes adequate perfusion? *J. Cardiovasc. Surg.*, **16**, 458–64.
Editorial (1982) Brain damage after open heart surgery. *Lancet*, **i**, 1161–3.
Ellison, N., Edmunds, L. H. Jr and Colman, R. W. (1978) Platelet aggregation following heparin and protamine administration. *Anaesthesiology*, **48**, 65–8.
Esposito, R. A., Culliford, A. T., Colvin, S. B., Thomas, S. J., Lackner, H. and Spencer, F. C. (1983) The role of the activated clotting time in heparin administration and neutralisation for cardiopulmonary bypass. *J. Thorac. Cardiovasc. Surg.*, **85**, 174–85.
Faichney, A., Davidson, K. G., Wheatley, D. J. and Walker, I. D. (1982) Prostacyclin in cardiopulmonary bypass operations. *J. Thorac. Cardiovasc. Surg.*, **84**, 601–8.
Ferguson, T. B., Burbank, A. and Burford, T. H. (1967) The disposable bubble oxygenator. Evaluation of an improved model. *Surgery*, **61**, 260.
Furness, A. and Wright, G. (1979) Detection of bubbles in blood vessels and extracorporeal circuits. (Letter to Editor) *Med. Biol. Eng. Comput.*, **17**, 534–5.
Galletti, P. M. and Brecher, G. H. (1962) *Heart Lung Bypass: Principles and Techniques of Extracorporeal Circulation.* Grune and Stratton, New York.
Gallagher, E. G. and Pearson, D. T. (1973) Ultrasonic identification of sources of gaseous microemboli during open heart surgery. *Thorax*, **28**, 295–305.
Goldstein, I. M. and Perez, H. D. (1980) Biologically active peptides derived from the fifth component of complement. *Progr. Haemostasis Thromb.*, **5**, 41–79.
Groom, T. C., Kraemer, M. and Reed, C. C. (1982) Use of a sweep gas in bubble oxygenators to obtain independent control of blood carbon dioxide levels. A preliminary report. *Proc. Am. Acad. Cardiovasc. Perf.*, **3**, 69–72.
Grulke, D. C., Marsh, N. R. and Mills, B. A. (1973) Measurement of microbubbles using the Coulter counter. *Br. J. Exp. Pathol.*, **54**, 684–91.
Hammerschmidt, D. E., Stroncek, D. F., Bowers, T. K. *et al.* (1981) Complement activation and neutropenia occurring during cardiopulmonary bypass. *J. Thorac. Cardiovasc. Surg.*, **81**, 370–7.
Hendriksen, L., Hjelms, E. and Lindeburgh, T. (1983) Brain hyperperfusion during cardiac operations. *J. Thorac. Cardiovasc. Surg.*, **86**, 202–8.
Hiberman, M., Myers, B. D., Carrie, B. J., Derby, G., Jamison, R. L. and Stinson, E. B. (1979) Acute renal failure following cardiac surgery. *J. Thorac. Cardiovasc. Surg.*, 77, 880–8.
Hill, J. D., Aguilar, M. J., Baranco, A., de Lanerolle, P. and Gerbode, F. (1969) Neuropathological manifestations of cardiac surgery. *Ann. Thorac. Surg.*, **7**, 409–14.
Hope, A. F., duP Henys, A. and Lotter, M. G. *et al.* (1981) Kinetics and sites of sequestration of indium 111-labeled human platelets during cardiopulmonary bypass. *J. Thorac. Cardiovasc. Surg.*, **81**, 880–6.
Jenevein, E. P. and Weiss, D. I. (1964) Platelet microemboli associated with massive blood transfusion. *Am. J. Pathol.*, **45**, 313–25.
Kemna, G. D. and Docherty, J. P. (1978) A comparison of the Bentley BOS 10, Shiley S-100 and Polystan Venotherm oxygenators during high flow perfusion and moderate hypothermia. *Proc. Am. Soc. Extracorp. Technol.*, **10**, 103–7.
Kolkka, R. and Hilberman, M. (1980) Neurological dysfunction following cardiac operation with low-flow, low pressure cardiopulmonary bypass. *J. Thorac. Cardiovasc. Surg.*, 79, 432–6.

Krebber, H. J., Hanrath, P., Janzen, R., Ritoff, M. and Rodewald, G. (1982) Gas emboli during open heart surgery. *J. Thorac. Cardiovasc. Surg.*, **30**, 401–4.

Kurusz, M., Christman, E. W., Williams, E. H. and Tyers, G. F. O. (1980) Roller pump induced tubing wear: another argument in favour of arterial line filtration, *J. Extracorp. Technol.*, **12**, 49–59.

Kurusz, M. (1981) Scanning electron microscopy of arterial line filters following cardiopulmonary bypass. *Proc. First World Congr. Extracorporeal Technology.* Brighton, Franklin Scientific Products, London.

Lee, W. H., Krumhaar, D., Fonkalsrud, E. W., Schjeide, O. A. and Maloney, J. V. (1961) Denaturation of plasma proteins as a cause of morbidity and death after intracardiac operations. *Surgery*, **50**, 29–39.

Lindberg, D. A. B., Lucas, F. V., Sheagren, J. and Malm, J. R. (1961) Silicone embolisation during clinical and experimental heart surgery employing a bubble oxygenator. *Am. J. Path.*, **39**, 129–35.

Longmore, D. B., Gueierrara, D. *et al.* (1979) Prostacyclin: a solution to some problems of extracorporeal circulation. *Lancet*, **ii**, 1002–5.

Loop, F. D., Szabo, J., Rowlinson, R. D. and Urbanek, K. (1976) Events related to microembolism during open heart surgery: Effectiveness of in-line filtration recorded by ultrasound. *Ann. Thorac. Surg.*, **21**, 412–20.

Lubbers, J. and van den Berg, J. W. (1976) An ultrasonic detector for microgasemboli in a blood flow line. *Ultrasound Med. Biol.*, **2**, 301–10.

Matsumoto, T., Wolferth, C. C. Jr and Perlman, M. H. (1981) Effects of pulsatile and non-pulsatile perfusion upon cerebral and conjunctival microcirculation in dogs. *Am. Surg.*, **37**, 61–4.

Matthews, A. J., Stead, A. L. and Abbott, T. R. (1984) Acid base control during hypothermia. *Anaesthesia*, **39**, 649–54.

McKenna, R., Bachman, F., Whittaker, B., Gilsen, J. and Weinberg, M. (1975) The haemostatic mechanism after open heart surgery II. Frequency of abnormal platelet function during and after extracorporeal circulation. *J. Thorac. Cardiovasc. Surg.*, **70**, 289–308.

McNamara, J. J., Burran, E. L. and Suehiro, G. (1972) Effective filtration of banked blood. *Surgery*, **71**, 594–7.

McNamara, J. J., Molet, M. D. and Strempie, J. F. (1970) Screen filtration pressure in combat casualties. *Ann. Surg.*, **172**, 334–41.

Miller, B. J., Gibbon, J. H., Greco, V. F., Cohn, C. H. and Allbritten, F. F. (1963) The use of a vent for the left ventricle as a means of avoiding air embolism to the systemic circulation during open cardiotomy with maintainance of the cardiorespiratory function of animals by a pump oxygenator. *Surg. Forum*, **4**, 29.

Moghissi, K., Machell, E. S. and Munday, K. A. (1969) Changes in renal blood flow and PAH extraction during extracorporeal circulation of short and long duration. Experimental study in dogs. *Cardiovasc. Res.*, **3**, 37–44.

Moseley, R. V. and Doty, D. B. (1970) Death associated with multiple pulmonary emboli soon after battle injury. *Ann. Surg.*, **171**, 336–46.

Moulinier, H. and Mausurel, G. (1979) Detection of bubbles in blood vessels and the evaluation of their flow. *Med. Biol. Eng. Comput.*, **16**, 585–8.

Newland, P. E., Pastoriza-Pinol, J. V., McMillan J., and Stirling, G. R. (1982) A report on the use of five bubble oxygenators for cardiopulmonary bypass surgery. *Anaesth. Intens. Care*, **10**, 45–9.

Newman, J. H. (1983) ARDS: new insights and unsolved problems. *Int. Care. Med.*, **9**, 303–6.

Nichols, H. T., Morse, D. P. and Hirose, T. (1958) Coronary and other embolism during open cardiac surgery. *Surgery*, **43**, 236.

Nicks, R. (1969) Air embolism in cardiac surgery: incidence and prophylaxis. *Aust. N.Z. J. Surg.*, **38**, 328.

Nishi, R. Y. (1972) Ultrasonic detection of bubbles with Doppler flow transducers. *Ultrasonics*, **10**, 173–9.

Page, U. S., Bigelow, J. C., Carter, C. R. and Swank, R. L. (1974) Emboli (debris) produced by bubble oxygenators. Removal by filtration. *Ann. Thorac. Surg.*, **18**, 161–71.

Parker, D., Delpy, D. T. and Hasall, D. N. (1983) A new approach to inline gas monitoring: development of an oxygen sensor. *Med. Biol. Eng. Comput.*, **21**, 134–7.

Patterson, R. H. Jr and Twitchell, J. B. (1971) Disposable filter for microemboli, use in cardiopulmonary bypass and massive transfusions. *J. Am. Med. Assoc.*, **215**, 76–8.

Patterson, R. H. Jr, Wasser, J. S. and Porro, R. S. (1974) The effects of various filters on microembolic cerebrovascular blockade following cardiopulmonary bypass. *Ann. Thorac. Surg.*, **17**, 464.

Pearson, D. T. (1981) Cardiotomy reservoirs and blood filters. In *Techniques in Extracorporeal Circulation* (ed. M. I. Ionescu), 2nd edn, Butterworths, London.

Pearson, D. T., Carter, R. F., Hammo, M. B. and Waterhouse, P. S. (1981) Gaseous microemboli during open heart surgery. In *Towards Safer Cardiac Surgery* (ed. D. B. Longmore), MTP, Lancaster, pp. 325–54.

Pearson, D. T., Holden, M. P., Poslad, S. J., Murray, A. and Waterhouse, P. S. (1985) A clinical evaluation of the gas transfer characteristics and gaseous microemboli production of two bubble oxygenators. *Life Support Systems*, **2**, 252–266.

Pearson, D. T., Holden, M. P., Waterhouse, P. S. and Clarke, I. (1983) Gaseous microemboli during open heart surgery. *Proc. Am. Acad. Cardiovasc. Perf.*, **4**, 103–9.

Pearson, D. T., Watson, B. G. and Waterhouse, P. S. (1978) An ultrasonic analysis of the comparative efficiency of various cardiotomy reservoirs and blood filters. *Thorax*, **33**, 352–8.

Preston, F. E., Martin, J. F., Stewart, R. M. and Davies-Jones, G. A. B. (1979) Thrombocytosis, circulating platelet aggregates and neurological dysfunction. *Br. Med. J.*, **2**, 156–8.

Radegran, K., Ahren, C. and Teger-Nilsson, A. C. (1982) Prostacyclin during extacorporeal circulation for coronary bypass. *J. Thorac. Cardiovasc. Surg.*, **60**, 205–11.

Ream, A. K., Reitz, B. A. and Silverberg, G. (1984) Temperature correction of PCO_2 and pH in estimating acid–base status. An example of the emperor's new clothes? *Anaesthesiology*, **56**, 41–4.

Reed, C. C., Romagnoli, A., Taylor, D. E. and Clark, D. K. (1974) Particulate matter in bubble oxygenators. *J. Thorac. Cardiovasc. Surg.*, **68**, 971.

Sakauye, L., Servas, F. M., O'Connor, K. B. and Cottonaro, C. (1982) An *in vitro* method to quantitate gaseous microemboli production of bubble oxygenators. *J. Extracorp. Technol.*, **14**, 445–52.

Sanderson, J. M., Wright, G. and Sims, F. W. (1972) Brain damage in dogs immediately following pulsatile and non-pulsatile blood flows in extracorporeal circulation. *Thorax*, **27**, 275–86.

Selman, M. W., McAlpine, W. A. and Ratan, R. D. (1967) The effectiveness of various heart lung machines in the elimination of microbubbles from the circulation. *J. Thorac. Cardiovasc. Surg.*, **53**, 613–17.

Semb, B. K. H., Pederson, T., Hatterland, K., Storstein, L. and Lilleaasen, P. (1982) Doppler ultrasound estimation of bubble removal by various arterial line filters during extracorporeal circulation. *Scand. J. Thorac. Cardiovasc. Surg.*, **16**, 55–62.

Senning, A. (1952) Ventricular fibrillation during extracorporeal circulation used as a method to prevent air embolism and to facilitate intracardiac operations. *Acta Chir. Scand.* (Suppl. 171).

Severinghaus, J. W. (1966) Blood gas calculator. *J. Appl. Physiol.*, **21**, 1108–16.

Slogoff, S., Girgis, K. Z. and Keats, A. S. (1982) Etiologic factors in neuropsychiatric complications associated with cardiopulmonary bypass. *Anaesth. Analag.*, **61**, 903–11.

Solis, R. T. and Gibbs, M. B. (1972) Filtration of microaggregates in stored blood. *Transfusion*, **12**, 245–50.

Solis, R. T., Goldfinger, D., Gibbs, M. B. and Zeller, J. A. (1974) Physical characteristics of microaggregates in stored blood. *Transfusion*, **14**, 538–49.

Solis, R. T., Kennedy, P. S., Beall, A. C., Noon, G. P. and DeBakey, M. E. (1975) Cardiopulmonary bypass. Microembolisation and platelet aggregation. *Circulation*, **52**, 103–8.

Solis, R. T., Noon, G. P., Beall, A. C. and DeBakey, M. E. (1974) Particulate microembolism during cardiac operation. *Ann. Thorac. Surg.*, **17**, 332–44.

Stockard, J. J., Bickford, R. G., Myers, R. R. *et al.* (1974) Hypotension induced changes in cerebral function during cardiac surgery. *Stroke*, **5**, 730–46.

Swank, R. L. (1961) Alteration of blood on storage: measurement of adhesiveness of 'ageing' platelets and leukocytes and their removal by filtration. *New Engl. J. Med.*, **265**, 728–33.

Swank, R. L. (1982) Platelet and platelet–neutrophil aggregates. Their genesis and pathophysiological effects. *Proc. Am. Acad. Cardiovasc. Perf.*, **4**, 95.

Taber, R. E., Maraan, B. M. and Tomatis, L. (1970) Prevention of air embolism during open heart surgery. A study of the role of trapped air in the left ventricle. *Surgery*, **68**, 685.

Tamari, Y., Aledort, L., Puszkin, E. *et al.* (1975) Functional changes in platelets during extracorporeal circulation. *Ann. Thorac. Surg.*, **19**, 639–47.

Taylor, K. M. (1982) Editorial: Brain damage during open heart surgery. *Thorax*, **37**, 873–6.

Taylor, K. M. (1983) Assessment of cerebral damage during cardiopulmonary bypass with particular reference to perfusion and microembolic damage. *Am. Acad. Cardiovasc. Perf.*, **4**, 110–13.

Taylor, K. M., Dawson, H., Desai, J., Jamieson, M. P. G., Brannan, J. J. and McKenna, J. M. (1983) The effect of methyl prednisolone pretreatment on brain damage in dogs during cardiopulmonary bypass. *J. Cardiovasc. Surg.*, **24**, 622–7.

Taylor, K. M., Devlin, B. J., Mittra, S. M., Gillan, J. G., Brannan, J. J. and McKenna, J. M. (1980) Assessment of cerebral damage during open heart surgery: A new experimental model. *Scand. J. Thorac. Cardiovasc. Surg.*, **14**, 197–203.

Ts'ao, C., Lin, C. Y., Glagov, S. and Replogle, R. L. (1973) Disseminated leucocyte injury during open heart surgery. *Arch. Pathol.*, **95**, 357–65.

Tufo, H. M., Ostfeld, A. M., Shekelle, R. (1970) Central nervous system dysfunction following open heart surgery. *J. Am. Med. Assoc.*, **212**, 1333–40.

Valentin, N. and Vilhelmsen, R. (1976) Blood and tissue silicone in extracorporeal circulation. *J. Cardiovasc. Surg.*, **17**, 20–6.

Van den Dungen, J. J. A. M., Karliczek, G. F., Brenken, U. and Wildevuur, C. R. H. (1982) Clinical study of blood trauma during perfusion with membrane and bubble oxygenators. *J. Thorac. Cardiovasc. Surg.*, **83**, 108–16.

Walker, I. D., Davidson, J. F., Faichney, A., Wheatley, D. J. and Davidson, K. G. (1981) A double blind study of prostacyclin in cardiopulmonary bypass surgery. *Br. J. Haematol.*, **49**, 415–23.

Walton, H. G., Sugden, E. H. and White, J. A. (1982) A look at the BOS-10 and H-1500 oxygenators. *J. Extracorp. Technol.*, **14**, 405–9.

Ward, C. A., Ruegsegger, B., Stanga, D. and Zingg, W. (1974) Reduction of platelet adhesion to biomaterial by the removal of gas nuclei. *Trans. Am. Soc. Artif. Int. Organs*, **20A**, 77–84.

Wellons, H. A. Jr and Nolan, B. F. (1973) Prevention of air embolism due to trapped air in filters used in extracorporeal circuits. *J. Thorac. Cardiovasc. Surg.*, **65**, 476–8.

Wilson, J. W. (1972) Prevention of pulmonary cellular damage with pharmacological doses of corticosteroid. *Surg. Gynaecol. Obstet.*, **13**, 675–84.

Woods, J. E., Kirklin, J. W., Owen, C. A., Thompson, J. H. and Taswell, H. F. (1967) Effects of bypass surgery of coagulation sensitive clotting factors. *Mayo Clin. Proc.*, **42**, 724–35.

Wright, G. and Sanderson, J. M. (1976) Cellular aggregation and destruction during blood circulation and oxygenation. *Thorax*, **31**, 405–9.

Wright, G. and Sanderson, J. M. (1979) Cellular aggregation and trauma in cardiotomy suction systems. *Thorax*, **34**, 621–8.

Young, J. A., Kisker, C. T. and Doty, D. B. (1978) Adequate anticoagulation during cardiopulmonary bypass determined by active clotting time and the appearance of fibrin monomer. *Ann. Thorac. Surg.*, **26**, 231–40.

19
Micropore filtration during cardiopulmonary bypass

L. BERMAN and F. MARIN

19.1 INTRODUCTION

Microembolic damage to vital organs, particularly the brain, is one of the recognized hazards associated with cardiopulmonary bypass (CPB) procedures. It has been shown that particulate and gaseous microemboli present prior to and generated during extracorporeal circulation may significantly influence the neurological status of cardiac surgery patients (Aberg and Kihlgren, 1977; Allardyce *et al.*, 1966; Branthwaite, 1973, 1975; Clark *et al.*, 1975b; Gervin *et al.*, 1974; Hill *et al.*, 1969; Kritikou and Branthwaite, 1977; Patterson *et al.*, 1974). Micropore filters were developed to prevent the perfusion of microemboli during cardiopulmonary bypass (CPB). It is the purpose of this chapter to review the use of micropore filters in the arterial, cardiotomy, cardioplegia and recirculation lines of the CPB circuit.

19.2 DEVELOPMENT OF CARDIOPULMONARY BYPASS FILTERS

19.2.1 Pioneering work

The development of extracorporeal blood filters began with two independent lines of investigation. In the early 1960s, Dr R. L. Swank of the University of Oregon Health Sciences Center observed that the microviscosity of stored blood was significantly greater than that of fresh blood. His subsequent analysis of this phenomenon lead to the discovery of microaggregates (Swank, 1961), composed of non-viable platelets and granulocytes, which accumulate in banked blood during storage. These particles range from 10 μm in size upwards. Microaggregate concentrations of 10^8/unit of stored blood have been reported (Solis *et al.*, 1974).

Swank developed the approach of using a dacron wool filter to remove microaggregates from blood. Its initial clinical use was in the cardiotomy line of the extracorporeal circuit, to remove particulate contamination before returning the blood to the main CPB circuit. Clinical studies provided evidence that removal of particulate contamination from cardiotomy blood reduced the level of cerebral vascular microembolization, and had a beneficial effect on the neurological status of patients undergoing CPB (Hill *et al.*, 1970; Osborn *et al.*, 1970).

Concurrently, Dr R. H. Patterson, at the Cornell University Medical College in New York City studied the effects of microemboli on cerebral function. He demonstrated the presence of both particulate and gas microemboli, and provided evidence that the oxygenator was an important source of microemboli (Kessler and Patterson, 1970; Patterson and Kessler, 1969). Dogs undergoing CPB exhibited depressed brain metabolism presumed to be due to cerebral microvascular embolization. Dr Patterson reinforced this evidence by designing and constructing a screen micropore filter which when placed in the arterial line reduced the number of perfused microemboli and very significantly improved the animals' neurological status following CPB (Patterson *et al.*, 1971). This 25 μm pore stainless-steel mesh filter proved unsuitable for human CPB as the necessarily higher flow rates produced an unacceptable degree of haemolysis.

19.2.2 Developments in the 1970s

The earliest commercially available filters for use in CPB were manufactured by Pioneer–Swank (dacron wool depth filter) and Pall Biomedical Products Corporation (polyester-mesh screen filter).

The Pioneer–Swank filter was originally provided for cardiotomy line use. A modified version was later made available for arterial line use. The Pall filter was designed for use in both the cardiotomy and arterial line. Several other manufacturers subsequently provided variants of the original depth and screen filters though the depth filtration approach for arterial line filters was discontinued by all but two manufacturers. (Discussion of contemporary products is found in Section 19.7)

19.3 ORIGINS OF PARTICULATE AND GASEOUS CONTAMINATION

19.3.1 Particulate contamination

(a) Intrinsic contamination

There are a variety of ways in which particulate contamination may be introduced into the CPB circuit prior to use. Stored blood, used in priming the circuit or administered during the surgical procedure, will contribute particulate contamination due to the microaggregates of degenerated platelets and granulocytes, fibrin and occasional red blood cells (Solis *et al.*, 1974; Swank, 1961). Inorganic particulate debris is inevitably generated within the various components of the circuit during manufacture and assembly. The amount of inorganic contamination depends upon both the manufacturer's attention to proper flushing of components and the user's care during assembly (Ashmore *et al.*, 1968; Clark *et al.*, 1975a; Dimmick *et al.*, 1975; Dutton and Edmunds, 1973; Pastoriza-Pinol *et al.*, 1979; Reed *et al.*, 1974).

(b) Extrinsic contamination

Particulate contamination is also generated during the bypass procedure. The cardiotomy reservoir is the most obvious source of particulate contamination in the bypass circuit. Bone and tissue fragments, and fat emboli present in the operating field are picked up in the suction line and passed into the main circuit. Flow turbulence and stagnation, blood–air interfaces, and mechanical trauma from roller pumps denature proteins and damage cellular blood components. These then aggregate, leading to the formation of potentially harmful particulate emboli.

Other aspects of extracorporeal circulation also generate particulate contamination. During CPB, blood is exposed to a large area of 'foreign' surface. Platelets and blood proteins react with this surface, leading to the formation of microaggregates. The blood–gas interface and flow turbulence in bubble oxygenators and cardiotomy lines also generate particulate contamination (Addonizio *et al.*, 1982; Allardyce *et al.*, 1966; Chenoweth *et al.*, 1981; deLeval *et al.*, 1975; Dutton *et al.*, 1974; Heiden *et al.*, 1975; Jacob and Hammerschmidt, 1981; Jones *et al.*, 1982; Kessler and Patterson, 1970; Loop *et al.*, 1976; Page *et al.*, 1974; Radegren *et al.*, 1982; Solen *et al.*, 1978; Solis *et al.*, 1975a,b; Van Den Dungen, *et al.*, 1982; Wright and Sanderson, 1979).

Due to the repeated compression of tubing in the pump race, roller pumps stress the inner wall of the tubing causing spallation. This process (spallation) relates to a number of factors, including the tubing material, duration and velocity of pumping, and the degree of pump head occlusion (Kurusz *et al.*, 1980).

19.3.2. Gaseous contamination

Generation of gaseous emboli in the bypass circuit may occur in two ways: creation of microbubbles and inadvertent massive air entry into the fluid flow path.

(a) Microbubbles

Microbubbles are continuously generated and entrained in the circulating blood during bypass. Bubble oxygenators are the most obvious source of microbubbles. Within the oxygenator, integral defoaming devices effectively eliminate large bubbles, but not microbubbles (Kessler and Patterson, 1970; Mollison and Streczyn, 1976; Patterson and Kessler, 1969; Pedersen *et al.*, 1982; Semb *et al.*, 1982). Membrane oxygenators, because of their mode of operation, do not normally generate high levels of microbubbles. However, small leaks in the membrane separating the gas and blood compartments, or insufficient pressure differentials between the blood and gas compartments may lead to microbubble formation.

A further list of inadvertent sources of microbubbles in the bypass circuit has been archived in the literature, including pin hole leaks in the arterial line proximal to the pump, kinking or clamping the arterial line, striking the oxygenator, vortexing in the arterial reservoir, and excessive or rapid warming of the circulating blood.

(b) Massive air embolism

The clinical occurrence of massive air embolism is a relatively rare, but life-threatening, event. A number of causes of massive air entry into the bypass circuit have been documented, including; rupture of arterial lines and connectors, oxygenator defects, and arterial reservoir run-dry due to insufficient venous return, or sudden acceleration of a roller pump (Christman and Jurusz, 1980; Kurusz *et al.*, 1979; Mills and Ochsner, 1980; Spampinato *et al.*, 1981; Stoney *et al.*, 1980).

The high morbidity and mortality related to these occurrences detailed in the clinical setting was reported by Stoney *et al.* (1980), and indicated the need for effective devices, such as arterial line micropore filters, to reduce the risk to patients. (Massive air embolism is discussed in detail in Chapter 21.)

19.4 MECHANISMS OF FILTRATION

Two distinctly different filtration mechanisms for blood exist. They are exemplified by the filters developed respectively by Swank and Patterson. The dacron wool Swank filter is a representative 'depth' type filter, the Patterson filter a 'screen' type filter.

19.4.1 Depth filters

Depth filters for blood filtration contain packed filter 'media' (filtering materials) which may be composed of either packed fibres ('wool') or porous plastic foam. These media provide (1) a tortuous path through which fluids must pass, and (2) a large wetted surface for particle adsorption. Very large particles are intercepted at the initial surface of the medium. Smaller particles are carried by the fluid flow into the medium. The fluid readily passes around the internal structure of the medium, while particles entrained in the fluid stream resist directional change, due to their inertial mass. The particles therefore move along a straighter path and tend to impact on the wetted internal surface of the medium. Adsorptive forces retain particles on the internal surfaces of the medium.

The particle removal efficiency of depth-type filters is a function of the amount of wetted surface area available for adsorption, the physicochemical nature of the particles and filter media, and the size of the passageways available for flow. The efficiency of particle removal increases as flow path becomes longer or narrower.

Certain functional characteristics must be considered when designing depth filters. Increased depth or decreased effective pathway diameter will lead to an increased pressure drop (resistance to flow) across the medium. Increased depth also increases blood–foreign surface contact area. During filter design these factors must be weighed against those in the previous paragraph, depending on the intended conditions of use.

Particles too large to enter the filter bed accumulate on the outer or 'first' surface of the medium (Fig. 19.1). If there are significant numbers of such particles, the effective life of the filter becomes limited by its available first surface area. In order to increase the first surface area of a depth filter, the total filter medium volume and, therefore, the total foreign surface contact area are increased significantly. Therefore a judicious balance must be made in the design of such filters.

Particle removal efficiency in depth filters depends not only on the probability of impaction, but also on the availability of adsorptive surface for particle removal. During use, the available adsorptive surface becomes coated with particles, and the adsorption of additional particles decreases. Eventually, saturation may occur and particles larger than the initial design limit of the filter can pass through the filter. This 'saturation-breakthrough' phenomenon is characteristic of any depth type of filter medium, and serves as a major determinant of the effective filtration capacity of depth filters.

19.4.2 Screen filters

Screen filters for blood have filter media composed of polymer threads woven into a fabric of defined porosity Fig 19.2. Particles larger than the pores are physically retained on the first surface of the filter. Particle removal is an absolute function of pore size. This mechanism is termed Direct Interception; adsorptive forces are not involved to any significant extent. Therefore, screen

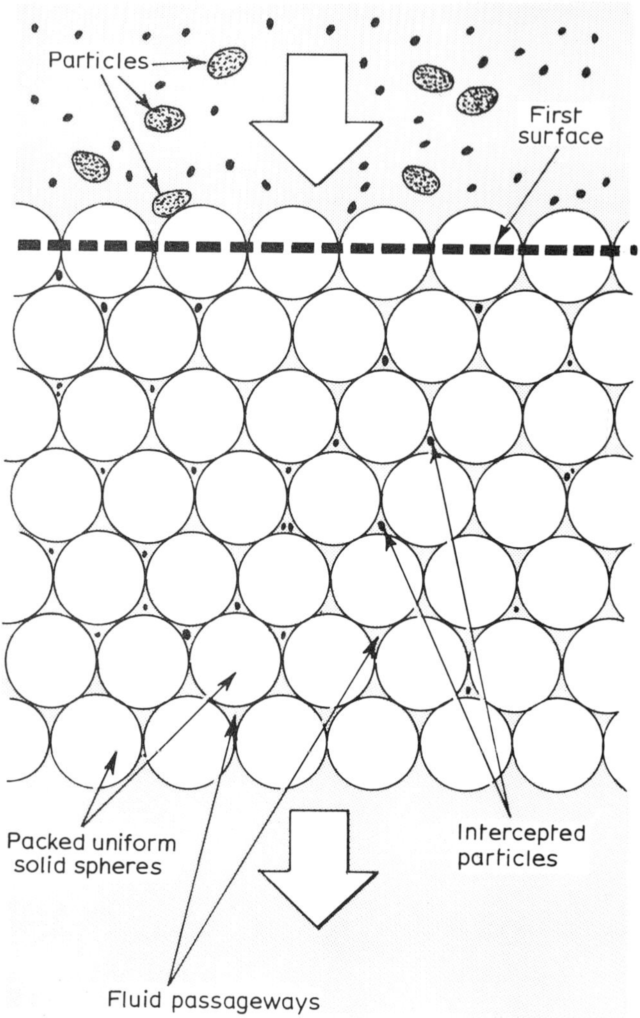

Fig. 19.1 Depth filter model.

filters will not allow particles larger than their pore size rating through the medium, even with prolonged use. Screen filter media present relatively small wetted foreign surface areas, compared with depth filters. Within a given volume of housing, the first surface area can be increased, by pleating the medium, thereby increasing capacity without inordinately increasing total foreign contact surface area. The large open surface area of screen filters reduces both the velocity of flow through and the pressure differential across the medium. Shear-induced damage to cellular blood components is thereby reduced or avoided.

19.5 MATERIALS USED IN MICROPORE FILTER CONSTRUCTION

Of all the parts of a filter, the greatest amount of 'foreign' surface area in contact with the blood is in the filter medium (screen or depth). Two types of materials are used in arterial filter screens: polyester and nylon. Recently, there has been interest in the effects of nylon on complement activation in perfused blood. Chenoweth *et al*., (1981) reported an increase in C3a and C5a fragments in perfused blood due to the nylon tricot in an oxygenator defoamer. Yellon *et al.* (1981) reported increased complement activation from the nylon mesh of an arterial line blood filter compared to a polyester mesh.

Clinical data may indicate a significant pathophysiological effect of this *in vitro* complement activation. The Emergency Care Research Institute reported a high incidence of clinical problems with a nylon medium filter (Berkowitz, 1980) and, in another study, psychometric testing of patients showed poorer postoperative test results when a nylon medium filter was used, compared to a polyester medium filter (Wellons and Nolan, 1973). The role of other factors, such as pore size and flow dynamics, has not yet been determined.

As to the aetiology of these effects, other work suggests a possible mechanism: electron micrography of clinically used filters has shown a heavy deposit of granulocytes on nylon fibre media, compared to polyester (Kurusz *et al.*). This heavy deposition may have been secondary to complement activation by the nylon medium (Jacob and Hammerschmidt, 1981).

Further research is needed to clarify fully the initial observations with respect to the biocompatibility of nylon in heparinized blood perfusion circuits.

19.6 GASEOUS EMBOLI RETENTION MECHANISMS OF MICROPORE FILTERS

In addition to removing particulate contaminants from blood, micropore filters can prevent the passage of both microbubbles and massive air emboli. This property is especially important in arterial line applications. Filter media are composed of materials which are relatively hydrophilic (water-loving). Hydrophilic substances interact strongly, at the molecular level, with water; in other words, such substances are 'wetted'. When a porous hydrophilic medium is wetted, *adhesive* forces act to hold a layer of water in intimate contact with the medium, and *cohesive* forces hold bulk water, not directly in contact with the medium, within the pores.

This combination of adhesive and cohesive forces resists displacement of liquid from the pores by gases. In a flow situation, this means that liquid will pass through the pores, but undissolved gas will be held back up to a limiting differential pressure (ΔP).

The actual amount of differential pressure required to force gas through a circular pore, is termed the 'bubble point pressure' (BPP) and can be approximated by the following equation:

$$BPP = \frac{4\gamma \cos \theta}{d}$$

where γ = surface tension of the liquid (a measure of cohesion); θ = wetting angle of liquid/solid interaction (a measure of adhesion); d = diameter of pore.

For a polyester screen filter with 40 μm pores, and plasma as the wetting agent, the bubble point pressure is approximately 37 mmHg (4.9 kPa). This may appear to be a low pressure when compared with the 200–250 mmHg (26.7–33.3 kPa) gauge pressure on the arterial line pressure. However, due to the large open area available in screen type arterial filter media, the ΔP across the medium is typically only a few mmHg, even at high flow rates, and even with peak systrolic pressure of pulsatile perfusions. Therefore, under normal conditions the ΔP across the medium is not sufficient to push microbubbles larger than the pore size through the filter medium.

Depth-type filters will also resist air passage by the same mechanisms. However, due to the irregular shape and varied sizes of the depth filter's passageways, the BPP is not readily predictable.

The ability of arterial line filters to prevent the passage of air protects the patient not only from microbubbles and small air boli, but also from the effects of massive air entry into the bypass circuit. Bulk air will not pass through the medium, unless the ΔP across the medium exceeds BPP. As stated earlier, when blood flow occurs through the total available surface area of the filter medium, the pressure drop at 5 l min^{-1} is only a few mmHg. Consider a hypothetical screen filter, with an upstream chamber volume of 100 ml, and a filter medium with area capable of providing a trans-screen pressure drop of 3 mmHg (0.4 kPa). Entry of 50 ml of air, due to whatever accidents or circuit malfunction, into the filter's upstream chamber, will occlude one half of the filter medium. The pressure drop across the medium would double to 6 mmHg (0.8 kPa). Further introduction of air will reduce the surface available for blood flow and increase the trans-screen pressure drop until the bubble point is finally exceeded. At high flow rates, this will provide additional seconds of response time for the perfusionist or surgeon (see Chapter 21, Fig. 21.3).

This margin of safety can be further enhanced by incorporating a vent-line between the filter's upstream chamber and a non-pressurized reservoir in the circuit, preferably the oxygenator (Fig. 19.3) Under these conditions, as air is pumped into the filter, it displaces blood from the vent-line as well as the upstream chamber of the filter. Once the vent-line is purged of blood, air will flow through the line at high rates preventing the build-up of excessive pressure on the upstream side of the screen, which might otherwise reach the BPP. The use of a vent-line is highly recommended due to the greatly increased margin of safety it provides. Employment of a vent-line of short length and with minimal flow constrictions, and placement of the filter as low as practical, relative to the patient, will provide significant protection from massive air embolism, depending on flow rates and other variables.

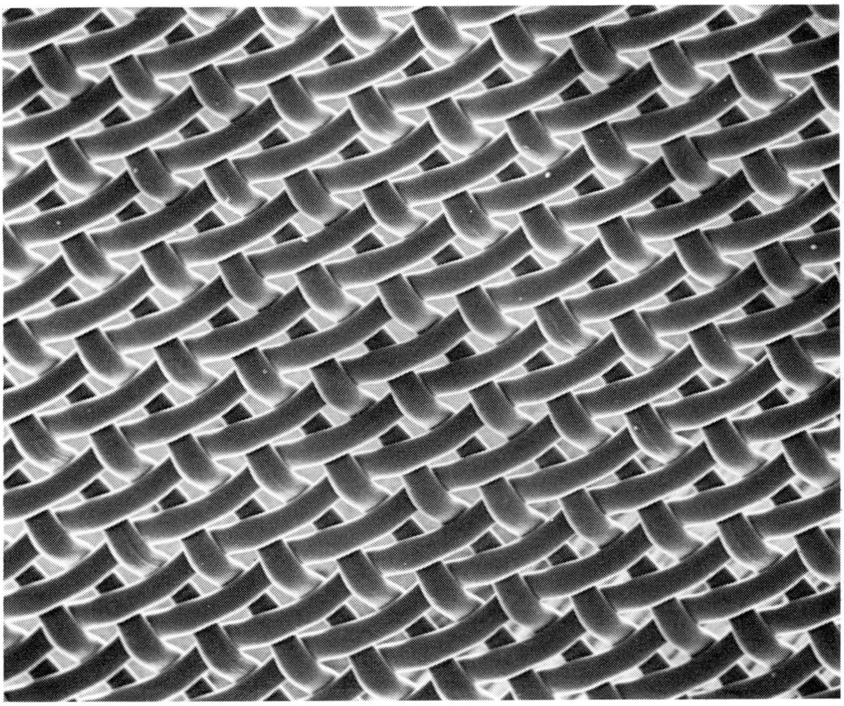

Fig. 19.2 Screen filter media.

19.7 CURRENT PRACTICE IN MICROPORE FILTRATION DURING CPB

Two recent surveys by Binford *et al.* (1981) and Kurusz *et al.* (1983) tabulated the use of micropore filters (and other equipment and techniques in perfusion) in the USA.

These surveys indicate the following trends in micropore filtration.

(1) Arterial line filters are being employed by an increasing majority of open-heart teams. Approximately 78% of perfusionists surveyed use arterial line filters. With respect to the need for arterial filters, 48% of respondents to the recent survey by Kurusz *et al.* (1983) reported having seen gross air emboli trapped or vented by their arterial line filter.
(2) The screen or direct interception filter is becoming dominant over depth filters for arterial line use (99% vs. 1%). Manufacturers introducing arterial line filters for the first time have chosen the screen type mechanism.
(3) The vast majority of perfusion circuits (97%) incorporate a cardiotomy line micropore filter, either in the line below the cardiotomy reservoir, or built into the reservoir.
(4) Almost all circuits (97%) incorporate an oxygen line filter.

Arterial line filters available in the US and/or Europe and their characteristics are listed in Table 19.1.

Table 19.1 Arterial line filters available in the US and Europe

Adult/pediatric, neonatal	*Brand and model*	*Media composition*	*Pore size/ rating (μm)*	*Screen or depth*
Adult	Bentley AF10	Nylon	25	Screen
Adult	Delta BT37	Nylon	37	Screen
Adult	Johnson & Johnson Intercept 1330	Nylon	20	Screen
Adult	Pall EC3840	Polyester	40	Screen
Adult	Bard (Harvey) H-625	Polyester	33	Screen
Adult	Viggo Swank HF6000	Dacron Polyester	13 nominal	Depth
Adult	Shiley SAF20	Nylon	20	Screen
Adult	Dideco Aggar D360	Nylon/Polyester	40	Screen/ Depth
Pediatric/ neonatal	Pall LPE1440	Polyester	40	Screen
Pediatric/ neonatal	Bentley AF5	Nylon	25	Screen
Neonatal	Delta K37	Nylon	37	Screen

The accompanying photograph (Fig. 19.4) shows many of those filters listed in Table 19.1.

The function of all the screen filters is similar in principle to the original 40 μm screen (Pall EC3840). As shown in Fig. 19.3, blood enters the filter housing through an inlet port and passes to the filter medium which it

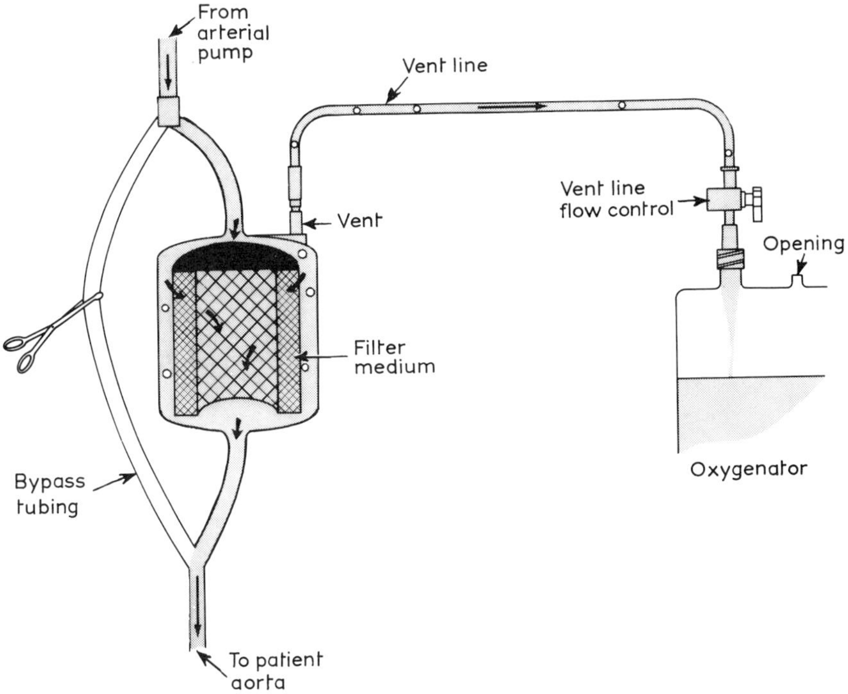

Fig. 19.3 Circuit connections for arterial line filtration during CPB.

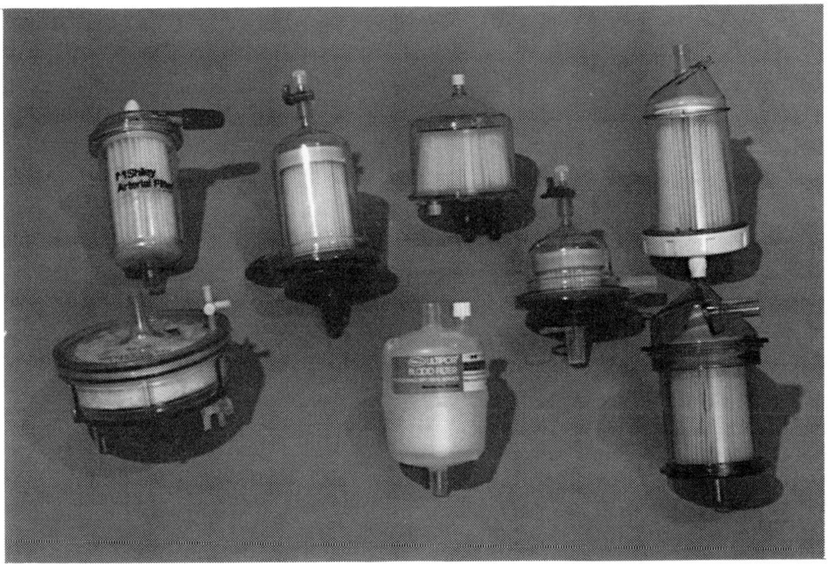

Fig. 19.4 A selection of arterial line filters for CPB.

penetrates from outside to inside. The screen filter medium is arranged in a cylindrical configuration. Gaseous and solid emboli are retained by the external surface of the screen, while the blood passes through to the inside of the cylinder and out of the filter housing through an outlet port.

Retained gas emboli tend to coalesce and rise to the top of the 'upstream' chamber. They will remain here during the perfusion (so long as the total gas volume retained does not occlude a large portion of the filter mesh). When the vent is left open throughout the perfusion (as recommended by these authors) gas emboli will automatically exit the vent and pass through the vent-line to a component of the circuit which is itself vented to the atmosphere. Vent-lines are included by 95% of perfusionists using arterial line filters (Kurusz *et al.*, 1983).

19.7.1 Venting of arterial line filters

When possible, the filter vent should lead to a chamber of the oxygenator which is constantly vented to atmosphere. In cases where the cardiotomy reservoir must be used to collect the vented fluid, it is essential never to pressurize the cardiotomy reservoir without first closing the vent flow control or utilizing an effective valve to ensure unidirectional flow. Otherwise, air could be forced retrograde from the pressurized cardiotomy reservoir into the filter and arterial line.

The arterial line filter vent port is often used, for convenience, for two other functions:

(1) Arterial line pressure monitoring (by 62% of respondents in the Kurusz survey).
(2) Sampling of arterial line blood for blood gas analysis.

These authors recommend that, if practical, these procedures should not interrupt the continuous flow through the vent (often called purge-line blood flow). A flow control valve which will allow both functions to occur simultaneously, has been developed for this purpose.

19.7.2 Priming of micropore filters

The goal when priming an arterial line filter is to remove all gas bubbles during the recirculation of priming fluid prior to CPB. Each manufacturer should provide priming instructions for his product. Many perfusionists (73% according to the Kurusz study) flush their circuit with medical grade CO_2 prior to priming. The higher solubility of CO_2 in the priming fluid, compared to the O_2 and N_2 normally present, provides a speedier debubbling of the circuit, including the filter (Wellons and Nolan, 1973).

19.7.3 Safety bypass line

Many manufacturers recommend the use of a safety bypass line around the arterial filter. A safety bypass line consists of 2 Y-connectors plus a length of tubing making an alternate flow path around the filter (Fig. 19.3). The safety bypass line is primed during pre-CPB recirculation and clamped off for the duration of the procedure. Should the perfusionist, for whatever reason, decide to discontinue flow through the filter, he removes the clamp from the bypass line and clamps off the inflow to and outflow from the filter. In practice, the use of this bypass line is rarely needed. Of perfusionists in the US using arterial line filters 93% include safety bypass lines in their perfusion circuits (Kurusz *et al.*, 1983).

19.8 ANCILLARY CPB CIRCUIT FILTERS

19.8.1 Pre-bypass filters

Pre-bypass filters were developed to deal with the problem of particulate contamination arising during manufacture and assembly of the CPB system. The presence of this type of particulate contamination has been well documented. Particles range in size from 5 to 500 μm. The number and composition of particles present in any given system are highly variable. Cotton and plastic fibres, hair, dust, plastic fragments, proteinaceous material and other unidentified solids have been described (Ashmore *et al.*, 1968; Clark *et al*, 1975a; Dimmick *et al.*, 1975; Dutton and Edmunds, 1973; Pastoriza-Pinol *et al.*, 1979; Reed *et al.*, 1974). There are currently at least four manufacturers of filters specifically intended for pre-bypass applications. These filters are designed to remove particles larger than 5 μm in diameter at flow rates up to 6 l min^{-1}. Because of the 5 μm removal rating, these filters are limited to use with crystalloid priming fluids only.

19.8.2 Cardioplegia filters

Cardioplegia solutions are employed to arrest cardiac activity and protect the myocardium from the effects of interrupted perfusion. These aims are accomplished by infusing a cold solution of varying composition through the coronary circulation. There are a number of potential risks present with this procedure, including the infusion of particulate contamination and air in the form of microbubbles or bolus into the coronary arteries (Mortensen *et al.*, 1981). Because of these potential risks, the use of a filter which removes particulate contamination and prevents perfusion of air is desirable (Hearse *et al.*, 1983). Filters specifically designed for cardioplegia infusion are beginning to appear commercially. One major distinction must be made; filters for cardioplegia solution containing blood will have different requirements than those intended for non-haemic cardioplegia solutions.

19.9 CLINICAL AND LABORATORY STUDIES OF MICROPORE FILTRATION

There are two primary concerns regarding any medical device. It must be both safe and efficacious in its proposed application. Various design factors interact and contribute to the overall performance of micropore filters and their effect on recirculating blood, including:

(1) The pore size through which the cellular components pass.
(2) The total area of wetted blood–surface contact.
(3) The degree of flow turbulence.
(4) The type and number of materials composing the filter and its medium.

It is often difficult to assess the specific contribution of individual design features. However, studies have been conducted which evaluate the overall performance of these devices in terms of safety and efficacy.

19.9.1 Safety

The primary safety factor is that blood components passing through the filter should not be damaged. A number of studies have examined the effects of arterial line filters on erythrocytes, platelets, leucocytes and plasma protein components.

Changes in plasma free-haemoglobin levels provide some measure of the extent of haemolysis during CPB. Some haemolysis inevitably occurs during CPB, whether or not a micropore filter is present, due to shear and other stresses generated by roller pumps, and more particularly to flow turbulence and blood–gas interfaces in cardiotomy circuits and bubble oxygenators (see Chapter 15). Patterson and Twichell (1971), Guidoin *et al.* (1976), and Skagseth *et al.* (1974) demonstrated that the insertion of a 40 μm screen micropore filter did not increase haemolysis. Guidoin found that haemolysis was increased by the presence of dacron wool or polyurethane foam depth filters but not with polyester screen filters.

Platelet, leucocyte, and fibrin levels often decrease during CPB, independent of filter use. Various factors, including blood–air interfaces, and foreign surface contact have been implicated in the denaturation and adsorption of serum proteins and the aggregation of platelets and leucocytes during CPB. A micropore filter, like any other component in the CPB circuit, has the potential to interact with blood components. However, studies have failed to demonstrate significant losses of blood components due to micropore filters

(Patterson *et al.*, 1971; Patterson and Twichell, 1971). Some early studies claimed that filters caused excessive protein loss or cell aggregation (Heimbecker *et al.*, 1976). These results probably reflect inadequate rinsing prior to fixation, inadequate coagulation control, or both, and have not been sustained by subsequent studies.

The bioreactivity of materials used for filter construction deserves serious consideration. A report by Chenoweth *et al.* (1981) showed that nylon is a potent activator of the complement cascade. Complement activation is known to enhance granulocyte aggregation and sequestration in the pulmonary microvasculature, with subsequent release of vasoactive substances (Jacob and Hammerschmidt, 1981). Studies by Kurusz *et al.* (1981) demonstrate greater leucocyte adherence to a nylon screen filter medium than to a polyester screen medium, suggesting that nylon is intrinsically more bioreactive than polyester. This raises concern among some investigators about the inclusion of nylon in oxygenators and micropore filters, although definitive studies of the clinical effects have not, as yet, been carried out.

19.9.2 Efficacy of micropore filters in clinical practice

A number of studies have been carried out *in vitro* to examine the efficacy of micropore filters in removing particulate and gaseous microemboli from circulating fluids. Although technically difficult to perform, all studies indicate that micropore filters are effective in removing particulate and gaseous microemboli (Loop *et al.*, 1976; Mollison and Streczyn, 1976).

More importantly, laboratory and clinical studies examining the efficacy of micropore filters in reducing patient morbidity and mortality during CPB are available. Hill *et al.* (1970) reported a decrease in patient mortality, from 19.8% to 6.5% following the inclusion of a micropore filter in the cardiotomy line. The incidence of non-fat cerebral embolization also declined from 31% to 4.2%. Branthwaite (1975), measuring changes in cerebral electrical activity among patients undergoing CPB found that serious postoperative neurological sequelae were associated with rapid depression of brain activity, particularly at the initiation of bypass. Minimizing hypotension and the inclusion of a 40 μm polyester screen micropore filter in the arterial line significantly reduced the incidence and severity of depressed brain activity. Carlson *et al.* (1973) examined the effect of inclusion of arterial line filters on the neurological status of patients undergoing bypass using pre- and postoperative Bender–Gestalt visual motor tests. Again, the presence of an arterial line filter provided significant protection of neurological function. An extensive study of the factors influencing the neurological effects of CPB was carried out by Aberg (1974), using a battery of perception/motor tests. Significantly better patient outcomes were associated with the use of arterial line micropore filters.

Recently, more direct measures of damage to central nervous tissue have been developed. These tests rely on measuring the presence, in the cerebrospinal fluid, of biochemical markers of brain injury, released by damaged tissue. Taylor has shown that the level of brain-specific creatine phosphokinase (CPK-B) increases significantly in dogs during CPB (Taylor *et al.*, 1980). Studies by Kjekshus *et. al.* (1980) have shown a strong correlation between the level of CPK-B in the cerebrospinal fluid and the degree of neurological damage caused by cerebral ischaemia. Aberg and Kihlgren (1977) studied the enzyme adenylate kinase as a marker for brain cell injury. The magnitude of changes in adenylate kinase levels in the cerebrospinal fluid correlate well with the degree of neurological dysfunction detected by standard psychomotor tests. Of relevance to this discussion is the observation by Taylor *et al.* (1980) that significant neurological protection was provided by the inclusion of a 40 μm polyester screen arterial filter in the bypass circuit. Whereas dogs perfused without an arterial filter had elevated cerebrospinal CPK-B levels, dogs perfused with an arterial filter had significantly lower levels of CPK-B.

Most studies, to date, have simply addressed the question of whether an arterial filter provided significant improvement in the patient's status post-surgery. Recently, however, the first study comparing the efficacy of two different arterial filters was reported. Willner *et al.* (1983) compared the neuropsychiatric performance of patients undergoing CPB with or without one of two brands of arterial filter. Their data indicate that neurological dysfunction was minimal among those patients undergoing procedures in which the 40 μm polyester screen filter was employed. Significant reductions were noted among matched patients undergoing procedures in which a 25 μm nylon screen filter was used. It is not, as yet, possible to assess specifically which design features (nylon vs. polyester, flow dynamics, pore size, etc.) might be contributing to this difference in performance.

19.10 DEVELOPMENTS IN MICROPORE FILTRATION DURING CPB

It is difficult to predict what the future will hold in terms of further development of arterial line filters. With respect to materials, we would hope that increased knowledge of blood–surface interactions will lead to materials and media with the least propensity for undesirable interactions with blood. With respect to ease of use, one looks forward to advances in technique to shorten the time required for priming and a more definitive indication of the completion of priming. Furthermore, the development of a fully automatic air venting system is another desirable advance. An integral indicator of transfilter pressure would be a useful practical feature to the perfusionist.

As typical in clinical practice, one may expect the needs of the user and patient to dictate the modification and improvement of existing products.

REFERENCES

Aberg, T. (1974) Effect of open heart surgery on intellectual function. *Scand. J. Thorac. Cardiovasc. Surg.* (Suppl. 15).

Aberg, T. and Kihlgren, M. (1977) Cerebral protection during open heart surgery. *Thorax*, **32**, 525–33.

Addonizio, V. P. , Strauss, J. F. , Chang, Li-F., Fisher, C. A. , Colman, R. W. and Edmunds, L. G. (1982) Release of lysosomal hydrolases during simulated extracorporeal circulation. *J. Thorac. Cardiovasc. Surg.*, **84**, 28.

Allardyce, D. B., Yoshida, S. H. and Ashmore, P. G. (1966) The importance of microembolism in the pathogenesis of organ dysfunction caused by prolonged use of the pump oxygenator. *J. Thorac. Cardiovasc. Surg.*, **52**, 706.

Ashmore, P. G., Suiter, V. and Ambrose, P. (1968) The incidence and effects of particulate aggregation and microembolism in pump-oxygenator systems. *J. Thorac. Cardiovasc. Surg.*, **55**, 691.

Berkowitz, D. A. (1980) Inspection and preventive maintenance of cardiopulmonary equipment and an overview of problems. *J. Extracorp. Technol.*, **12**, 68.

Binford, J. M., Miller, D. W. and Hessel, E. A. (1981) Results of a survey of the professional activities of 811 cardiopulmonary perfusionists in North America. *Proc. Am. Acad. Cardiovasc. Perf.*, **2**, 102.

Branthwaite, M. A. (1973) Detection of neurological damage during open-heart surgery. *Thorax*, **28**, 464–72.

Branthwaite, M. A. (1975) Prevention of neurological damage during open-heart surgery. *Thorax*, **30**, 258–61.

Carlson, R. G., Lande, A. J., Landis, B., Rogoz, B., Baxter, J., Patterson, R. H., Stenzel, K. and Lillehei, C. W. (1973) The Lande–Edwards membrane oxygenator during heart surgery. *J. Thorac. Cardiovasc. Surg.*, **66**, 894.

Chenoweth, D. E., Cooper, S. W., Hugli, T. E., Stewart, R. W., Blackstone, E. H. and Kirklin, J. W. (1981) Complement activation during cardiopulmonary bypass: Evidence for generation of C3a and C5a anaphylatoxins. *New Engl. J. Med.*, **304**, 497.

Christman, E. W. and Kurusz, M. (1980) Preventing massive gas embolism during cardiopulmonary bypass: A review of safety devices. *J. Extracorp. Technol.*, **12**, 115.

Clark, R. E., Dietz, D. R. and Miller, J. G. (1975a) Continuous detection of microemboli during cardiopulmonary bypass in animals and man. *Circulation*, **54**, III-74–III-78.

Clark, R. D., Margraf, H. W. and Beauchamp R. A. (1975b) Fat and solid filtration in clinical perfusions. *Surgery*, **77**, 216–24.

deLeval, M. R., Hill, J. D., Mielke, C. H., Macur, M. F. and Gerbode, F. (1975) Blood platelets and extracorporeal circulation. *J. Thorac. Cardiovasc. Surg.*, **69**, 144.

Dimmick, J. E., Bove, K. E., McAdams, A. J. and Benzino, G. E. (1975) Fiber embolization – A hazard of cardiac surgery and catheterization. *N. Engl. J. Med.*, **292**, 685.

Dutton, R. C. and Edmunds, L. H. (1973) Measurement of emboli in extracorporeal perfusion systems. *J. Thorac. Cardiovasc. Surg.*, **65**, 523.

Dutton, R. C., Edmunds, L. H., Hutchinson, J. C. and Roe, B. B. (1974) Platelet aggregate emboli produced in patients during cardiopulmonary bypass with membrane and bubble oxygenators and blood filters. *J. Thorac. Cardiovasc. Surg.*, **67**, 258.

Gervin, A. S., McNeer, J. F., Wolfe, W. G., Puckett, C. L. and Silver, D. (1974) Ultrapore hemofiltration during extracorporeal circulation. *J. Thorac. Cardiovasc. Surg.*, **67**, 237–43.

Guidoin, R., Laperche, Y., Martin, L., Awad, J. and Winchester, J. (1976) Disposable filters for microaggregate removal from extracorporeal circulation. *J. Thorac. Cardiovasc. Surg.*, **71**, 502.

Heiden, D., Mielke, C. H., Rodvien, R. and Hill, J. D. (1975) Platelets, hemostasis, and thromboembolism during treatment of acute respiratory insufficiency with extracorporeal membrane oxygenation. *J. Thorac. Cardiovasc. Surg.*, **70**, 644.

Heimbecker, R., Robert, A. and McKenzie, F. N. (1976) The extracorporeal pump filter – saint or sinner? *Ann. Thorac. Surg.*, **21**, 55.

Hill, J. D., Aguilar, M. J., Baranco, A., deLanorelle, P. and Gerbode, F. (1969) Neuropathological manifestations of cardiac surgery. *Ann. Thorac. Surg.*, **7**, 409.

Hill, J. D., Osborn, J. J., Swank, R. L., Aguilar, M. J., deLanerolle, P. and Gerbode, F. (1970) Experience using a new dacron wool filter during extracorporeal circulation. *Arch. Surg.*, **101**, 649–52.

Jacob, H. S. and Hammerschmidt, D. E. (1981) Complement induced granulocyte aggregation importance in myocardial infarction and shock lung. *J. Am. Med. Assoc.*, **245**, 2013.

Jones, H. M., Matthews, N., Vaughan, R. S. and Stark, J. M. (1982) Cardiopulmonary bypass and complement activation: involvement of classical and alternative pathways. *Anaesthesia*, **37**, 629.

Kessler, J. and Patterson, R. H. Jr. (1970) Production of microemboli by various blood oxygenators. *Ann. Thorac. Surg.*, **9**, 221–4.

Kjekshus, J. K., Vaagenes, P. and Hetland, O. (1980) Assessment of cerebral injury with spinal fluid creatine kinase (CSF-CK) in patients after cardiac resuscitation. *Scand. J. Clin. Lab. Invest.*, **40**, 437.

Kritikou, P. E. and Branthwaite, M. A. (1977) Significance of changes in cerebral electrical activity at onset, of cardiopulmonary bypass. *Thorax*, **32**, 534–8.

Kurusz, M., Schneider, B., Brown, J. and Conti, V. (1983) Filtration during open heart surgery devices techniques, opinions and complications. *Acad. Cardiovasc. Perf.*, **4**, 123–9.

Kurusz, M., Christman, E. W., Williams, E. H. and Tyler, G. F. O. (1980) Roller pump induced tubing wear: another argument in favor of arterial line filtration. *J. Extracorp. Technol.*, **12**, 49.

Kurusz, M., Schneider, B., Conti, V. R. and Williams, E. H. (1981) Scanning electron microscopy of arterial line filters following clinical cardiopulmonary bypass. Proc. First World Congress on Open Heart Technology. Franklin Scientific Projects, London.

Kurusz, M., Shaffer, C. W., Christman, E. W. and Tyers, G. F. O. (1979) Runaway pumphead: new cause of gas embolism during cardiopulmonary bypass. *J. Thorac. Cardiovasc. Surg.*, **77**, 792.

Loop, F. D., Szabo, J., Rowlinson, R. D. and Urbanek, K. (1976) Events related to microembolism during extracorporeal perfusion in man: effectiveness of in-line filtration recorded by ultrasound. *Ann. Thorac. Surg.*, **21**, 412.

Mills, N. L. and Ochsner, J. L. (1980) Massive air embolism during cardiopulmonary bypass. *J. Thorac. Cardiovasc. Surg.*, **80**, 708.

Mollison, D. R. and Streczyn, M. V. (1976) In depth evaluation of arterial line filtration of air emboli in bubble and membrane oxygenators. *AmSect Proc.*, 99.

Mortensen, J. D., Yates, W. G. and Schoenberg, A. A. (1981) *Cardiopulmonary Bypass Systems: A Study of Safety and Performance.* TR5534-010, 2, April 1981. Contract 223-80-5081 Between UBTL Division of UURI and Bureau of Medical Devices of Food and Drug Administration, University of Utah Research Institute, 520 Wahara Way, Salt Lake City, Utah 84108.

Osborn, J. J., Swank, R. L., Hill, J. D., Aguilar, M. J. and Gerbode, F. (1970) Clinical use of a dacron wool filter during perfusion for open heart surgery. *J. Thorac. Cardiovasc. Surg.*, **60**, 575–81.

Page, U. S., Bigelow, J. C., Carter, C. R. and Swank, R. L. (1974) Emboli (debris) produced by bubble oxygenators: removal by filtration. *Ann. Thorac. Surg.*, **18**, 164.

Pastoriza-Pinol, J. V., McMillan, J., Smith, B. F., Sandy, M., Lancucki, C., Stirling, G. R. and Newland, P. E. (1979) An analysis of microembolic particles originating in the extracorporeal circuit before bypass. *J. Extracorp. Technol.*, **11**, 211.

Patterson, R. H. and Kessler, J. (1969) Microemboli during cardiopulmonary bypass detected by ultrasound. *Surg. Gyn. Obstet.*, **129**, 505–10.

Patterson, R. H. Jr, Kessler, J. and Bergland, R. M. (1971) A filter to prevent cerebral damage during experimental cardiopulmonary bypass. *Surg. Gyn. Obstet.*, **132**, 71–4.

Patterson, R. H. and Twichell, J. B. (1971) Disposable filter for microemboli use in cardiopulmonary bypass and massive transfusion. *J. Am. Med. Assoc.*, **215**, 76.

Patterson, R. H. Jr, Wasser, J. S. and Porro, R. S. (1974) The effect of various filters on microembolic cerebrovascular blockade following cardiopulmonary bypass. *Ann. Thorac. Surg.*, **17**, 464–9.

Pedersen, R., Hatteland, K. and Semb, B. K. H. (1982) Bubble extraction by various arterial filters measured in vitro with doppler ultrasound techniques. *Ultrasound Med. Biol.*, **8**, 71.

Radegren, K., Aren, C. and Teger-Nilsson, A. C. (1982) Prostacyclin infusion during extracorporeal circulation for coronary bypass. *J. Thorac. Cardiovasc. Surg.*, **83**, 205.

Reed, C. C., Romangnoli, A., Taylor, D. E. and Clark, D. K. (1974) Particulate matter in bubble oxygenators. *J. Thorac. Cardiovasc. Surg.*, **68**, 971.

Semb, B. K. H., Pederson, T., Hatteland, K., Storstein, L. and Lilleaasen P. (1982) Doppler ultrasound estimation of bubble removal by various arterial line filters during extracorporeal circulation. *Scand. J. Thorac. Cardiovasc. Surg.*, **16**, 55.

Skagseth, E., Floysaker, T. and Refsum, S. B. (1974) Disposable filter for microemboli in cardiopulmonary bypass. *J. Cardiovasc. Surg.*, **15**, 318.

Solen, K. A., Whiffen, J. D. and Lightfoot, E. N. (1978) The effect of shear, specific surface and air interface on the development of blood emboli and hemolysis. *J. Biomed. Mat. Res.*, **12**, 381.

Solis, R. T., Beall, A. C., Noon, G. P. and DeBakey, M. E. (1975a) Platelet aggregation: effects of cardiopulmonary bypass. *Chest*, **67**, 558.

Solis, R. T., Goldfinger, D., Gibbs, M. B. and Zeller, J. A. (1974) Physical characteristics of microaggregates in stored blood. *Transfusion*, **14**, 538–50.

Solis, R. T., Kennedy, P. S., Beall, A. C., Noon, G. P. and DeBakey, M. E. (1975b) Cardiopulmonary bypass: microembolization and platelet aggregation. *Circulation*, **52**, 103.

Spampinato, N., Stassano, P., Gagliardi, C., Tufano, R. and Iorio, D. (1981) Massive air embolism during cardiopulmonary bypass: successful treatment with immediate hypothermia and circulatory support. *Ann. Thorac. Surg.*, **32**, 602.

Stoney, W. S., Alford, W. C., Burrus, G. R., Glassford, D. M. and Thomas C. S. (1980) Air embolism and other accidents using pump oxygenators. *Ann. Thorac. Surg.*, **29**, 336.

Swank, R. L. (1961) Alterations of blood on storage: measurement of adhesiveness of 'aging' platelets and leukocytes and their removal by filtration. *New. Engl. J. Med.*, **265**, 728–33.

Taylor, K. M., Devlin, B. J., Mittra, S. M., Gillan, J. G., Brannan, J. J. and McKenna, J. M. (1980) Assessment of cerebral damage during open-heart surgery – a new experimental model. *Scand. J. Thorac. Cardiovasc. Surg.*, **14**, 197.

Van Den Dungen, J. J. A. M., Karliczck, G. F., Brenken, U., Homan Van Der Heide, J. N. and Wildevuur, C. R. H. (1982) Clinical study of blood trauma during perfusion with membrane and bubble oxygenators. *J. Thorac. Cardiovasc. Surg.*, **83**, 108.

Wellons, H. A. and Nolan, S. P. (1973) Prevention of air embolism due to trapped air in filters used in extracorporeal circuits. *J. Thorac. Cardiovasc. Surg.*, **65**, 476–8.

Willner, A. E., Caramonte, L., Garvey, J. W., Wolpowite, A., Weisz, D., Rabiner, C. J. and Wisoff, B. G. (1983) The relationship between arterial filtration during open heart surgery and mental abstraction ability. *Proc. Am. Acad. Cardiovasc. Perf.*, **4**, 56.

Wright, G. and Sanderson, J. M. (1979) Cellular aggregation and trauma in cardiotomy suction systems. *Thorax*, **34**, 621.

Yellon, R. F., Vernick, S., and Golub, A. (1981) Effect of blood microfilters on complement activity in human blood. *Transfusion*, **21**, 610.

20
Myocardial protection – hypothermia and cardioplegia

M. V. BRAIMBRIDGE

In recent years there has been a fundamental shift in emphasis in myocardial protection away from coronary artery perfusion in its various modes towards cold cardioplegic arrest. Cardioplegic arrest allows a still, bloodless operating field, yet protects the myocardium from the effects of ischaemia by reduction of its metabolism to a minimum by coronary infusion of cold chemical cardioplegic solutions. Alternative techniques for coronary artery surgery had been ventricular fibrillation with the coronary arteries continuously perfused via the aorta, local haemostasis at the anastomotic sites being obtained by stitches or obturators, intermittent aortic occlusion or, in aortic valve surgery, continuous perfusion of the coronary arteries by cannulae. The great majority of centres – 99% in the USA – prefer cardioplegia.

Compared with valve and congenital cardiac surgery, coronary artery disease adds specific hazards to myocardial protective procedures. Distribution of blood or cardioplegic solution from the aortic root depends on residual flow through narrow arteries or collateral vessels. The myocardium may already be compromised by ischaemia or a previous episode of infarction, a situation known to be associated with greater difficulties in myocardial protection (Rosenkranz *et al.*, 1982; Balderman *et al.*, 1982). On the other hand, the ventricle is seldom hypertrophied unless hypertension or valve disease is also present.

20.1 PRETREATMENT OF THE MYOCARDIUM

The concept of pretreating the myocardium by building up its energy stores or modifying its metabolism to enable it better to withstand ischaemia is not new. Potassium, glucose and insulin (Berggren *et al.*, 1982; Lolley *et al.*, 1978), calcium antagonists (Bretschneider *et al.*, 1975; Starnes *et al.*, 1982), steroids (Goldman *et al.*, 1978; Toleda-Pereya and Jara, 1979), adenosine triphospate (Peyton *et al.*, 1982) and beta blocking agents (Boudoulas *et al.*, 1978) have all been tried. Evidence of dysrhythmia improvement is shown by many of these measures but improvement in myocardial protection is more difficult to substantiate, particularly clinically. Few units regularly pretreat their patients with the specific object of reducing ischaemic myocardial damage (Berggren *et al.*, 1982; Lolley *et al.*, 1978): most continue up to the day of surgery with the pre-operative drugs that the patient has received as his medical regimen (Boudoulas *et al.*, 1978).

Pre-operative explanation of the surgical procedure, effective premedication and quiet induction of anaesthesia by a skilled anaesthetist may be more effective in preventing operative myocardial damage than days of medication and instrumentation before anaesthesia begins (see Chapter 3 and 4).

20.2 CARDIOPLEGIA OR INTERMITTENT AORTIC OCCLUSION?

Controversy is not yet over as to whether cardioplegia or intermittent aortic occlusion is preferable for myocardial protection during cardiac surgery and a few units in the world still use coronary artery perfusion for aortic valve surgery.

Intermittent aortic occlusion has the advantage of operative simplicity, the aortic crossclamp being applied after the coronary artery has been opened and removed after the distal anastomosis has been completed when a normal beat is resumed. Mitral valve surgery may be similarlv performed. Most anastomoses can be completed within the arbitrarily set limits of 10 minutes each, and the time taken to complete three anastomoses by a trained surgeon in a patient with a good ventricle is within the limits of myocardial tolerance (Pepper *et al.*, 1982; Roberts *et al.*, 1981). Problems arise when a longer time for the procedure becomes necessary (Pepper *et al.*, 1982). The occurrence of unexpected technical difficulty may complicate any operation.

Inherent objections to intermittent aortic occlusion in terms of myocardial protection are two. A heart rendered ischaemic for a period resumes beating but, unless coronary flow returns to normal, does not repay its oxygen debt (Becker *et al.*, 1981). A beating heart does not therefore necessarily imply a fully oxygenated heart in the presence of coronary artery disease as full myocardial perfusion only occurs when all the proximal anastomoses are completed and, if some branches are not revascularised, not even then.

The second objection is the 'stunned heart' concept (Braunwald and Kloner, 1982). Serial intermittent ischaemic episodes of 5–15 min are cumulative in their infarction potential (Geft *et al.*, 1982), even with apparently adequate periods of reperfusion. These episodes aggravate the 'stunned' myocardium which follows any ischaemic interval (Braunwald and Kloner, 1982). Prolongation of ischaemic time therefore makes a technique that is adequate for rapid surgery unsafe if the total ischaemic period becomes prolonged (Pepper *et al.*, 1982).

Cold chemical cardioplegia eliminates obsession with speed as a major consideration. An unprotected heart deteriorates as a direct function of time of ischaemia (Geft *et al.*, 1982; Jones *et al.*, 1981) but cardioplegic protection removes the statistical relationship between occlusion time and myocardial damage (Pepper *et al.*, 1982; Conti *et al.*, 1978). The heart becomes still, totally relaxed, empty and manipulable. Many series, both clinical and experimental, have shown cardioplegia to be superior overall to intermittent aortic occlusion (Adappa *et al.*, 1978; Brower *et al.*, 1982; Craver *et al.*, 1978; Follette *et al.*, 1978; Hjelms and Steiness, 1982; Kirklin *et al.*, 1979; Weisel *et al.*, 1978). There are series in which intermittent aortic occlusion is equivalent in protection to cardioplegia for short periods of occlusion and in patients with good left ventricular function (Pepper *et al.*, 1982; Roberts *et al.*, 1981). There are no communications showing superiority of intermittent aortic occlusion over cardioplegia in terms of myocardial protection.

Continuous coronary perfusion via cannulae held or stitched into the coronary ostia is rarely used today. It has the fundamental disadvantages of interfering with the operative field, of maintaining tone in the heart and so limiting access, of being rarely, for technical reasons, continuous, but, of greater importance, of failing to protect adequately the inner half of the myocardium (Braimbridge *et al.*, 1977).

20.3 CARDIOPLEGIC MYOCARDIAL PROTECTION

Cardioplegic myocardial protection demands attention to detail if its full potential is to be realised. Such protection is an integral part of cardiopulmonary bypass technique. Consideration therefore needs to be given to the pump/oxygenator equipment, arterial and venous cannulation and perfusion protocols as well as cardioplegic solutions and infusion methods, maintenance of myocardial hypothermia and the problems of reperfusion when the aortic clamp is removed. The term 'infusion' is applied to the initial infusion of cardioplegic solution, 'reinfusion' to subsequent boluses and 'reperfusion' to resumption of normal aortic perfusion when the crossclamp is removed.

The three components of myocardial protection by cardioplegia are the choice of an effective solution, the maintenance of electromechanical inactivity and the use of profound topical hypothermia. Each needs consideration if maximal protection is to be achieved.

20.3.1 Cardiopulmonary bypass considerations

The conduct of cardiopulmonary bypass affects myocardial protection procedures and consideration needs to be given to systemic flow, core temperature and composition of the priming fluid. (Priming fluid composition is discussed in detail in Chapter 14.)

(a) Perfusion flow rates

Systemic arterial flow in most centres is set at $2.4\,l\,min^{-1}\,m^{-2}$. This flow is continued if intermittent aortic occlusion is chosen. Many centres also maintain this flow with cardioplegic myocardial protection. Such a flow increases non-coronary collateral flow, whereby blood reaches the coronary arteries via mediastinal vessels at the pericardial reflections, rewarming the heart and causing it to beat or fibrillate, so destroying the metabolic advantage of electromechanical inactivity (Buckberg, 1979). Non-coronary flow may be as much as $400\,ml\,min^{-1}$ in severe coronary disease (Hetzer *et al.*, 1980), which may induce recurrence of electrical activity a few minutes after cardioplegic infusion.

Reducing systemic flow to $1.5\,l\,min^{-1}\,m^{-2}$ reduces this non-coronary flow by two thirds (Warnecke *et al.*, 1983) and the myocardium remains cooler and longer in asystole (Hearse *et al.*, 1981). Reducing the systemic flow to this level was a critical component of Shumway's technique of topical hypothermia and its neglect resulted in his results often not being reproducible in other units (Griepp *et al.*, 1973). That such a flow reduction is adequate at 25°C for organ perfusion was shown at St Thomas' Hospital by there being no increase in the dose of sodium bicarbonate required to control acidosis on bypass: nor was there a higher incidence of cerebral or renal complications compared with perfusion at $2.4\,l\,min^{-1}\,m^{-2}$. The systemic pressure generated by this flow varies with the state of the systemic vascular resistance, particularly if adjusted with vasodilating drugs (Tucker *et al.*, 1979).

(b) Core temperature

It is not possible to abolish totally either non-coronary collateral flow or rewarming of the heart directly from the adjacent tissues. The colder these tissues and the systemic blood are, the easier it is to keep the heart cold and so improve myocardial protection (Grover *et al.*, 1981). On the other hand, reducing the temperature too far prolongs cardiopulmonary bypass time unnecessarily. A temperature of around 25°C has been found to be a good compromise (Kirklin, 1983) with maximum protection for the myocardium combined with minimal effect on bypass time and bleeding following surgery.

Lower temperatures of 20°C have also been advocated (Robicsek, 1982; Goor *et al.*, 1982).

20.3.2 Cardioplegia solutions

Ideally a solution should be used only if each of its components has been selectively studied with dose–response curves at different temperatures to determine its maximal effect in relation to the other components and it should include only those substances that have been clearly demonstrated to have a positive protective action. Only the St Thomas' solution has been so studied (Hearse *et al.*, 1981). Nevertheless, many different solutions are in experimentally and clinically successful use. Their composition falls into two main groups: those containing blood as the cardioplegic vehicle and those which are entirely crystalloid. The latter can again be roughly subdivided into those crystalloid solutions which aim to be basically close to extracellular fluid ionic concentrations with added components, e.g. the St Thomas' solution, and those where cardiac arrest is achieved by absence of the calcium ion, a low sodium concentration and the addition of procaine with the osmolality being made up with another substance such as a mannitol, e.g. Bretschneider's solution (Bretschneider, 1980).

(a) **Blood cardioplegia**

Blood as the vehicle for cardioplegia is associated with the name of Buckberg (1979). It is essentially oxygenated blood from the arterial line of the pump oxygenator, cooled and diluted with the cardioplegic solution to produce a solution which is alkaline at a pH of 7.7, has a raised concentration of potassium to produce cardiac arrest and a reduced calcium level and haematocrit, produced by adding 26 mmol of potassium to 1 litre of a 16% blood plasma/dextrose saline solution buffered with Tris buffer (Follette *et al.*, 1978). It is cooled to 10–16°C and has to be re-infused every 20 min for optimum protective effect (Takamoto *et al.*, 1980). Its main theoretical advantage is its oxygenating potential during infusion, and particularly during re-infusion. The ability to modify its components and temperature has advantages and Rosenkranz *et al.* (1982) noted that a warm induction technique, i.e. warm cardioplegic infusion prior to cold, improved myocardial protection in poorly contractile hearts.

Another advantage of blood cardioplegia is the buffering potential of the plasma. The alkaline pH of Buckberg's blood cardioplegia, however, conflicts with Fleckenstein's finding that an acid pH favoured myocardial recovery. The work of Nugent *et al.* (1982) showed that alkalinity conferred no benefit and that a pH of around 7.1 was probably optimum.

The temperature at which blood cardioplegia is administered is critical.

Buckberg (1979) originally used 16–20°C; McGovern *et al.* (1982) showed it to be most effective at 20°C and much less so at 4°C, with crystalloid cardioplegia at 4 or 10°C proving to be as effective as blood cardioplegia at 20°C. The increased viscosity of blood at lower temperatures also reduces its potential for cooling areas of the myocardium beyond major coronary stenoses via collateral vessels.

Experimentally blood cardioplegia meticulously administered every 20 min can be shown to be more protective than some crystalloid solutions (Takamoto *et al.*, 1980). Most clinical studies show no advantage of blood over crystalloid cardioplegia though there is a suggestion from Roberts *et al.* (1982) that it may be helpful for long ischaemic periods and in poor ejection fraction patients.

In practical terms blood cardioplegia is necessarily more complex and certainly more expensive in equipment used than crystalloid cardioplegia as there has to be a separate circuit and reservoir. This, however, also offers the most important advantage of blood cardioplegia in that the equipment can be used in perfusion of the aortic root immediately prior to the removal of the aortic clamp, so modifying the reperfusion period, an area of myocardial protection that has not yet been fully characterised.

(b) Crystalloid cardioplegia

Crystalloid 'asanguinous' cardioplegic solutions are historically and currently the most widely used solutions. They may conventionally be divided into 'intracellular' and 'extracellular' solutions.

(i) 'Intracellular' solutions

'Intracellular' solutions are based on the concept of producing cardiac arrest by reducing ionic gradients across the cell membrane. Bretschneider's (1980) solution has a low sodium ($15\,mmol\,l^{-1}$)and absent calcium, contains mannitol and is buffered with histidine Table 20.1. Kirsch's Cardioplegin was a bolus of magnesium aspartate and procaine which was modified by

Table 20.1 Formulation of Bretschneider cardioplegic solution (mmol/l)

NaCl	15
KCl	8
$MgCl_2$	8
Histidine	180
Tryptophon	2.0
Mannitol	20
pH	7.2

Rodewald who added a larger volume and some calcium, while reducing the magnesium concentration (Bleese *et al.*, 1979).

'Intracellular' solutions have the theoretical disadvantage of producing the calcium paradox, with myocardial damage occurring on reperfusion with calcium-containing blood, though clinically this is unlikely as most water used for making solutions is 'contaminated' by some calcium and non-coronary collateral flow brings calcium into the myocardium. Hypothermia also minimises the risk. The practical disadvantage is the necessity for prolonged (8–10 min) low flow and pressure infusion necessary for ionic equilibrium with the myocardium.

(ii) 'Extracellular' solutions

Cardioplegic solutions based on extracellular ionic concentrations produce asystole primarily by their raised potassium concentration.

1. *High potassium solutions.* Adding 20–40 mmol potassium to Ringer's lactate or Normosol ensures extracellular ionic concentrations of most components, including, importantly, calcium. Such solutions have been popular in the USA. Many variants, including omission of calcium or magnesium and including different buffers, are used.

2. *High magnesium and potassium solutions.* Following the demonstration in the isolated rat heart that the addition of 16 mmol l^{-1} of magnesium chloride significantly improved myocardial protection, the St Thomas' cardioplegic solution was introduced clinically in 1975. 16 mmol of both

Table 20.2 Formulation of St. Thomas' Hospital cardioplegic solution No2 (Plegisol) (mmol/l)

Na^+	110
K^+	16
Ca^{2+}	1.2
Mg^{2+}	16
Cl^-	160
Sodium bicarbonate	10
pH	7.8
Osmolality (mosmol/kg H_2O)	320

magnesium and potassium chloride with 1 mmol procaine in a 20 ml ampoule were added to 1 l of 4°C Ringer's solution (Braimbridge *et al.*, 1977). This solution has recently been modified by reducing the calcium and potassium concentrations and adding sodium bicarbonate as a buffer (Plegisol®, Abbott Laboratories, Chicago) (Table 20.2).

(iii) Additional components in crystalloid solutions

Steroids, popular in earlier solutions for their potential for membrane stabilisation, have largely been abandoned because of lack of evidence for their efficacy. Glucose and insulin can be shown experimentally to have an adverse effect when added to a cardioplegic solution (Hearse *et al.*, 1978) and clinically could not be shown to improve results significantly.

Local anaesthetics such as procaine and lignocaine have been used in 1–11 mM concentration in various solutions. The 7.4 mM concentration in Bretschneider's original solution is an essential component in the production of rapid cardiac arrest: the 1 mM concentration of the original St Thomas' solution had been shown experimentally to add significantly to its protective effects, partly through prevention of the vasoconstrictive effects of the particle content of commercial intravenous solutions (Robinson *et al.*, 1984) and partly also due to an inherent additive effect in filtered solutions (Yamamoto *et al.*, 1983).

Calcium antagonists (nifedipine, verapamil, diltiazem) significantly improve myocardial protection when added to some cardioplegic solutions (Boe *et al.*, 1982; Clark *et al.*, 1982; Flameng *et al.*, 1981; McGovern *et al.*, 1981; Vouhe *et al.*, 1982). Experimentally this effect is maximal at normal temperatures and can be shown to be largely abolished at lower temperatures (Nayler, 1982; Yamamoto *et al.*, 1983). Nifedipine, like procaine, abolishes the particle vasoconstrictor effect of coronary infusates and its clinical protective enhancement may therefore be mediated by improving distribution of the cardioplegic solution in coronary artery disease.

(c) Choice of cardioplegic solution

Several studies indicate that blood potassium cardioplegia, the histidine-based Bretschneider solution and the St Thomas' cardioplegic solution allow safe cardiac arrest for periods in excess of 3 hours. Crystalloid cardioplegia is basically simple, cheap and effective and allows for user errors. Blood cardioplegia, well conducted, ensuring distribution to all areas of the myocardium with frequent reinfusions is also effective but is more complex and expensive in terms of equipment. The technique of administration of cardioplegia is today as important a factor in ensuring optimum myocardial protection as the choice of cardioplegic solution.

20.3.3 Temperature of cardioplegic solutions

Blood cardioplegia is usually infused at 10–16°C. Crystalloid cardioplegia is infused at 4°C, having been kept overnight in the blood refrigerator: a normal refrigerator has compartments that are usually too warm or too cold. In the presence of coronary artery disease, the temperature of areas of the myocardium distal to 100% occlusions is monitored. If this remains warm, which is rare with adequate volumes of 4°C crystalloid solutions, a bypass graft is constructed to that vessel first and the graft infused with 200 ml of 4°C solution. Fibrous aneurysms, however, remain warm.

20.3.4 Volume and infusion pressure for cardioplegic solutions

Volumes vary depending on whether it is an initial or a subsequent infusion.

(a) Initial infusion

Large volumes are required, particularly in coronary surgery, if the whole heart is to be rendered uniformly cold. A litre of solution is given ideally if the solution has been shown to be effective regardless of the volume used (e.g. the St Thomas' solution) (Jynge *et al.*, 1977). With calcium-free solutions (e.g. the Bretschneider solution) care has to be taken to infuse a specific volume (30 ml kg^{-1}) over a specific time (9 min) ensuring that the infusion pressure in the aorta does not rise above 40 mmHg (5.3 kPa) (Bretschneider, 1980). Neglect of volume or flow rate restrictions may otherwise cause myocardial damage (Jynge *et al.*, 1977). Engelman *et al.* (1982) showed that very large volumes, e.g. 4 l, of calcium-containing solutions can safely be given and may be advantageous compared with smaller volumes.

Such large volumes cannot be used unless total bypass is established with caval snares and the coronary effluent discarded from the right atrium or unless a haemoconcentrator is used in the cardiopulmonary bypass circuit. Consequently the average initial infusion around the world is nearer 500 ml that 1 l. Some surgeons continue infusion until cardiac arrest and relatively uniform hypothermia is achieved, thereby using a variable volume: others, including the author, infuse 1 l routinely even if asystole is achieved immediately.

If 1 l is infused over 2–3 min and the coronary arteries are normal, the aortic root pressure is approximately 40 mmHg (5.3 kPa). With coronary artery disease, this pressure is significantly higher. So long as the pressure is below 150 mmHg (20 kPa) and the cardioplegic solution contains calcium, pressure itself is unimportant (Johnson *et al.*, 1982) and higher pressure has the advantage of increasing distal flow via collateral vessels in 100% occlusions of main coronary arteries. With blood cardioplegia and its greater viscosity, infusion pressure will tend to be higher.

(b) Subsequent infusions

Apart from any inherent advantage of renewing the cardioplegic solution's effect on the myocardium, re-infusions serve to recool the heart, which will have warmed towards ambient and core temperatures, reinforce asystole and wash out metabolites (Walls *et al.*, 1982). The last is of significant benefit. The optimum frequency of re-infusion has not been finally established. Single or hourly infusions, regardless of aortic occlusion time, were usual in the earlier applications of cardioplegia in the 1970s (Darracott-Cankovic, 1983). Buckberg (1979) showed that, with blood cardioplegia, 20 min infusions were better than single infusions in maintaining myocardial integrity. Clinically, 20–30 min intervals are most commonly used and appear optimum in relation to surgical convenience.

The same solution as that used initially is usually re-infused but a reduced potassium content with each re-infusion has been recommended. Clinically it is more convenient to use the same solution until harder evidence is available.

The volume used at each re-infusion is less, usually half, of the original cardioplegic infusion. In coronary disease 500 ml at each re-infusion ensures optimum, though not necessarily uniform, distribution.

20.3.5 Filtration of solution

Commercial solutions for intravenous use have a maximum limit for size and number of particles prescribed by the British and US Pharmacopoeias. These solutions have been the basis for the great majority of cardioplegic solutions with no assessment having been made of the effect of these particles when infused into arteries. Robinson *et al.* (1984) have shown vasoconstriction, a progressive fall in coronary flow and myocardial damage following direct infusion of intravenous solutions intra-arterially. These effects can be prevented by filtering the solution through a 0.8 μm filter or by incorporating vasodilators such as procaine or nifedipine. It is advisable therefore to filter all cardioplegic solutions through a 0.8 μm filter before coronary infusion if no vasodilator component is used.

20.3.6 Infusion route and equipment

A wide-bore needle in the aortic root, inserted through a purse-string suture and connected to an intravenous infusion bag, is the simplest method of infusing a cardioplegic solution. The needle needs to be 2 mm in diameter to allow at least 1 l to flow in in 2 min and ideally has a side hole and a flange for fixation so that it can be also used as a left heart vent and for removal of air when the aortic clamp is removed (Braimbridge, 1979; Catinella *et al.*, 1982). If there is any aortic regurgitation, a 3 mm needle is required to allow for the extra flow while maintaining an adequate aortic root pressure for proper myocardial distribution. DeBakey coronary and other commercial cannulae are equally effective.

If the aortic valve is to be replaced, the aorta will be opened and the individual coronary arteries infused with separate cannulae. These may be handheld metal cannulae to allow for ease of placement (Braimbridge, 1979) or plastic coronary cannulae held with forceps. Each cannula can be connected separately to infusion bags or joined with a Y connector to a single bag. The latter allows a common pressure to distribute the solution to both arteries.

The infusion pressure can be generated by hand pressure, by a blood pressure cuff around the bag, by an infusion pump or by gravity. The last is suitable for the long, slow infusion of intracellular solutions, e.g. Bretschneider, but is inadequate for the more rapid infusion of the extracellular solutions. The infusion pressure in the aortic root can be monitored directly via a needle, assessed manually or ignored. The first is ideal, the second adequate, the third usual.

Retrograde infusion of cardioplegic solutions via the coronary sinus is an alternative infusion which may obviate the effect of 100% stenoses of the coronary arteries (Gundry and Kirsh, 1982; Lessana, 1982; Menasche *et al.*, 1982; Saylam *et al.*, 1982). Careful monitoring of infusion pressures to avoid oedema, placement of the cannula without a balloon immediately at the coronary sinus orifice to avoid occlusion of an adjacent branch and evacuating the effluent adequately from the aortic root are essential parts of the protocol. While efficient distribution of the fluid to the myocardial bed can be shown, the disadvantage is that, unlike the dog, the anatomy in the human veins varies with up to 20% of venous return being directed into the cardiac chambers, particularly from the right ventricle. This complication is obviated by filling the entire right atrium, rather than the coronary sinus about. Comparison of retrograde and antegrade protection shows little difference however (Menasche *et al.*, 1982).

20.4 MAINTENANCE OF HYPOTHERMIA

Following the initial infusion of cardioplegic solution, the energy requirements of the myocardium need to be reduced to the lowest possible level for the entire period of aortic occlusion by keeping it cold and arrested throughout. It has been suggested by Tyers *et al.* (1977) from work on the isolated rat heart that a temperature below 10°C is positively deleterious to the myocardium. Subsequent work on both rat and dog heart has shown that hypothermia as low as 0.5°C not only causes no damage but is in fact protective in direct relation to the temperature (Shragge *et al.*, 1978; Kao *et al.*, 1982; Rosenfeldt, 1982). There is no advantage in terms of oxygen provision in cooling blood cardioplegia below 20°C because the shift in the oxygen dissociation curve makes it less effective than 4 or 10° crystalloid solution in protecting the myocardium (McGovern *et al.*, 1982).

20.4.1 Technique of hypothermia

The components of cardiac rewarming have been analysed by Rosenfeldt and Watson (1979). The most important factor in rewarming is the return of blood to the heart from pulmonary, bronchial and mediastinal non-coronary collaterals (Johnson *et al.*, 1982), with, if the patient remains on partial bypass, systemic venous return to the right heart (Kao *et al.*, 1982). Conduction of heat from the surrounding tissues across the pericardium – liver, lungs and mediastinum (Goor *et al.*, 1982) – heat radiation from operating room lights and heat uptake from room air are also significant. Even assistants' hands holding the heart may be important (Borst, 1982).

(a) Core temperature

Reduction of the systemic core temperature will minimise heat gain from blood returning to the heart and from conduction from surrounding tissues. The optimum temperature is probably 25°C taking into account time on bypass and bleeding problems if a lower temperature is used (Kirklin, 1983). If the core temperature is to be returned to near normal at the time that the aortic clamp is removed, other measures have to be accentuated to counteract the greater rewarming potential in the myocardium during the last 15 minutes.

(b) Insulation of ventricles

Heat gain from adjacent liver, lung and mediastinum is reduced by isolating the ventricles from the parietal pericardium. The ideal insulating material will be thin and supple to prevent displacement of the heart and corrugated to allow cooling fluid to flow to the posterior surface of the left ventricle. Corrugated soft latex rubber, of the type usually used for abdominal drains, answers these criteria. Also used have been sponges and nylon mesh and refrigerated pads with circulating coolants (Bonchek, 1982), all of which cause displacement of the heart to a greater or lesser extent.

In coronary artery surgery such insulation is less important because the ventricle is displaced during performance of the distal anastomoses but becomes relevant if the proximal anastomoses are performed with the aortic clamp in position (Salerno, 1982) and if valve replacement is performed in addition.

(c) Pericardial cooling (topical hypothermia)

The areas of the heart most at risk from increased oxygen demand as the heart slowly rewarms are the outer half of the left ventricle (Braimbridge *et al.*,

1978), particularly on its posterior aspect (Borst and Iversen, 1980; Van Way *et al.*, 1982), the right ventricle (Braimbridge and Darracott-Cankovic, 1980) and the atria. The Shumway technique (Griepp *et al.*, 1973) of running cold fluid over the surface of the heart inside the insulative material via a multiple-holed catheter is effective in cooling the ventricles and left atrium. The technique can be accelerated by inserting a pump into the system (Rosenfeldt *et al.*, 1981; Wheeldon *et al.*, 1976). Suction of fluid from the pericardium is best performed with a roller pump because it is quieter than wall suction. The cooling catheter can be arranged appropriately during distal coronary anastomoses. Commercial coolant pads are difficult to position.

The cooling fluid run over the myocardium is usually Ringer's lactate (Hartmann's) or saline except in 'intracellular' cardioplegic solution centres where the sodium content is undesirable (Bleese *et al.*, 1979). Ice saline slush is effective but may cause phrenic paralysis. Topical cooling is particularly important in coronary artery surgery where every area may not cool uniformly from the cardioplegic infusion (Laschinger *et al.*, 1982).

Topical cooling has been shown to enhance myocardial protection particularly in the presence of coronary artery stenoses (Laschinger *et al.*, 1982).

(d) **Right heart cooling**

The surgeon's natural preoccupation with the left ventricle has diverted attention from the right heart. The right atrium and ventricle are thin, exposed to operating room lights and, on partial bypass, have systemic venous blood within their cavities (Van Way *et al.*, 1982). Deterioration of the right ventricle while the left remains well protected by cardioplegia has been documented both cytochemically and physiologically (Braimbridge and Darracott-Cankovic, 1980; Chiu *et al.*, 1980). Deterioration of the right atrium may be assumed from the occurrence of supraventricular dysrhythmias and heart block.

The addition of right heart cooling by ensuring that cooling fluid flows over the right, as well as the left, ventricle and specifically cooling the right atrium by a catheter inserted alongside the superior vena caval cannula through the released atrial appendage snare will ensure SA and AV node hypothermia with reduction in the incidence of supraventricular dysrhythmias (Hearse *et al.*, 1981) and of A-V nodal conduction delay (Smith *et al.*, 1983).

(e) **Left heart venting**

Removal of bronchial return and non-coronary collateral flow rather than letting it pool in the left heart will aid maintenance of myocardial hypothermia. Bronchial venous return is considerable in cyanotic congenital heart disease and non-coronary collateral flow may be as much as 400 ml min^{-1} in patients with severe coronary artery disease and minimal angina (Hetzer *et al.*, 1980). Left heart vents are not essential for coronary artery surgery, or for that matter valve surgery either, but they reduce myocardial re-warming and oxygen consumption (Kanter *et al.*, 1982; Salerno and Charette, 1979). The left heart may be vented from the left ventricle, left atrium or aorta. A left ventricular vent inserted through the apex is the most effective, but in coronary artery surgery it may interfere with access to the coronary arteries, may dislodge apical clot and entails displacing the ventricle for its removal during the recovery phase. A ventricular vent inserted via the pulmonary vein or left atrium avoids these disadvantages, but may cause problems in closing the insertion site. The simplest technique is to use the cardioplegic infusion needle in the aorta to vent the left heart. For this purpose it needs to be relatively blunt and fixed to the aorta by a flange (Braimbridge, 1979; Catinella *et al.*, 1982). A small air bleed from a fine needle in the suction line avoids sucking the tubing flat.

20.4.2 St Thomas' Hospital myocardial protection protocol

Initial infusion with 1 l of 4°C St Thomas' solution routinely reduces the myocardial temperature below 15°C in coronary disease and to 8–10°C with normal coronary arteries. Hypothermia is maintained by reducing core temperature to 25°C and systemic flow to 1.5 l $min^{-1} m^{-2}$ to cool and minimise non-coronary collateral flow and rewarming from adjacent tissues. The ventricles are isolated from the pericardium with a tailored sheet of corrugated latex rubber. An infant feeding catheter with multiple side holes is stitched to the pericardium across the right ventricle in valve operations and appropriately positioned in coronary surgery with a small sponge to spread the 4°C Hartmann's solution evenly. A second catheter tied to the superior caval cannula and inserted into the right atrium via the released appendage snare allows right atrial cooling with 4°C Hartmann's solution. Reinfusion of 500 ml of the St Thomas' solution is performed every 30 min. Core rewarming begins 15 min before the projected time for removal of the aortic clamp to allow core temperature to reach 37°C. The systemic pressure is reduced to 20 mmHg (2.7 kPa) to minimise froth and coronary air embolism as the aortic clamp is removed and full flow of 2.4 l $min^{-1} m^{-2}$ at normal temperatures reinstituted.

20.5 REPERFUSION OF THE MYOCARDIUM

The term 'reperfusion' of the myocardium is confined here to myocardial reperfusion with systemic blood at the end of the ischaemic period.

20.5.1 Prevention of reperfusion injury

There is a difference between injury caused by ischaemia becoming evident during reperfusion and reperfusion injury caused by perfusing an ischaemic area with blood. If myocardial protection has been adequate, neither will occur. If it has been inadequate, certainly the first and possibly the second may happen.

Follette *et al.* (1981), from Buckberg's laboratory, proposed perfusing the myocardium below the aortic clamp at the end of the ischaemic interval with cold blood containing reduced calcium, a high potassium, an alkaline pH and mannitol. Recovery from an hour's ischaemia was improved thereby. This approach has led many units using crystalloid cardioplegia to remove the aortic clamp at a low systemic temperature and pressure and keep them low for some minutes, even though the absence of blood cardioplegia equipment prevents adoption of the full Follette protocol. Rousou *et al.* (1982) and Brown *et al.* (1982) have shown experimentally that normal temperatures and pressures of normal blood are optimal for preventing reperfusion injury and Darracott-Cankovic (1984) and McDonagh and Laks (1982) have demonstrated that oedema of the myocardium only occurs if myocardial protection has been inadequate. Engelman *et al.* (1976), however, showed improved recovery with anti-oedema compounds. Adding glutamate to the reperfusion blood was suggested to improve recovery by Rosenkranz *et al.* (1982). Engelman *et al.* (1982) were unable to confirm this finding with blood, though it did improve recovery after crystalloid cardioplegia.

Return of the temperature and pressure to normal, without oncotic or other manipulation of the perfusing blood, as soon as possible after removal of the aortic clamp is therefore experimentally justifiable and certainly the simplest protocol for centres using crystalloid cardioplegia. Modification of the reperfusion period is not yet fully characterised either clinically or experimentally and time will tell whether a more complex approach is justified.

20.5.2 Avoidance of air embolism

Coronary air embolism significantly depresses myocardial contractility at a time when good function is most required. Air is most likely to enter the coronary arteries when the aortic occlusive and sidebiting clamps are removed.

Air embolism is best prevented by avoiding production of froth in the aortic root which occurs when a high pressure jet of blood is forced by a high systemic pressure through a slowly opened clamp. Such froth is difficult to remove quickly through a needle. If the systemic pressure is reduced to 20 mmHg (2.7 kPa) by temporarily turning off the arterial pump and the aortic clamp rapidly removed, air rather than froth is rapidly expelled or sucked from the aortic root. The cardioplegia infusion needle is ideal for this purpose, particularly if it is has already been in use as a left heart vent. Coronary bypass grafts are occluded by bulldog clamps and secondarily needled, as are the left and right ventricles.

20.5.3 Avoidance of over-distension of the left ventricle in the reperfusion phase

The cardioplegic ventricle regains its tone rapidly after resumption of warm coronary perfusion with oxygenated blood, but does not immediately result in a powerful coordinated contraction (Roberts *et al.*, 1981). This period will be prolonged by poor pre-operative function or intermittent serial episodes of ischaemia (the 'stunned' ventricle) (Braunwald and Kloner, 1982; Geft *et al.*, 1982). If there is delay, particularly if aortic regurgitation is also present, the ventricles will overdistend with subsequent reduction of contractility and cardiac output (Lucas *et al.*, 1981). Subendocardial myocardial perfusion is compromised by the raised end-diastolic pressure.

Monitoring the left atrial pressure at this time records any diastolic pressure rise and allows remedial action to be taken. If no vent has been used, the heart may be defibrillated, emptied manually or a pulmonary artery vent rapidly inserted if these measures fail. Such measures will prevent depression of left ventricular function from overdistension and reduce its oxygen consumption (Kanter *et al.*, 1982).

20.5.4 Discontinuation of cardiopulmonary bypass

The delay in return of effective myocardial contraction following cardioplegia demands patience on the part of the surgeon and experience in deciding when to discontinue cardiopulmonary bypass. When the QRS complex has narrowed, the ventricles have become uniformly pink and visually contract well and the left ventricle is ejecting on partial bypass with an acceptable left atrial pressure against the systemic pressure, bypass may safely be discontinued. Premature discontinuation results in the spiral of ventricular distension and falling output. A guide is to continue supportive bypass for 10 min for every hour of aortic occlusion.

20.6 MYOCARDIAL PROTECTION FOR SPECIFIC CLINICAL PROBLEMS

Standard myocardial protection procedures have necessarily to be modified under certain conditions such as the use of differing sequences of coronary anastomoses, valve replacement and coronary surgery, ascending aortic replacement or congenital anomalies.

20.6.1 Differing sequences of coronary anastomoses

With intermittent aortic occlusion, each distal anastomosis is performed with the aortic clamp applied. The clamp is removed between grafts and the heart allowed to resume beating. Proximal anastomoses are constructed with sidebiting clamps and the heart beating either before or after the distal grafts. This sequence has been largely carried over into cardioplegic myocardial protection with all distal anastomoses performed with cardioplegia and the proximal areas with sidebiting clamps and a beating heart.

Buckberg's work showing that a beating heart with coronary artery narrowings does not become ischaemic while it is perfused, but cannot repay an oxygen debt following a period of ischaemia (Becker *et al.*, 1981) has led some surgeons, including the author, into performing all anastomoses, both proximal and distal, with a single application of the aortic clamp (Salerno, 1982). Myocardial protection is assumed to be better with maximal cardioplegic protection followed by immediate total and adequate reperfusion when the aortic clamp is removed, than beating while each graft is applied, leaving the area of the last graft unable to repay its oxygen debt until it is completed. Under these circumstances, the most severely narrowed artery is bypassed first and the proximal end is attached to the aorta immediately. Subsequent cardioplegic reinfusions then reach the area beyond the block. The sequence is repeated with the next most severely narrowed artery and so on. Internal mammary grafts are left till last. If non-coronary collateral flow is considerable into the aortic root when no left heart vent is used and interferes with the anastomosis, suction can be applied to the cardioplegia needle.

20.6.2 Valve replacement and coronary surgery

If mitral or aortic valve replacement is to be performed, the left ventricle may be hypertrophied and is therefore particularly at risk if coronary stenoses restrict proper distribution of the cardioplegic solution. A thermistor probe is ideally used after the initial cardioplegic infusion to check each area of the myocardium supplied by the narrowed arteries. If any area is above 15°C after infusion of 1 litre of solution, the distal saphenous vein graft to that artery is performed first and the graft infused with solution each time the aortic root or main coronary arteries are re-infused. Performing all proximal anastomoses with a single application of the aortic clamp is particularly suited to aortic valve replacement with coronary surgery, especially when the aorta is short or atheromatous because it can be closed and the proximal ends applied without using sidebiting clamps which dislodge atheroma and can be awkward to site with the aortic suture line (Salerno, 1982).

20.6.3 Ascending aortic replacement

Cardioplegia has transformed technical facility and mortality in ascending aortic replacement with or without resiting of the coronary ostia. The initial infusion is given into the coronary ostia after opening the aorta and the proximal anastomosis of the aortic graft performed and the coronary ostia attached with re-infusion if necessary. Occluding the distal end of the graft around the cardioplegia infusion line after evacuating air and distending it under pressure performs the last re-infusion of the ostia and, in addition, tests for leaks at anastomoses that are difficult to reach after the distal end of the graft is anastomosed and blood perfuses the aorta.

20.6.4 Congenital heart surgery

Cardioplegia is particularly suited to complex congenital heart surgery because of the safe ischaemic time allowed and the clear, relaxed operating field. The main problem is the considerable bronchial venous and non-coronary return to the heart in cyanotic heart disease which may obscure the field and restart the heart. The volume of cardioplegic solution used may also be considerable in relation to the pump prime.

Reducing systemic blood flow at low core temperatures minimises the first problem with appropriately sited vent suction removing intracardiac blood. Total bypass with removal of cardioplegic solution from the right atrium prevents excessive haemodilution.

20.7 COMPLICATIONS OF CARDIOPLEGIA

The introduction of cardioplegia saw a marked reduction in myocardial dysfunction and ventricular dysrhythmias following open-heart surgery. It also saw an increase in other, though relatively minor, complications such as the risk of haemodilution and more frequent, though temporary, supraventricular dysrhythmias and heart block.

20.7.1 Haemodilution

The larger volumes of cardioplegic solution, over 2 litres, that are desirable particularly in coronary surgery and longer operations may cause excessive haemodilution of the extracorporeal circulating volume. This is most simply avoided by establishing total bypass with caval snares and evacuating the solution from the right atrium. Incorporating a haemoconcentrator is a more expensive alternative (see Chapter 17). Reducing the initial volume and the frequency of re-infusion is a common but unsatisfactory method of avoiding the problem.

20.7.2 Supraventricular dysrhythmias and temporary heart block

Maintenance of right heart integrity is frequently neglected in units using cardioplegia and the right atrium begins to beat as it rewarms under the operating room lights and with systemic venous return entering it. Right atrial cooling reduces or abolishes A-V conduction delay (Smith *et al.*, 1983) and lowers the incidence of supraventricular dysrhythmias (Hearse *et al.*, 1981). Rewarming the core temperature to 37°C before removing the aortic clamp has proved the most effective simple measure in the avoidance of temporary heart block at St Thomas' Hospital.

REFERENCES

Adappa, M. G., Jacobson, L. B., Hejtzer, R., Hill, M. D., Kam, B. and Kerth, W. J. (1978) Cold hyperkalemic cardiac arrest versus intermittent aortic crossclamping and topical hypothermia for coronary bypass surgery. *J. Thorac. Cardiovasc. Surg.*, **75**, 171–8.

Balderman, S. C., Bhayana, J. N., Masud, A. Z., Michalek, S. and Gage, A. A. (1982) Perioperative protection of the myocardium in patients with impaired ventricular function. *Ann. Thorac. Surg.*, **33**, 445–52.

Becker, H., Vinten-Johansen, J., Buckberg, G. D., Follette, D. M. and Robertson, J. M. (1981) Critical importance of ensuring cardioplegic delivery with coronary stenoses. *J. Thorac. Cardiovasc. Surg.*, **81**, 507–15.

Berggren, H., Ekroth, R., Heilitz, J., Hjalmarson, A., Waldenstrom, A., Waldenstrom, J. and William-Olsson, G. (1982) Improved myocardial protection during cold cardioplegia by means of increased myocardial glycogen stores. *Thorac. Cardiovasc. Surg.*, **30**, 389–92.

Bleese, N., Doring, V., Kalmar, P., Krebber, H. J., Pokar, H. and Rodewald, G. (1979) Clinical application of cardioplegia in aortic crossclamping periods longer than 150 minutes. *Thorac. Cardiovasc. Surg.*, **27**, 390–92.

Boe, S. L., Dixon, C. M., Sakert, T. A. and McGovern, G. J. (1982) The control of calcium sequestration with nifedipine cardioplegia. *J. Thorac. Cardiovasc. Surg.*, **84**, 678–84.

Bonchek, L. I. (1982) Discussion of Laschinger *et al.* (1982). *J. Thorac. Cardiovasc. Surg.*, **84**, 807–14.

Borst, H. G. (1982) Discussion of Laschinger *et al.* (1982). *J. Thorac. Cardiovasc. Surg.*, **84**, 807–14.

Borst, H. G. and Iversen, S. E. (1980) Myocardial temperatures in clinical cardioplegia. *Thorac. Cardiovasc. Surg.*, **28**, 29–33.

Boudoulas, H., Snyder, G. L., Lewis, R. P., Kates, R. E., Karayannacos, P. E. and Vasko, V. S. (1978) Safety and rationale for continuation of propranolol therapy during coronary bypass operations. *Ann. Thorac. Surg.*, **26**, 222–7.

Braimbridge, M. V. (1979) Equipment for inducing cold cardioplegic arrest. *J. Thorac. Cardiovasc. Surg.*, **77**, 323–4.

Braimbridge, M. V. and Darracott-Cankovic, S. (1980) Assessment of right ventricular preservation during cold cardioplegic arrest. In *Cardiovascular Surgery* (eds W. Bircks, J. Ostermeyer and H. D. Schulte) Springer Verlag, Berlin, pp. 625–8.

Braimbridge, M. V., Chayen, J., Bitensky, L., Hearse, D. J., Jynge, P. and Cankovic-Darracott, S. (1977) Cold cardioplegia or continuous coronary perfusion? *J. Thorac. Cardiovasc. Surg.*, **74**, 900–6.

Braimbridge, M. V., Darracott, S., Clement, A. J., Bitensky, L. and Chayen, J. (1978) Cold cardioplegia versus continuous coronary perfusion: clinical and cytochemical assessment. In *Modern Cardiac Surgery* (ed. D. B. Longmore) MTP, Lancaster, pp. 285–98.

Braunwald, E. and Kloner, R. A. (1982) The stunned myocardium: prolonged postischemic ventricular function. *Circulation*, **66**, 1146–9.

Bretschneider, H. J. (1980) Myocardial protection. *Thorac. Cardiovasc. Surg.*, **28**, 295–302.

Bretschneider, H. J., Hubner, G., Knoll, D., Lohr, B., Nordbeck, H. and Spieckermann, P. G. (1975) Myocardial resistance and tolerance to ischemia: physiological and biochemical basis. *J. Cardiovasc. Surg.*, **16**, 241–60.

Brower, R. W., de Jong, J. W., Haalesbos, M., Simoons, M. L., Bos, A. V., de Jong, D. S., Bos, E., Hugenholtz, P. G. (1982) Evaluation of cardioplegia in coronary artery bypass surgery. In *Kalziumantoginisten zur Kardioplegie und Myokardprotektion in der offenen Herzchirurgie* (eds H. Just, A. Tchirkov, and V. Schlosser) George Thieme Verlag, Stuttgart, pp. 69–83.

Brown, A. H., Morritt, G. N. and Hammo, M. (1982) Avoidance of reperfusion injury after cardioplegia. *Thorax*, **37**, 275–9.

Buckberg, G. D. (1979) A proposed solution to the cardioplegic controversy. *J. Thorac. Cardiovasc. Surg.*, **77**, 803–15.

Catinella, F. P., Knopp, E. A., Cunningham, J. N. and Adams, P. X. (1982) A simplified method for delivery of cold blood cardioplegia and aortic root venting during coronary artery bypass. *J. Cardiovasc. Surg.*, **23**, 163–5.

Catinella, F. P., Nathan, I. M., Paone, G., Adams, P. X. and Cunningham, J. N. (1982) An on-line system for delivery of blood cardioplegia. *J. Cardiovasc. Surg.*, **23**, 252–5.

Chiu, R. C. J., Brown, P. R., Rabinovich, M. A., Mulder, D. S. and Burgess, J. H. (1980) Right heart protection in cold cardioplegia. *Proc. Symp. Cardioplegia, the First Quarter Century*. London, pp. 180–2.

Clark, R. E., Christlieb, I. V. and Clark, B. K. (1982) Nifedipine in cardiovascular surgery: experimental and clinical results. In *Kalziumantagonisten zur Kardioplegie und Myokardprotektion in der offenen Herzchirurgie* (eds H. Just, A. Tchirkov and V. Schlosser) George Thieme Verlag, Stuttgart, pp. 43–68.

Conti, V. R., Bertranou, E. G., Blackstone, E. H., Kirklin, J. W. and Digerness, S. B. (1978) Cold cardioplegia versus hypothermia for myocardial protection. *J. Thorac. Cardiovasc. Surg.*, **76**, 577–86.

Craver, J. M., Sams, A. B. and Hatcher, C. R. (1978) Potassium induced cardioplegia: additional protection against ischaemic myocardial injury during coronary revascularization. *J. Thorac. Cardiovasc. Surg.*, **76**, 24–7.

Darracott-Cankovic, S., Braimbridge, M. V., Kyosola, K., Bitensky, L. and Chayen, J. (1984) Use of microscope interferometry for measuring changes in water content of small samples of tissue. *Cell Biochem. Function*, **2**, 57–61.

Engelman, R. M., Chandra, R., Baumann, F. G. and Goldmann, R. A. (1976) Myocardial reperfusion, a cause of ischemic injury during cardiopulmonary bypass. *Surgery*, **80**, 266–76.

Engelman, R. M., Dobbs, W. A., Rousou, J. H. and Meeran, M. K. (1982) Myocardial high-energy phosphate replenishment during ischemic arrest: aerobic vs. anaerobic metabolism. *Ann. Thorac. Surg.*, **33**, 453–9.

Engelman, R. M., Rousou, J. H. and Lemeshou, S. A. (1982) High volume crystalloid cardioplegia – an improved method of myocardial preservation. *Circulation*, **66** (Suppl. II), 150.

Flameng, W., Daenen, W., Borgers, M., Thone, F., Xhonneux, R., van der Water, A. and van Belle, H. (1981) Cardioprotective effects of Lidoflazine during 1 hour normothermic global ischemia. *Circulation*, **64**, 796–807.

Follette, D. M., Fey, K., Buckberg, G. D., Helly, J. J., Steed, D. L., Foglia, R. P. and Maloney, J. V. (1981) Reducing postischemic damage by temporary modification of reperfusate calcium potassium pH and osmolarity. *J. Thorac. Cardiovasc. Surg.*, **82**, 221–38.

Follette, D. M., Mulder, D. G., Maloney, J. V. and Buckberg, G. D. (1978) Advantages of blood cardioplegia over continuous coronary perfusion or intermittent ischemia: experimental and clinical study. *J. Thorac. Cardiovasc. Surg.*, **76**, 604–17.

Geft, I. L., Fisbein, M. C., Ninomiya, K. Hashida, J., Chaux, E., Yano, J., Y-Rit, J., Genov, T., Shell, W. and Ganz, W. (1982) Intermittent brief periods of ischemia have a cumulative effect and may cause myocardial necrosis. *Circulation*, **66**, 1150–8.

Goldman, R. A., Schaff, H. V., Flaherty, J. T., Bulkley, B. H., Brawley, R. K., Donahoo, J. S and Gott, V. L. (1978) Failure of methyl prednisolone to protect myocardial function or prevent myocardial edema following ischemic cardiac arrest. *J. Surg. Res.*, **24**, 477–87.

Goor, D. A., Mohr, R. and Lavee, J. (1982) Enhanced protection of myocardial function by systemic deep hypothermia during cardioplegic arrest in multiple coronary bypass grafting. *J. Thorac. Cardiovasc. Surg.*, **84**, 237–42.

Griepp, R. B., Stinson, E. B. and Shumway, N. E. (1973) Profound local hypothermia for myocardial protection during open-heart surgery. *J. Thorac. Cardiovasc. Surg.*, **66**, 731–46.

Grover, F. L., Fewel, J. G., Ghidoni, J. J. and Trinkle, J. K (1981) Does lower systemic temperature enhance cardioplegic myocardial protection. *J. Thorac. Cardiovasc. Surg.*, **81**, 11–20.

Gundry, S. R. and Kirsh, M. M. (1982) A comparison of retrograde cardioplegia versus antegrade cardioplegia in the presence of coronary artery obstruction. *Circulation*, **66** (Suppl II), 152.

Hearse, D. J., Braimbridge, M. V. and Jynge, P. (1981) Protection of the ischemic myocardium. *Cardioplegia*. Raven Press, New York.

Hearse, D. J., Stewart, D. A., and Braimbridge, M. V. (1978) Myocardial protection during ischemic cardiac arrest: deleterious effects of glucose and mannitol in cardioplegic infusates. *J. Thorac. Cardiovasc. Surg.*, **76**, 16–23.

Hetzer, R., Warnecke, H., Wittrock, H., Engel, H. J. and Borst, H. G. (1980) Extracoronary collateral myocardial blood flow during cardioplegic arrest. *Thorac. Cardiovasc. Surg.*, **28**, 191–6.

Hjelms, E. and Steiness, E. (1982) Myocardial protection in coronary artery bypass surgery. A study comparing cold cardioplegia and intermittent aortic cross clamping. *J. Cardiovasc. Surg.*, **23**, 403–6.

Johnson, R. E., Dorsey, L. M., Moye, S. J., Hatcher, C. R. and Guyton, R. A. (1982) Cardioplegic infusion: the safe limits of pressure and temperature. *J. Thorac. Cardiovasc. Surg.*, **83**, 813–23.

Jones, R. N., Attarian, D. E., Currie, W. D., Olsen, C. O., Hill, R. C., Sink, J. D. and Wechsler, A. S. (1981) Metabolic deterioration during global ischemia as a function of time in the intact normal dog heart. *J. Thorac. Cardiovasc. Surg.*, **81**, 264–73.

Jynge, P., Hearse, D. J. and Braimbridge, M. V. (1977) Myocardial protection during ischemic cardiac arrest. A possible hazard with calcium-free cardioplegic infusates. *J. Thorac. Cardiovasc. Surg.*, **73**, 846–55.

Kanter, K. R., Schaff, H. V., Gott, V. L. and Gardner, T. J. (1982) Reduced oxygen consumption with effective left ventricular venting during postischemic reperfusion. *Circulation*, **66** (Suppl. I), 50–4.

Kao, R. L., Conti, W. R. and Williams, E. H. (1982) Effect of temperature during potassium arrest on myocardial metabolism and function. *J. Thorac. Cardiovasc. Surg.*, **84**, 243–9.

Kirklin, J. B. (1983) Cardiopulmonary bypass. Delivered at International Symposium of Cardiac Surgery. Erice, February.

Kirklin, J. W., Conti, V. R. and Blackstone, E. H. (1979) Prevention of myocardial damage during cardiac operations. *New Engl. J. Med.*, **301**, 135–41.

Laschinger, J. C., Catinella, F. P., Cunningham, J. N., Knopp, E. A., Nathan, I. M. and Spencer, F. C. (1982) Myocardial cooling: beneficial effects of topical hypothermia. *J. Thorac. Cardiovasc. Surg.*, **84**, 807–14.

Lessana, A. (1982) Discussion of Laschinger *et al.* (1982). *J. Thorac. Cardiovasc. Surg.*, **84**, 808–14.

Lolley, D. M., Ray, J. F., Myers, W. O., Sheldon, G. and Sautter, R. D. (1978) Reduction of intraoperative myocardial infarction by means of exogenous anaerobic substrate enhancement: preoperative randomised study. *Ann. Thorac. Surg.*, **26**, 515–23.

Lucas, S. K., Schaff, H. V., Flaherty, J. T., Gott, V. L. and Gardner, T. J. (1981) The harmful effects of ventricular distension during postischemic reperfusion. *Ann. Thorac. Surg.*, **32**, 486–94.

McDonagh, P. F. and Laks, H. (1982) Use of cold blood cardioplegia to protect against coronary microcirculatory injury due to ischemia and reperfusion. *J. Thorac. Cadiovasc. Surg.*, **84**, 609–18.

McGovern, G. J., Dixon, C. M. and Burkholder, J. A. (1981) Improved myocardial protection with nifedipine and potassium based cardioplegia. *J. Thorac. Cardio vasc. Surg.*, **82**, 239–44.

McGovern, G. J., Flaherty, J. T., Gott, V. L., Bulkley, B. H. and Gardner, T. J. (1982) Failure of blood cardioplegia to protect myocardium at lower temperatures. *Circulation*, **66** (Suppl. II), 60–7.

Menasche, P., Kural, S., Fanchet, M., Lavergnae, A., Commin, P., Bercot, M., Touchot, B., Georgiopoulos, G. and Piwnica, A. (1982) Retrograde coronary sinus perfusion: a safe alternative for ensuring cardioplegic delivery in aortic valve surgery. *Ann. Thorac. Surg.*, **34**, 647–58.

Nayler, W. G. (1982) Protection of the myocardium against postischemic reperfusion damage: the combined effect of hypothermia and nifedipine. *J. Thorac. Cardiovasc. Surg.*, **84**, 897–905.

Nugent, W. C., Levine, F. H., Liapis, C. D., LaRaia, P. J., Tsai, C. H. and Buckley, M. J. (1982) Effect of pH of cardioplegic solution on postarrest myocardial preservation. *Circulation*, **66** (Suppl. II), 68–72.

Pepper, J. R., Lockey, E., Darracott-Cankovic, S. and Braimbridge, M. V. (1982) Cardioplegia versus intermittent ischaemic arrest in coronary bypass surgery *Thorax*, **37**, 887–92.

Peyton, R. B., Van Trigt, P., Pellom, G. L., Jones, R. N., Sink, J. D. and Wechsler, A. (1982) Improved tolerance to ischemia in hypertrophied myocardium by preischemic enhancement of adenosine triphosphate. *J. Thorac. Cardiovasc. Surg.*, **84**, 11–15.

Roberts, A. J., Moran, J. M., Sanders, J. H., Spies, S. M., Lichtenthal., P. R., Kaplan,

K. J. and Michaelis, L. L. (1982) Clinical evaluation of the relative effectiveness of multidose crystalloid and cold blood potassium cardioplegia in coronary artery bypass graft surgery: a non-randomized matched-pair analysis. *Ann. Thorac. Surg.*, **33**, 421–33.

Roberts, A. J., Sanders, J. H., Moran, J. M., Kaplan, K. J., Lichtenthal, P. R., Spies, S. M. and Michaelis, L. L. (1981) Non-randomized matched pair analysis of intermittent ischemic arrest versus potassium crystalloid cardioplegia during myocardial revascularization. *Ann. Thorac. Surg.*, **31**, 502–11.

Roberts, A. J., Spies, S. M., Sanders, J. H., Moran, J. M., Wilkinson, C. J., Lichtenthal, P. R., White, R. L. and Michaelis, L. L. (1981) Serial assessment of left ventricular performance following coronary artery bypass grafting. Early postoperative results with myocardial protection afforded by multidose hypothermic potassium crystalloid cardioplegia. *J. Thorac. Cardiovasc. Surg.*, **81**, 69–84.

Robicsek, F. (1982) Myocardial protection during coronary surgery. Getting the maximum advantage of both cardioplegia and hypothermia. *Thorac. Cardiovasc. Surg.*, **3**, 187–8.

Robinson, L., Braimbridge, M. V. and Hearse, D. J. (1984) The potential hazard of particulate contamination of cardioplegic solutions. *Thorac. Cardiovasc. Surg.* **87**, 48–58.

Rosenfeldt, F. L. (1982) The relationship between myocardial temperature and recovery after experimental cardioplegic arrest. *J. Thorac. Cardiovasc. Surg.*, **84**, 656–66.

Rosenfeldt, F. L., Fambiatos, A., Pastoriza-Pinol, J. and Stirling, G. R. (1981) A recirculating cooling system for improved topical cardiac hypothermia. *Ann. Thorac. Surg.*, **32**, 401–5.

Rosenfeldt, F. L. and Watson, D. A. (1979) Interference with local myocardial cooling by heat gain during aortic crossclamping. *Ann. Thorac. Surg.*, **27**, 13–16.

Rosenkranz, E., Okamoto, F., Buckberg, G. D., Vinten-Johansen, J., Edwards, H. and Bugyi, H. (1982) Advantages of glutamate-enriched cold blood cardioplegia in energy depleted hearts. *Circulation*, **66** (Suppl. II), 151.

Rosenkranz, E. R., Vinten-Johansen, J., Buckberg, G. D., Okamoto, F., Edwards, H. and Bugyi, H. (1982) Benefits of normothermic induction of blood cardioplegia in energy depleted hearts, with maintenance of arrest by multidose cold cardioplegic infusions. *J. Thorac. Cardiovasc. Surg.*, **84**, 667–77.

Rousou, J. H., Dobbs, W. A., Meeran, M. K. and Engelman, R. M. (1982) The temperature dependence of recovery of metabolic function following hypothermic potassium cardioplegic arrest. *J. Thorac. Cardiovasc. Surg.*, **83**, 117–21.

Salerno, T. A. (1982) Single aortic cross-clamping for distal and proximal anastomoses in coronary surgery: an alternative to conventional techniques. *Ann. Thorac. Surg.*, **33**, 518–20.

Salerno, T. A. and Charette, E. J. P. (1979) Elimination of venting in coronary artery surgery. *Ann. Thorac. Surg.*, **27**, 340–3.

Saylam, A., Aytac, A., Andac, O., Tuncer, I. and Aslan, A. (1982) Retrograde coronary sinus perfusion of cold cardioplegic solutions in the presence of coronary arterial occlusions. Experimental study. *Thorac. Cardiovasc. Surg.*, **30**, 378–82.

Shragge, B. W., Digerness, S. B. and Blackstone, E. H. (1978) Complete recovery of myocardial function following cold exposure. *Circulation* (Suppl. II), 56–97.

Smith, P. K., Buhrman, W. C., Levett, J. M., Ferguson, T. B., Holman, W. L. and Cox,

J. L. (1983) Supraventricular conduction abnormalities following cardiac operations. *J. Thorac. Cardiovasc. Surg.*, **85**, 105–15.

Starnes, V., Hammon, J. W., Lupinetti, F. M., Olson, R. D., Boncek, R. J. and Bender, H. W. (1982) Functional and metabolic preservation of the immature myocardium with verapamil following global ischemia. *Ann. Thorac. Surg.*, **34**, 58–65.

Takamoto, S., Levine, F. H., La Raia, P. J., Adzick, N. S., Fallon, J. T., Austin, W. G. and Buckley, M. J. (1980) Comparison of single-dose and multiple-dose crystalloid and blood potassium cardioplegia during prolonged hypothermic aortic occlusion. *J. Thorac. Cardiovasc. Surg.*, **79**, 19–28.

Toleda-Pereya, L. H. and Jara, F. M. (1979) Myocardial protection with methyl prednisolone. Evaluation of variability of hearts subjected to warm ischemia before transplantation. *J. Thorac. Cardiovasc. Surg.*, **71**, 619–21.

Tucker, W. Y., Ellis, R. J., Mangano, D. T., Ryan, C. J. and Ebert, P. A. (1979) Questionable importance of high potassium concentrations in cardioplegic solutions. *J. Thorac. Cardiovasc. Surg.*, **71**, 183–90.

Tyers, G. F. O., Williams, E. H., Hughes, H. C. and Todd, G. J. (1977) Effect of perfusate temperature on myocardial protection from ischemia. *J. Thorac. Cardiovasc. Surg.*, **73**, 766–71.

Van Way, C. W., Hood, A. G., Leonard, S., Bohus, R. W. and Gentry, S. D. (1982) Thermokinetics of cold cardioplegic arrest. *J. Cardiovasc. Surg.*, **23**, 297–304.

Vouhe, P. R., Helias, J., Robert, P. and Grondin, C. M. (1982) Myocardial protection through cold cardioplegia with potassium or diltiazem. Experimental evidence that diltiazem provides better protection even when coronary flow is impaired by a critical stenosis. *Circulation*, **63**, 1078–85.

Walls, J. T., Nasser, F. N., Baron, D. W., Tinker, J. H. and Harrison, C. E. (1982) Beneficial effects of multidose coronary artery washout during elective cardiac arrest and cardiopulmonary bypass: biochemical and hemodynamic evaluation. *J. Thorac. Cardiovasc. Surg.*, **83**, 772–8.

Warnecke, H., Iversen, S., Hetzer, R., Wittrock, H. and Borst, H. G. (1983) Improved safety of hypothermic cardioplegic arrest by low flow bypass. *Thorac. Cardiovasc. Surg.*, **31**, 12.

Weisel, R. D., Goldman, B. S. and Lipton, I. H. (1978) Optimal myocardial protection. *Surgery*, **84**, 812–16.

Wheeldon, D. R., Bethune, D. W., Gill, R. D. and English, T. A. H. (1976) A simple cooling circuit for topical cardiac hypothermia. *Thorax*, **31**, 565–71.

Yamamoto, F., Braimbridge, M. V., Manning, A. S. and Hearse, D. J. (1983) Cardioplegia and slow calcium channel blockers. *J. Thorac. Cardiovasc. Surg.*, **86**, 252–61.

21
Safety during cardiopulmonary bypass

D. R. WHEELDON

21.1 BYPASS SAFETY

The concept of safety is very subjective. Figures published by the Royal Society for the Prevention of Accidents (RoSPA) show that of the deaths resulting from accidents in Great Britain in 1980 45% were due to transport accidents and 43% resulted from accidents in the home. Although efforts are made to improve the safety of both these aspects of our everyday life (witness the new safety belt law) we still regard both as being relatively 'safe'. In the same year there were 98 reported deaths due to surgical and medical misadventure (0.5%) but this is probably an underestimate since apart from the comprehensive reports on obstetric mortality (HMSO, 1973) and the studies by the Association of Anaesthetists (Lunn and Mushin, 1982), there is considerable resistance to this type of medical audit in this country.

In 1981 there were 12 990 patients who underwent open cardiac surgery in National Health Service hospitals in the UK, of whom 948 (7.3%) died within 30 days of operation (Cardiac Surgical Register, 1981). Two recent UK surveys revealed that a fatal perfusion accident occurred once per 1800 procedures and that a serious incident occurred once per 130 procedures (Wheeldon, 1979, 1981). Similar figures were obtained by a recent American survey (Stoney *et al.*, 1980). Although these figures are relatively low when compared with the national mortality figures of 73 deaths per 1000 perfusions they conceal a much wider morbidity, the true scale of which can only be a matter for conjecture.

During the past two decades of cardiac surgery much progress has been made, particularly with regard to myocardial preservation, the development of a wider range of efficient and convenient perfusion products, and the development of better perfusion techniques. This has resulted in hospital mortalities being reduced from the 30% level in the early 1970s to less than 10% today (Fig. 21.1). The advent of coronary artery surgery has produced a very large increase in the number of patients undergoing cardiac surgery, and, many people are now turning their attention to qualitative aspects of overall patient care, the goal being that a patient should enjoy a better quality of life after open-heart surgery. After all, if he has had the right operation carried out with the correct technical expertise and we have adequately preserved the functional integrity of his organs whilst surgical intervention has taken place, then there is no good reason why this should not be so.

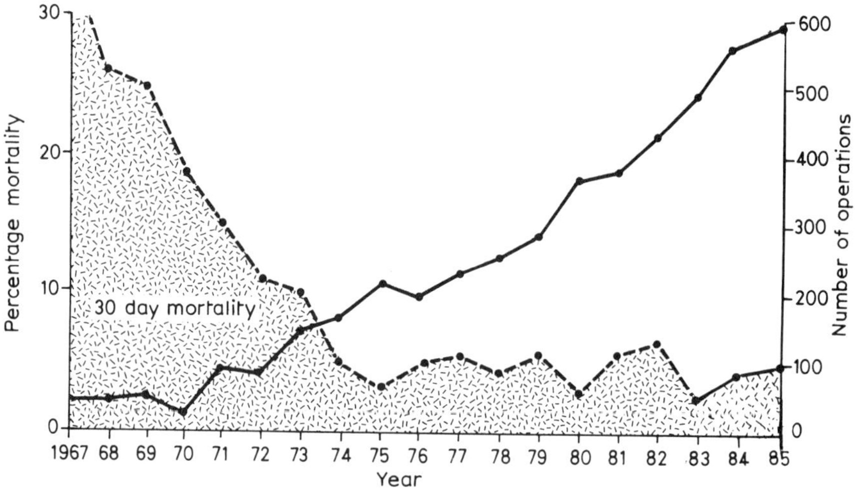

Fig. 21.1 Cardiac surgery – Papworth Hospital (1967–85). 30 day mortality statistics.

The Wessex Regional Cardiothoracic Unit has undertaken two recent surveys into the quality of life after operation (Ross *et al.*, 1976; Monro *et. al.*, 1983). In this series of 3000 consecutive operations patients have been followed up from one to 8.5 years. A high proportion have returned to work and enjoy a normal life and 80% of the 3000 patients were alive at the time of the review. These results must have been most gratifying. However, there was no analysis of those patients who did not benefit or who were worse as a result of the treatment.

21.2 ORGANIZATIONAL ASPECTS

The First World Congress on Open Heart Technology (in 1981) devoted an entire session to the organizational aspects of an open-heart surgical unit.

This was entirely appropriate since this is a most important and fundamental aspect of cardiac surgery. Aspects discussed included the required components of an open-heart unit, together with the qualities required of the unit members and their respective responsibilities. Attention was also focused on the wider organizational aspects with respect to the community which the unit serves. The point was emphasized that for cardiac surgery to be successful it must be performed by a smoothly functioning team. There must be co-operation, co-ordination and effective communication among the disciplines and each speciality must have a clearly defined area of responsibility and authority. Optimum patient care also requires that these individuals work together regularly and frequently.

Attemps to discover the nature and effectiveness of team work in the UK by survey revealed little consensus of opinion about individual responsibilities, which may either indicate lack of serious consideration of this matter or a deficiency of the questionnaire in its ability to elucidate the way in which units approach this problem. There does, however, now seem to be a greater acceptance of the importance of the team approach.

21.2.1 Departmental organization

The *Health and Safety at Work* Act, built upon the recommendations of the Robens Committee, came into being in July 1974. Although it will still be some time before the Act is fully effective in the Health Service it would be as well for perfusion departments to implement their own organizational safety guidelines before regulations are arbitrarily imposed on them. Health Devices (1980) published an excellent early review of perfusion equipment problems together with a very useful check list for inspection and preventative maintenance.

On the electrical safety side, new safety standards do exist. In 1963 the Ministry of Health published its own code, HTM8. In 1969, Technical Committee TC62 of the International Electrotechnical Commission (IEC) commenced work on an International Standard for the safety of medical equipment, leading to the publication of IEC601/1.

Several countries have now adopted IEC601/1 as a national standard. In Britain the adoption was through the publication of BS5724 part I. IEC601/1 will be used in Directives on Electromedical Equipment and X-ray Equipment throughout the European community. BS5724 part I provides general requirements for the safety of medical electrical equipment. Part II will specify the special safety requirements for particular types of equipment, whilst part III will specify appropriate performance requirements.

Although BS5724 was intended to guide manufacturers there are implications for NHS users. Whilst manufacturers are asked whether their equipment meets BS5724 or IEC601/1 on the Supplies Questionnaire Form

EMQ1, a manufacturer's reply refers to a type test. Thus, the purchaser must satisfy himself that the particular equipment he has received is safe and functionary. This is the responsibility of the District Works Office, either using his own EMBE technicians, or the hospital Medical Electronics Department. In exceptional cases, the British Standards Institute Test House can provide a limited service.

21.2.2 Perfusion department safety organization

The following list is intended as a general guide towards implementing organizational safety features into a perfusion department.

(a) General

Establishment of equipment records:

(1) Identification and location of each individual device.
(2) Record of maintenance and repairs to each device.
(3) Establishment of routine preventative maintenance protocols.

The above are probably best achieved by collaboration with the District Works Office and hospital Medical Physics Workshops.

(b) Faults book

Establish a record for all equipment failures and malfunctions. Record details and circumstances of all equipment failures.

(c) Perfusion protocol

Establish agreed protocols to be followed by all perfusionists in the following procedures:

(1) Basis for selection of equipment to be deployed in all the various clinical situations likely to be encountered.
(2) Pre-operative machine checks.
(3) Priming solutions and techniques for all circuits used.
(4) Case records which should include:
  (a) Patient statistics
  (b) Equipment used
  (c) Fluids and drugs used
  (d) Measured parameters
  (e) Frequency of entries
(5) Pre-bypass check list.

(6) Basic guidelines for perfusion management:
   (a) Blood flows
   (b) Pressure limits
   (c) Fluid replacement
   (d) Blood gas and electrolyte limits
   (e) Anti-coagulation
   (f) Temperature control
(7) Procedures to be followed in the event of equipment failure:
   (a) Electrical power
   (b) Mechanical pump failure
   (c) Oxygenator failure
   (d) Reservoir failure
   (e) Gas supply failure
   (f) Temperature control
   (g) Circuit rupture

Ensure that all perfusionists are capable of effecting emergency action in the event of any of the above equipment failures, in the minimum time and using a method which has been established as representing the minimum risk to the patient. All perfusionists should be required to demonstrate this ability once every three months.

(8) Team responsibility and communications.
   Establish agreed areas of responsibility and systems of communication. Establish a procedure in the event of failure situations.
(9) Establish a protocol for cleaning and de-contamination of all non-disposable equipment especially with respect to contamination with specific pathogens.

21.2.3 Patient specific safety protocols

It is useful to develop standard forms on which the following information can be recorded and which act as a check list.

(1) Identification of patient
   (a) Patient statistics
   (b) Diagnosis
   (c) Pre-operative haematology, biochemistry, drug therapy.
   (d) Cardiac investigative results
   (e) Any other relevant cardiac history
   (f) Proposed operation
(2) Selection of equipment according to protocol.
(3) Machine checks
   (a) Availability of alternative systems
   (b) Calibration checks

(c) Occlusion checks
(4) Circuit components
(a) Sterility
(b) Visual check for defects
(c) Availability of alternatives
(5) Prime according to protocol
Double check (two people) all fluids and drugs.
(6) Institute case record
(7) Ensure record of identification data on equipment and fluids used.
(8) Follow protocol for cleaning and decontamination.

The above procedures may appear to be unnecessary and impractical in a busy cardiothoracic unit, particularly where there is only one perfusionist available per case, however, I do believe them to be a necessary component of safe perfusion practice. In our unit we always employ two perfusionists per case, who work as a team and who are responsible for the perfusion, theatre monitoring, ACT monitoring and blood gas determinations, as well as record keeping. This provides for good integration, better job satisfaction and the desired degree of backup for safety.

21.3 ACCIDENTS

RoSPA describes an accident as being the consequence of a sequence of random events, always involving multiple causal factors, with chance alone often determining the resultant severity. Where clear causations are involved it is difficult to define the event as a true accident. Human failure, rather than environmental and mechanical defects, is a clearly defined factor in 80% of all accidents. RoSPA also gives a list of causations for accidents which occur in the general community at work and play (Table 21.1) most of which are also relevant to cardiothoracic surgery.

Table 21.1 Causes of accidents (RoSPA)

Non-human elements	
	Mechanical defects
	Environmental factors
	Lighting conditions
Human factors	
	Adventurous spirit
	Inadequate training
	Negligence and irresponsibility
	Fatigue
	Stress
	Impatience
	Carelessness
	The ageing process!

The results obtained from the two UK Perfusion Surveys are summarized in Fig. 21.2. The first obvious difference between the two surveys is the marked increase in the number of reported incidents. How much this reflects the nature of the questionnaire (since the first survey was a retrospective one ranging back over six years) and how much this is a real difference is difficult to say but I would suspect that at least some of the increase in reported incidents is real. Consumptive coagulopathies and arterial line air embolism remain major problems. The donor blood and prime incidents represent a few unfortunate cases but, nevertheless, demonstrate the serious consequences of not making use of careful procedures.

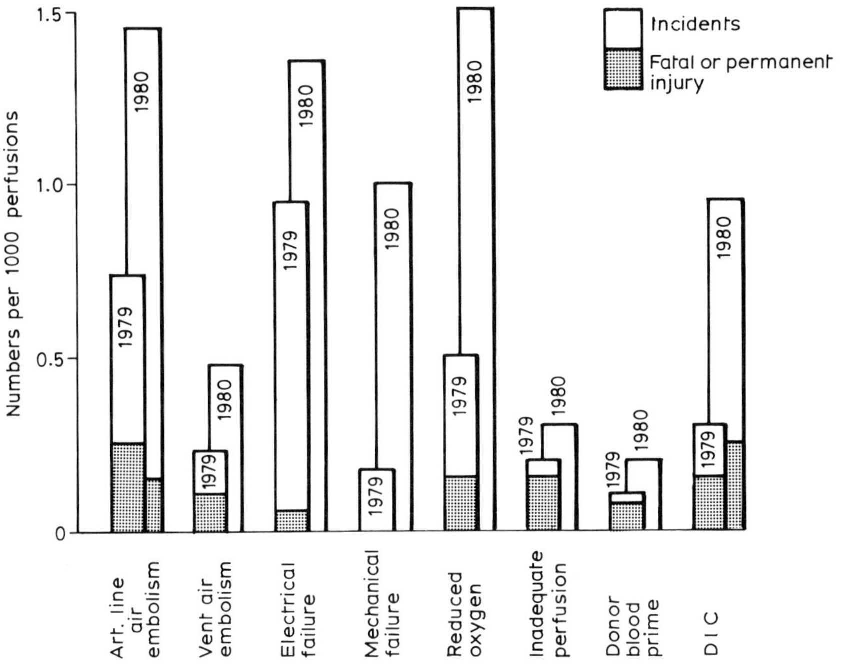

Fig. 21.2 Major causes of perfusion accidents.

21.3.1 Reduced oxygenation

This was reported as being the most frequent incident. Many modern hard shell bubble oxygenators make use of gas spargers which are placed in such a position that they are subjected to relatively high hydrostatic pressures, particularly during priming when the bubble column contains little foam. Excessive hydrostatic pressure may also be created by failing to vent the oxygenator during priming in addition to having little or no gas supply to the sparger. This results in fluid entering the core of the sparger which then requires high pressures to overcome the 'bubble point' and clear the gas channels. This may result in bypass being established with a sparger which is partially blocked. Most manufacturers specify a minimum gas flow of about $2\,l\,min^{-1}$ during priming to overcome this problem. We employ a priming technique in our unit which avoids introducing fluid into the bubble column at any stage prior to the initiation of bypass. This avoids sparger 'soaking' as well as keeping the PO_2 of the prime low. Should this situation occur the best treatment is to drain the bubble column into the cardiotomy reservoir and then to connect high pressure vacuum to the gas supply line for a few minutes in order to dry the sparger out. Depending on the nature of the priming fluid this will partly resolve the situation. If the patient requires blood flows towards the limits of the oxygenator capacity it may be more prudent to substitute a new oxygenator.

There may be a variety of causes for reduced oxygenation of membrane oxygenators. The spiral wound silicone membranes are prone to membrane displacement, particularly if the prime is circulated against a low resistance. Other factors include poor shim pressure control and variable exhaust back pressure in the case of parallel plate membranes. In addition, the gas delivery system may develop a leak or blockage resulting in a potentially confusing situation. There has also been a report of a cracked gas line filter leading to hypoxia at the onset of bypass (Schwartz *et al.*, 1980).

Should the problem reside in the particular oxygenator being used then the perfusionist will have to assess the relative risks of continuing with the defective oxygenator or changing to a new oxygenator on bypass. Emergency changing of oxygenators is not difficult if the perfusionist has practised the procedure at regular intervals and the necessary equipment is available at short notice (McMillan *et al.*, 1979). There is also something to be said for having a standard replacement oxygenator available for such a purpose. We use a VT 5000 which has connections already in place – since this oxygenator can be primed without a gas flow and the ports can be sealed by hand for rapid connection.

The other major reason for reduced oxygen delivery during bypass hinges on perfusion management. A full understanding of the mechanisms affecting oxygen supply to the major organs during CPB still eludes us. The various factors which influence oxygen delivery are often contradictory during perfusion and it is only by increasing our understanding of the dynamics of oxygen delivery during perfusion that we can design systems which adequately provide for oxygen needs. The recent progress in the production of servo-regulated gas supply devices for CPB use will help in this respect. This subject is covered elsewhere in this book (Chapter 10) and there is also a recent comprehensive treatment of the subject by Moores (1982).

21.3.2 Arterial line air embolism

Probably the most sudden and distressing incident which may occur during cardiopulmonary bypass is massive arterial air embolism, yet the attitude of perfusionists towards the use of devices designed to minimize this hazard varies enormously. At one extreme are those who seem to feel that the use of low level alarms somehow undermines their technical virility. At the other are those who believe in multiple servo-regulating devices. It has been interesting to note from both UK surveys that all the fatalities occurred in units where no alarms of any kind were used, as did almost all the incidents reported. My own feeling is that a level alarm is a useful aid as long as it is used as an aid and does not become a substitute for proper vigilance. Figure 21.3 demonstrates the consequences of total venous obstruction on a variety of different oxygenators with and without an arterial line filter and the effect of a shut-off valve on the arterial outlet. (These traces were obtained using an ultrasonic bubble detector (TM8) placed on the arterial line.) It can be seen that the valve closes positively after allowing a small volume of air through, whilst the arterial reservoir on the VT5000 collapses without letting any air through although foam is formed in the line. The inclusion of an arterial line filter

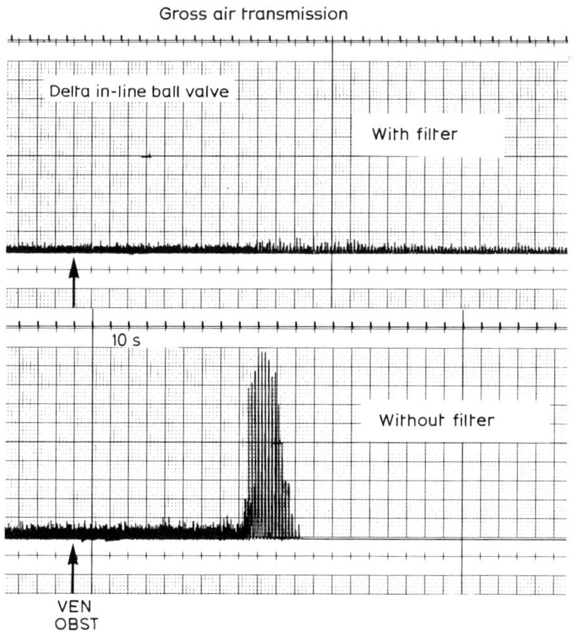

Fig. 21.3 Gross air transmission detected by arterial line ultrasound monitoring with and without a Utilipor arterial line filter.

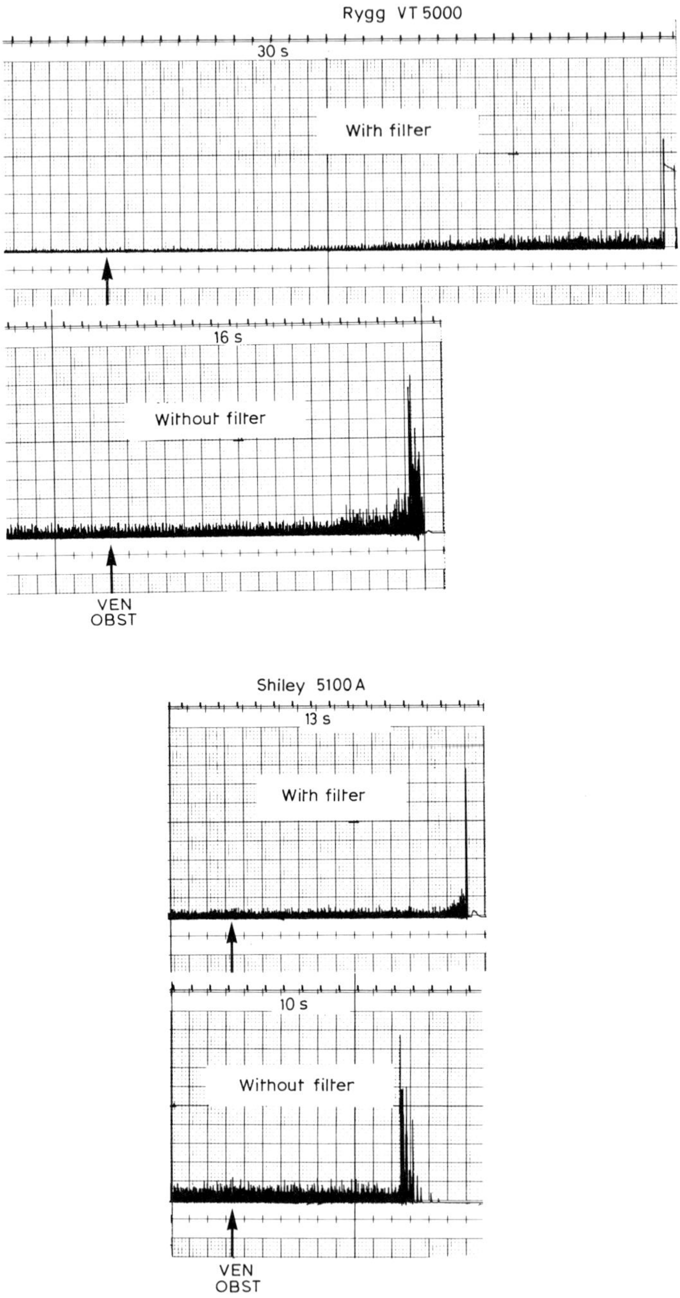

Fig. 21.3 *continued.*

extends the time delay by 30–80% depending on the oxygenator employed. The perfusionist should also note that, at best, he would have 30 s to react to this situation under these average conditions and, at worse, only 10 s.

The possibility of gross air embolism was a concern to those who designed some of the early heart–lung machines many of which were considerably more sophisticated than many modern machines. The most popular concept used for film and disc oxygenators was that of a constant volume device which servo-regulated the arterial or venous pump or both. Sensing devices consisted of oxygenator level sensing electrodes, level floats, tubing diameter sensors and those that directly monitored oxygenator weight (Galletti and Brecher, 1962).

21.3.3 Anti-gas embolism devices

These may be divided into four categories (Christman and Kurusz, 1980)

(1) Oxygenator-based devices.
(2) Pre-pump devices.
(3) Modified pump systems.
(4) Distal arterial line devices.

Commercial examples of these devices are listed in Table 21.2.

(1) Of the oxygenator level sensing devices the capacitance type is probably the most reliable (Page, 1977), and the reflectance infra-red devices the most unreliable (Stoney, *et al.*, 1980). Devices which continuously monitor oxygenator weight were used by Polystan and a modern version is also available from Advanced Med-Science. This devices is also useful for monitoring oxygenator volume but requires a fairly careful set up procedure. Another possible device of the same sort involves the connection of a pressure transducer to the arterial sample port.
(2) A mechanical ball valve placed at the arterial outlet is a very effective device for limiting gross air embolism (Burgess, 1977). The same effect can be achieved using small PVC reservoirs designed to collapse as the fluid is evacuated from them.
(3) One manufacturer currently offers a centrifugal pump (Biomedicus) which effectively becomes deprimed by gross air and we have shown that this pump will transmit far fewer microbubbles than a standard roller pump.
(4) There are several arterial line filters and bubble traps which have been shown to function as effective gas embolism traps and several workers have compared the effectiveness of these devices in this respect (Streczyn, 1977; Abts *et al.*, 1978; Siposs, 1981). One manufacturer also produces a distal in-line photo-cell micro-bubble detector which is reportedly

Table 21.2 Anti-gas embolism devices

Manufacturer	*Type*	*Alarm*	*Servo shut off*
1. Attached to oxygenators			
A. Advanced Med. Science	Non-invasive oxygenator weight monitor	Yes	Yes
B. American Optical	Non-invasive photocell	Yes	Yes
C. Cardiovascular Instruments	Non-invasive photocell	Yes	Yes
D. Cobe/Stockert	Non-invasive IR sensor	Yes	Yes
E. Delta Medical	Non-invasive capacitance	Yes	Yes
F. Sarns	Non-invasive photocell	Yes	Yes
Some manufacturers can provide sensors customized for a number of different oxygenators.			
2. Proximal devices			
E. Delta Medical	Invasive in line ball valve	No	No
F. Sarns	Non-invasive IR sensor	Yes	Yes
3. Pumps			
G. Bio-Medicus	Invasive pump head	No	No (Yes)
4. Distal Devices			
E. Delta Medical	Invasive in line valve system for vent line		
H. William Harvey/Bard	Invasive in line valve system for vent line		
I. Gish Biomedical	Invasive in line valve for arterial filter purge		
J. Biomedical Systems	Non-invasive positive pressure relief valve for cardiotomy reservoirs		

A. Advanced Med. Science Inc., Needham Heights, MA 02194 USA
UK Agents: Unknown.
B. American Optical Medical Division, Bedford, MA 01730 USA
UK Agents: British American Optical, 820 Yeovil Rd, Slough, Bucks.
C. Cardiovascular Instruments Inc., Wakefield, MA 01880 USA
UK Agents: Unknown.
D. Cobe Laboratories Inc., Lakewood, CO 80215 USA
UK Agents: Cobe Laboratories, Eastern Avenue, Gloucester, GL4 7SN.
E. Delta Medical Industries Inc., Costa Mesa, CA 92626 USA
UK Agents: Athrodex Ltd, Telford Rd, Bicester, Oxon. OX5 0TZ.
F. Sarns Inc., Ann Arbor, MI 48103 USA
UK Agents: Biomedical Systems, Bothwell, Strathclyde, Scotland.
G. Bio-Medicus Inc., Minnetonka, MN 55343 USA
UK Agents: C. F. Thackray Ltd, Park Street, Leeds LS1 1RQ.
H. Bard Cardiopulmonary Division, 1425 S Village Way, Santa Ana, CA 92705 USA
UK Agents: Bard International, Pennywell Estate, Sunderland, SR4 9EE.
I. Gish Biomedical Inc., 1800 E Carnegie Ave., Santa Ana, CA 92705 USA
UK Agents: Biomedical Systems Ltd, Bothwell, Strathclyde, Scotland.
J. Biomedical Systems Ltd, Bothwell, Strathclyde, Scotland.

accurate in detection of bubbles 1 ml in volume or greater (Vivian *et al.*, 1980). Other similar arterial line sensors have recently been developed, with automatic pump switch-off if 1 ml gas bubbles are detected.

21.3.4 Other perfusion-related causes of gross air embolism

The following lists are of other causes of gross air embolism reported in the literature related to the oxygenator, the pump, and the cardiotomy reservoir. I have not included those due to poor surgical technique.

(a) Oxygenator related

(i) Break in integrity of oxygenator connections
It is prudent to place the oxygenator in a position where it is protected from any theatre traffic.

(ii) Detachment of oxygenator from holder
The oxygenator holder should be of adequate design and well secured to the machine and oxygenator.

(iii) Non-venting of oxygenator
A systematic set-up procedure and pre-bypass check list should guard against the possibility of an unopened vent.

(iv) Clotted oxygenator (Mills and Ochsner, 1980; Stoney et al., *1980).*
Anticoagulant monitoring should now be mandatory.

(b) Pump related

(i) Runaway arterial pump head
Runaway arterial pump head can be caused by faulty electronic speed control – most modern pumps should be designed in such a way that component failure will result in the pump stopping rather than running out of control. Other causes are ergonomic in that they involve the potential for accidental increase in speed. An added potential danger involves servo inputs to pumps (usually from pulsatile modules) which can in certain fault situations cause a stationary pump to switch on.

(ii) Reversal of arterial pump
Directional controls, particularly on older pumps are not generally well designed but adherence to rigid check procedures should ensure against accidents of this kind, as well as accidents involving ruptured pump boots due to over-occlusion or foreign bodies entering the pump head, and accidental switch on (Kurusz *et al.*, 1979; Stoney *et al.*, 1980).

(iii) Occluded line proximal to arterial pump head

(iv) Reversal of vent pump
Accidents involving the retrograde passage of air via the vent system can also be guarded against by the use of in-line one-way valves which are currently available.

(c) Cardiotomy reservoir related

Accidents involving cardiotomy reservoirs have almost always involved the production of a positive pressure at the input to the reservoir. This has sometimes been deliberate so as to force blood through the filters or more commonly inadvertent and due to either a very high input without adequate venting or due to plugging of the filters. Accidents have included:

(1) Air forced back up an arterial filter bleed line and hence into the arterial line.
(2) Air forced back along a vent system through a non-occlusive pump or via a vent overflow system.
(3) Large amounts of air entrained in the cardiotomy return to the oxygenator forming large stable, nitrogen containing bubbles in the system (Mandl and Reilly, 1976; Duvall and Dearing, 1978; Pfefferkorn *et al.* 1981; Mills and Ochsner, 1980; Pearson *et al.*, 1981).

In our unit we are very particular in the way in which we use cardiotomy reservoirs. Our system (Fig. 21.4) involves employing a low pressure vacuum to the post-filtration side of the reservoir and we fit a positive pressure relief valve, of our own design, to the pre-filtration side of the reservoir. This ensures that pressure in excess of 1 mmHg (0.13 kPa) cannot be generated at input flows of up to 8 l min^{-1}. Return to the oxygenator is by way of a roller pump. This system encourages blood transit through the cardiotomy filter and return to the oxygenator is controlled and gas free without having to alter the position of the cardiotomy reservoir. Figure 21.5 shows the compliance of four hard shell cardiotomy reservoirs vented as suggested by the manufacturers. It can be seen that relatively high input pressures can be generated quite quickly by modest flows.

One other, and sometimes concomitant, hazard with cardiotomy reservoirs is filter blockage. I am not aware of any reservoir currently on the market which incorporates a filter overflow or bypass. Should filter blockage occur it may be difficult to detect in some devices until the situation has become very serious (Duval and Dearing, 1978). Times of greatest risk for this particular hazard include the emergency institution of bypass without adequate heparinization and the emergency re-institution of bypass after protamine reversal.

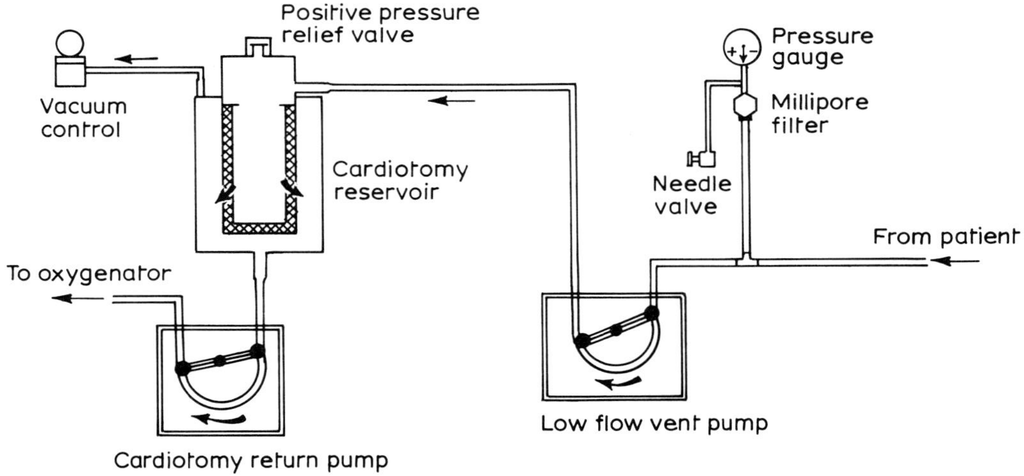

Fig. 21.4 Cardiotomy suction system – circuit diagram.

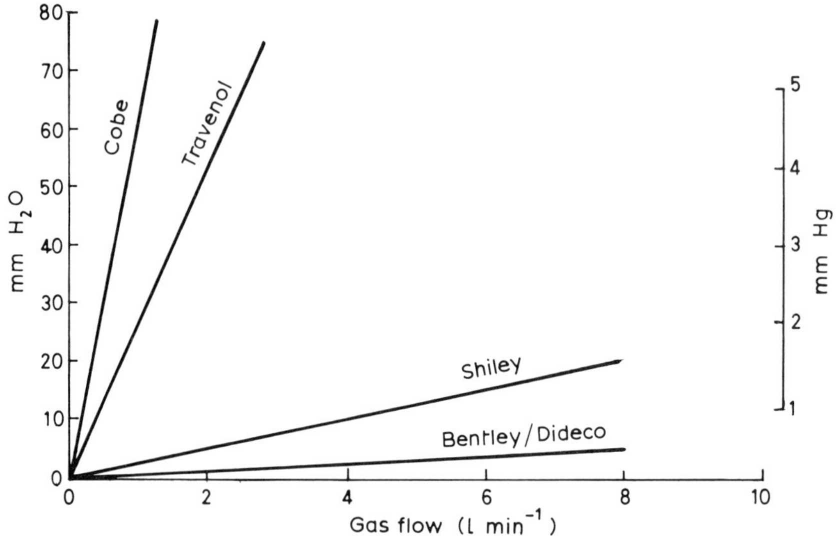

Fig. 21.5 Compliance of 4 hard-shell cardiotomy reservoirs vented according to manufacturer's instructions at incremental gas flows.

21.3.5 Management of gross air embolism

The incidence of systemic air embolism during cardiac operations has been variously reported as being 0–11.7% (Nicks, 1967; Silverstein and Krieger, 1960; Allen, 1963; Wheeldon, 1979, 1981; Doyle, 1978). However, the vast majority of instances are unreported and quietly ignored mainly due to a fear of litigation.

The control of air embolism obviously lies in prevention, as discussed previously. However, it is incumbent upon each open-heart team to be prepared to deal with the situation should it occur. The belief that this only happens to other teams is not an effective deterrent. Guidelines for this and other emergency procedures should be set up and practised by the perfusionist team.

The management of gross air embolism should include:

(1) The arterial pump is immediately stopped and the venous line clamped.
(2) The patient is placed in a steep head-down position.
(3) The aortic cannula is removed and the arterial circuit purged of air.
(4) The arterial cannula is connected to the venous line to facilitate retrograde perfusion. Alternatively, the atrium can be cannulated separately.
(5) Retrograde perfusion at a flow of 1 to 2 l min^{-1} and at a temperature of

20°C is carried out with the flow directed up the SVC. This is continued for a few minutes with the suction system being used to retrieve blood exiting from the aortotomy.

(6) The anaesthetist exerts pressure on the carotids and retrograde perfusion is continued until the arterial system is cleared of air. In extreme cases air may have entered the abdominal and femoral vessels and retrograde perfusion via the IVC may also be required.

(7) Standard bypass is resumed with hypothermia and attention is turned toward removing any air which may have entered the coronary system, by pharmacological elevation of the perfusion pressure and small needle puncture of the distal coronary system.

(8) Dexamethasone and antiplatelet agents are administered and the operative cardiac procedure completed as quickly as possible. Re-warming is accomplished slowly to a core temperature of 35°C and bypass is discontinued in the usual fashion.

(9) The patient is ventilated on 100% oxygen and the induction of deep barbiturate anaesthesia may also prove to be beneficial.

(10) Finally, hyperbaric treatment has been shown to be very effective particularly if initiated early after injury and good results have been obtained when instituted up to 48 hours after injury (Stoney, 1979; Takita *et al.*, 1968; Steward *et al.*, 1977; Kindwall, 1973; Winter *et al.*, 1971 and Pierce, 1981). However, this facility is not available in the majority of centres.

Patient management should be continued as follows.

Mean arterial pressure is maintained at 100–130 mmHg (13.3 kPa) with low right atrial pressures. The patient is ventilated with full muscle paralysis, and PCO_2 controlled between 30 and 40 mmHg (4–5.3 kPa). Initial FIO_2 is 100% for 6 hours and then reduced to 60% over the following 6 hours. The value of steroid therapy is unproven but may be beneficial. Therefore, give initial adult dose of 8 mg dexamethazone followed by 4 mg 6 hourly for 72 hours.

Hyperosmolar and diuretic therapy ideally should be managed with intracranial pressure monitoring but the potential benefits are so great as to warrant this therapy even without pressure monitoring. A loading dose of 0.5 g kg^{-1} 20% mannitol is followed by a continuous infusion at 0.1 g kg^{-1} for 72 hours. Add frusemide or ethacrynic acid at 0.5–1 mg kg^{-1} and twice daily thereafter. Check serum osmolality and do not exceed 320 mosmol kg^{-1} H_2O. Slow rewarming from 34°C to normothermia should be accomplished over 24 hours using a water blanket. Barbiturate therapy may be contra-indicated if cardiac function is severely depressed. Low dose thiopentone (1–3 mg kg^{-1}) has been used satisfactorily. Anti-platelet therapy should ideally be continued over 24 hours.

21.4 COAGULOPATHIES

Coagulopathies were the fourth most frequent source of serious incidents reported in the two UK surveys. Despite frequent references to its existence, there has not been a well-documented case of disseminated intra-vascular coagulation (DIC) resulting from cardiopulmonary bypass (CPB) in the literature. Inadequate anticoagulation during CPB (extra corporeal intra-vascular hyper-coagulability) associated with active coagulation, factor consumption and secondary fibrinolysis, however, may occur producing a coagulopathy similar to DIC and these are probably the patients recorded in the surveys.

Differing opinions exist regarding heparin dosage during CPB. The subject is discussed in detail in Chapter 16 and by Young (1982). Using the activated clotting time (ACT) to monitor adequacy of anticoagulation, the lowest 'safe value' would seem to be 400 s with a value of 450–500 s optimum which is consistent with the recommendations of Bull *et al.* (1975).

Patients who merit particularly careful attention with regard to heparinization are: children – who require relatively larger loading doses of heparin to achieve the same prolongation of clotting time; patients who have received pre-operative heparin therapy who exhibit significant heparin resistance (Eposito *et al.*, 1983); and patients where emergency re-institution of bypass is necessary following protamization.

The two UK perfusion surveys revealed that only about 60% of open-heart units in this country routinely employ anti-coagulation monitoring (Wheeldon, 1981) whilst about 80% of the 811 perfusionists surveyed by Binford *et al.* (1981) in the USA employed some form of heparin monitoring. There is no doubt in my mind that under-heparinization has been a significant, if poorly recognized, cause of morbidity associated with CPB and that too many surgical teams are reluctant to recognize this fact.

21.5 MECHANICAL AND ELECTRICAL FAILURES

Although electrical and mechanical failures are reported as frequent incidents the associated morbidity is very low, probably because most hospitals having active open-heart surgical programmes are of sufficient size to have adequate back-up facilities.

Mechanical failures are potentially more serious. However, most units would seem to be sufficiently well prepared to cope with these incidents without serious consequences.

21.6 PERFUSION MANAGEMENT

The subject of perfusion management is fully covered elsewhere in this book, however, a few points related to safety are relevant. Even after 25 years of CPB we still do not have a reliable means of monitoring the adequacy of whole body perfusion. Many guidelines have been proposed from the monitoring of arterio-venous saturation differences and developing acidosis (Ceislak, 1977; Streczyn, 1977), to the use of oxygen consumption plateauing (Mandl and Motley, 1979), with and without the use of pump-side computer aids. However, the fact remains that oxygen delivery to the vital organs depends on a multi-faceted interaction of perfusion conditions and there are no easily measured indicators of adequacy available to us in the operating theatre, as is evident from the literature on post-perfusion organ dysfunction and failure.

One recent trend is the use of 'low flow perfusion', that is indexed blood flows of less than $1.8\ l\ min^{-1}$. Low flow perfusion together with body cooling down to about 25°C provides better conditions for myocardial preservation and the advent of more efficient heat exchangers has meant that there is sufficient time for adequate re-warming whilst the proximal anastomoses are made. However, low flow perfusion without simultaneous active vasodilatory therapy can be dangerous and result in a disadvantageous distribution of available blood flow. An additional advantage of active vasodilation is the reduction of collateral circulation to the heart which results in better operating conditions. Inadequate perfusion was thought to be a significant factor in perfusion morbidity and mortality by respondents to both UK perfusion surveys.

21.7 PERFUSION SYSTEMS

The CPB machine, patient and perfusionist constitute a system which performs in a way which is not merely a summation of its constituent parts. Systems Performance is a science which has been employed by such diverse agencies as the Atomic Energy Commission and NASA, and from the perfusionist's point of view it is important that the fundamental principles of systems performance are recognized and allowed for. The characteristics of different circuits are probably more influenced by the type of oxygenator used than any other single component. However, substituting any new component can alter the balance of what should be a familiar system to the perfusionist in a way which provides new opportunities for misadventure.

The FDA sponsored study conducted by the University of Utah (Mortensen *et al.*, 1981) identified four broad areas as the causes of unsatisfactory perfusion. These were:

(1) Current state of the art of bypass perfusion – by which they meant the inadequacy of current perfusion management techniques.

(2) Pre-bypass pathological problems existing in the patient – this forms an ever-present variant in the system all too often over-looked.
(3) By-pass device inadequacy or failure.
(4) User's errors – which account for about 80% of all serious incidents.

The Utah study also made the point that the majority of perfusionists employ hybrid perfusion systems – that is systems which are constituted by a wide range of components from different manufacturers, all of which may have differences in their approach to the subject. Perfusionists are also frequently exposed to commercial pressures to try out new devices in the clinical setting with the temptation merely to substitute a new device for an existing one without any preliminary testing or even careful thought as to the possible consequences on the existing system. Although laboratory facilities may not be available to all units a new device should always be very carefully assessed before including in the clinical setting, no matter how trivial this may seem, particularly with regard to the way in which this device may differ in its relationships to the rest of the system.

21.8 DISCUSSION

It is probably reasonable to assume that the results of the surveys into perfusion accidents represent a considerable underestimation of the true number of serious incidents which occur.

The UK surveys would seem to indicate that the frequency of these incidents is increasing at a faster rate than the increase in the number of operations performed and that this represents a disturbing trend which prejudices the safety and well-being of patients undergoing CPB. This is unfortunate since other improvements in technique have resulted in considerably improved results over the past few years. Most accidents are due to human error so our efforts need to be directed towards minimizing this by careful preparation and the establishment of check lists and procedural protocols together with the use of electromechanical aids such as low level alarms.

Some trends which may be exacerbating this problem are worth mentioning. Firstly, the trend within the oxygenator industry to produce hard shell, hybrid bubble oxygenators with reduced priming volume is, I believe, a potent factor. Because of the integrated design of these devices changes in venous return flow are not evident until the blood enters the arterial reservoir, which represents a considerable time delay. In addition the reservoir is essentially 'open' so allowing free flow of air into the system, and the outlet design in some devices can lead to partial vortex formation and hence air entrainment. Secondly, the volume of work in most cardiothoracic units has increased enormously over the past few years and the perfusionist has often become involved in running auxiliary systems producing topical cooling or cardioplegia, hence potentially increasing the risks of distraction and complication. Inevitably such increases in workload encourage techniques of expedience rather than excellence. Thirdly, many units now use much more rapid cooling and rewarming aided by the increased efficiency of most modern inbuilt heat exchangers, which may produce problems of agglutination and protein denaturation. However, an encouraging trend is seen in some of the newer membrane oxygenator systems, the design of which provides much more protection against the possibilities of air embolism.

Finally, the importance of the development of a critical systematic approach, the constant attention to detail and the relentless pursuit of quality of the whole team, as a team, cannot be over-emphasized.

21.9 SAFETY FOR THE PERFUSIONIST AND SURGICAL TEAM

Awareness of safety factors related to Hepatitis B infection and the HTLV virus associated with Acquired Immune Deficiency Syndrome (AIDS) has prompted concern for the perfusionist and surgical team performing cardiac surgery in affected patients. Protection of health care staff has been the subject of management guidelines in patients known to be hepatitis B carriers. Avoidance of skin, mucus membrane and skin puncture contact with affected blood are routinely practised for hepatitis B patients. Although HTLV virus has relatively low infectivity, similar guidelines governing the safety for health care workers have recently been published. Further information may be obtained from the following available publications:

Department of Health and Social Security. *Guidance for Health Care Personnel Dealing with Patients Infected with Hepatitis B Virus*. CMO (84) 11. DHSS 1984, London.
Advisory Committee on Dangerous Pathogens. *Acquired Immune Deficiency Syndrome (AIDS) – Interim Guidelines*. DHSS 1984, London.

REFERENCES

Abts, L. R., Gough, J. D., Karon, D. C., Martin, J., Massmino, R. J., McGill, A. M. and Karlson, K. E. (1978) The efficiency of the removal of microparticles by the Johnson and Johnson arterial line filter. *AmSECT Proc.*, **4**, 14

Allen, P. (1963) Central nervous system emboli in open heart surgery. *Can. J. Surg.*, **6**, 332–7.

Berg, E. and Rygg, I. (1981) Organisational aspects of an open heart surgical unit. *Proc. First World Congress on Open Heart Technology*, Franklin Scientific Projects, London.

Binford, J. M., Miller, D. W. and Hesse, E. A. (1981) Results of a survey of the professional activities of 811 cardiopulmonary perfusionists in North America,

Proc First World Congress on Open Heart Technology. Franklin Scientific Projects, London.

BS 5724 (1979) Specification for safety of medical electrical equipment. Part I: General Requirements. British Standards Institution, London.

Bull, B. S., Korpman, R. A., Huse, W. M. and Briggs, B. D. (1975) Heparin therapy during extracorporeal circulation. Problems inherent in existing heparin protocols. *J. Thorac. Cardiovasc. Surg.*, **69**, 674.

Burgess, F. M. (1977) A new anti-air embolism device. *AmSECT Proc.*, 5, 23.

Cardiac Surgical Register (1981) Administered by The Society of Thoracic and Cardiovascular Surgeons of Great Britain.

Ceislak, F. C. (1977) Adequate tissue oxygenation during cardiopulmonary bypass. *AmSECT Proc.*, **5**.

Christman, E. W. and Kurusz, M. (1980) Preventing massive gas embolism during cardiopulmonary bypass: A review of safety devices. *J. Extracorp. Technol.*, **12**, 115–19.

DHSS (1963 Rev. 1969) Safety Code for Electro-Medical Apparatus. Hospital Technical Memorandum No 8. DHSS, London.

Doyle, D. L. (1978) *The Prevalence of Gross Air Embolism during Cardiopulmonary Bypass*. AmSECT 16th International Conference, San Diego, 1–3 March.

Duvall, R. M. and Dearing, J. P. (1978) Unrecognised plugging of a Bentley cardiotomy reservoir with three stage microporous filter. *J. Extracorp. Technol.*, **10**, 2.

Eposito, R. A., Culliford, A. T., Colvin, S. B., Thomas, S. J., Lackner, H. and Spencer, F. C. (1983) Heparin resistance during cardiopulmonary bypass. *J. Thorac. Cardiovasc. Surg.*, **85**, 346–53.

Galleti, P. M. and Brecher, G. A. (1962) *Heart–lung bypass. Principles and Techniques of Extracorporeal Circulation*. Grune and Stratton, New York.

Health Devices (1980) ECRI V9, 3.

Health Equipment Information (1981) Code of Practice for Acceptance Testing of Electrical Equipment. HEI No 95 DHSS, London.

HMSO (1973) Report on Confidential Enquiries into Maternal Deaths in England and Wales. HMSO, London.

IEC 601–1 (1977) Specification for the Safety of Electrical Equipment used in Medical Practice, Part I: General Requirements. International Electrotechnical Commission, Geneva.

Kindwall, E. P. (1973) Massive surgical air embolism treated with brief recompression to six atmospheres followed by hyperbaric oxygen. *Aerosp Med.*, **44**, 663–6.

Kurusz, M., Shaffer, C. W., Christman, E. W. and Tyers, G. F. O. (1979) Runaway pump head: New cause of gas embolism during cardiopulmonary bypass. *J. Thorac. Cardiovasc. Surg.*, **77**, 5.

Lunn, J. N. and Mushin, W. W. (1982) *Mortality Associated with Anaesthesia*. Association of Anaesthetists of Great Britain and Ireland, The Nuffield Provincial Hospitals Trust.

Mandl, J. P. and Reilly, J. B. (1976) Hazard of an unvented cardiotomy reservoir and an unoccluded left heart sump head. *AmSECT Proc.*, **IV**, 84.

Mandl, J. P. and Motley, J. R. (1979) Oxygen consumption plateauing: A better method of achieving optimum perfusion. *J. Extracorp. Technol.*, **11**, 2.

McMillan, J., Smith, B. F., Gooper, E., Newland, P. E. and Stirling, G. R. (1979) Emergency changing of an oxygenator during total cardiopulmonary bypass. *Anaesth. Intensive Care*, **VII**, 271–3.

Miller, S. S. and Mandl, J. P. (1977) Comparison of the effectiveness of various extracorporeal filters at reducing gaseous emboli. *AmSECT Proc.*, **5**, 55.

Mills, N. L. and Ochsner, J. L. (1980) Massive air embolism during cardiopulmonary bypass. *J. Thorac. Cardiovasc. Surg.*, **80**, 708–17.

Monro, J. L., Ross, J. K., Manners, J. H., Edwards, J. C., Lewis, B., Hyde, I., Ogilvie, B. C., Keeton, B. R., Conway, N. and Johnson, A. M. (1983) Cardiac Surgery in Wessex. *Br. Med. J.*, **286**, 361–5.

Moores, W. Y. (1982) Oxygen delivery during cardiopulmonary bypass. In *Pathophysiology of Cardiopulmonary Bypass* (ed. J. Utley), Williams and Wilkins, Baltimore.

Mortensen, J. D., Yates, W. G., Schoenberg, A. A., Baker, C. D., Grahn, A. R., Toronto, A. F. and Schapp, R. N. (1981) Final Report: Cardiopulmonary bypass systems: A study of safety and performance. University of Utah Research Institute. UBTL 5534–010

Nicks, R. (1967) Arterial air embolism. *Thorax*, **22**, 320.

Page, P. A. (1977) Clinical evaluation of a new non-invasive electromagnetic oxygenator blood level sensor. *AmSECT Proc.*, **5**, 50.

Pearson, D. T., Carter, R. F., Hammo, M. B. and Waterhouse, P. S. (1981) Gaseous micro-emboli during open heart surgery. *Towards Safer Cardiac Surgery*. MTP, Lancaster.

Pfefferkorn, R. O., Rose, M. W. and Pfefferkorn, S. P. (1981) An unreported pathway for the introduction of air emboli from an unvented hardshell cardiotomy reservoir. *Proc. First World Congress on Open Heart Technology*. Franklin Scientific Projects, London.

Pierce, E. (1981) Cerebral gas embolisation in heart surgery with special reference to patient management. *Proc. First World Congress on Open Heart Technology*. Franklin Scientific Projects, London.

Rainer, W. G. (1981) Organisational aspects of an open heart surgical unit. *Proc. First World Congress on Open Heart Technology*. Franklin Scientific Projects, London.

RoSPA (1980) The facts about accidents (SE 62) The Royal Society for the Prevention of Accidents, Birmingham, UK.

Ross, J. K., Monro, J. L. and Manners, J. M. (1976) Cardiac Surgery in Wessex: Review of 1000 consecutive open heart procedures. *Br. Med. J.*, Vol. 2 1485–9.

Schwartz, A. J., Howse, J., Ellison, N. and Widner, S. (1980) The gas line filter: A cause of hypoxia. *Anaesth. Analg.*, **59**, 617.

Silverstein, A. and Krieger, H. P. (1960) Neurologic complications of cardiac surgery. *Arch. Neurol.*, **3**, 601–5.

Siposs, G. G. (1981) A new disposable arterial line bubble trap. *Proc. First World Congress on Open Heart Technology*. Franklin Scientific Projects, London.

Steward, D., Williams, W. G. and Freedon, R. (1977) Hypothermia in conjunction with hyperbaric oxygenation in the treatment of massive air embolism during cardiopulmonary bypass. *Ann. Thorac. Surg.*, **24**, 591–3.

Stoney, W. S., Alford, W. C., Burrus, G. R., Glassford, D. M. and Thomas, C. S. (1980) Air embolism and other accidents using pump oxygenators. *Ann. Thorac. Surg.*, **29**, 336–40.

Streczyn, M. V. (1977) Gas emboli arterial line filtration efficiencies of the Pall and J and J filters under stress condition. *AmSECT Proc.*, **5**, 6.

Systems Performance, The Open University Technology 3rd Level Course No: TD 3421.

Takita, H., Olszewski, W., Schinert, G. and Lamphier, E. H. (1968) Hyperbaric treatment of cerebral air embolism as a result of open heart surgery. *J. Thorac. Cardiovasc. Surg.*, **55**, 682–5.

Vivian, W. A., Malloy, K. P., Hackett, J. E., Clark, D. K. and Reed, C. C. (1980) Clinical evaluation of an air embolism detection device. *Cardiovasc. Dis. Bull.* 7, 4, Texas Heart Institute.

Wheeldon, D. R. (1979) Can cardiopulmonary bypass be a safe procedure? In *Towards Safer Cardiac Surgery*, MTP, Lancaster.

Wheeldon, D. R. (1981) Safety during cardiopulmonary bypass. *Proc. First World Congress on Open Heart Technology.* Franklin Scientific Projects, London.

Winter, P. M., Alvis, J. H. and Gage, A. A. (1971) Hyperbaric treatment of cerebral air embolism during cardiopulmonary bypass *J. Am. Med. Assoc.*, **215**, 1786–8.

Young, J. A. (1982) Coagulation abnormalities with cardiopulmonary bypass. In *Pathophysiology of Cardiopulmonary Bypass* (ed. J. Utley), Williams and Wilkins, Baltimore.

Index